Nurses of Los Angeles
Uncapping the Mystery, 2nd Edition

Cynthia Broze

Semper Publishing
Phoenix, AZ

© 2024 Cynthia Broze

All rights reserved. No part of this book may be used or reproduced in any manner without written permission from the publisher.

Publisher's Cataloging-in-Publication
Broze, Cynthia 1953-
    Nurses of Los Angeles: Uncapping the Mystery, 2nd Edition/ Cynthia Broze
    pages 394
    Includes bibliographic references and index
    ISBN (softcover) 9780982650912
    LCCN 2024924639
    First softcover of the second edition

1. Nursing schools—California—Los Angeles—History.
2. Nurses—California—Los Angeles—Biography.
3. Nurses—California—Los Angeles—Reference
    BISAC: Medical/History, Medical/Biographies, Medical/Nursing/ Reference
    DCC: 610.73092–dc23

Published by Semper Publishing
Phoenix, California
Contact: semperpublishing.com
Printed in the United States of America

Every reasonable attempt has been made to identify owners of copyright. Errors or omissions will be corrected in future editions.

Dedicated to Eva Broze

Other books by Cynthia Broze

Aerial Nurse Corps of America: Lauretta Schimmoler and Leora Stroup
Pilot-In Air Evac

Contents

Acknowledgements and Preface viii

Introduction 11

1. Nurses Arrive in Los Angeles: 1856–1894 13
2. The Great Decade: 1895–1913 33
3. The History of Graduate Pins 99
4. The Great War to the Great Depression: 1914–1929 107
5. Nurses Take Off: 1930–1941 135
6. Girls Who Dreamt to Become a Nurse 159
7. World War II: 1942–1945 163
8. Everything but the Utility Sink 195
9. Baccalaureates, Associates, Theorists: 1946–1987 257
10. Books to Protest and Collect 293
11. Practitioners, Scientists, Organizations: 1970–1996 299
12. Anniversaries and Roses: 1997–2013 323
13. Los Angeles Schools of Nursing & Graduate Pins: 1897-2024 . 331

Notes 351

Bibliography 379

Index 383

About the Author 393

Acknowledgements

Every image in this book required someone to search through old files. I could not have completed this without the assistance of those individuals who searched for me. Thanks to everyone who gave me photographs and encouragement. I sincerely appreciate each unique image I received.

A few individuals extended their efforts and I would to thank them by name: Kathy Koch from the AANA, Sr. Marie Therese, Britta Granrud at the Women's Memorial Foundation, Susan Carr and Janell Mithani who cared to make the photo as good as possible, Suzanne Ward, and Janet Hobbs. Ethel Pattison and Vicy Young told me endless stories from the United Airlines archives, Lowell Irwin from the Good Samaritan Hospital Archives, Mary Telo, Theresa Johnson at UCLA, Ruth Lynch, and Landon Bennett.

Thanks to Amber Alvarado, Olivia Solis, Carol Marroquin, Edgar via Aimie Pak, Gayane Stepanyan, Judy Olausen, Laura Travis, and Phyllis Esslinger for photos of pins. Kudos to Kathleen Chai for her decades of knowledge about the Statewide Nursing Program. Gratitude to Diane Harris Hara for her assistance and encouragement. And an abundance of appreciation to Judy Olausen for the hours of tedious proofing.

Mostly, I want to thank the nurses who allowed me to interview them. I realize it's not an easy task to tell your story to a stranger and trust it will be written correctly. I enjoyed hearing your histories and I hope I conveyed each one as it was intended.

Preface

Who started the first nursing school in Los Angeles?

This was the first mystery I sought to uncover. Its name, The College Training School for Nurses, had not been disputed; its ownership had. County Hospital said they owned it, that they started the first training school. My research revealed that doctors at the College of Medicine, University of Southern California, initiated and funded the idea. They asked the County Supervisors for permission to use County Hospital as a training site but told them the County would incur no costs.[1] The first class began in 1896 and graduated in 1897 (a two-year program, but they granted the first class a one-year credit for their clinical work history). Good Samaritan Hospital also started a program in 1896, but the first class didn't graduate until 1898. The College Training School for Nurses was not a hospital-based school—unusual for that time. When the College Training School closed, Dr. Barber moved it to County.

What's new in the second edition?

- The first edition included schools in the City of Los Angeles. I've added a chapter with photographs of graduate nurse pins from all sixty-four schools in the entire County of Los Angeles, 1897 to 2024.

- I colorized or used original color photographs. I enjoyed the black and white photos, but I realized color made people look more like people instead of like art. Colorization software made it feasible to color 400 photos. However, all photos required correction of many elements resulting in a blend of my hand and the software (notated with a C). Colors might not be historically accurate due to lack of information.

- I added items: Johanna Von Wagner, first L.A. Nurse Housing Inspector; Edith Bryan, first PhD nurse in the U.S.; the Western Conservancy of Nursing History organization; the fascinating story of the Statewide Nursing Program; other historical tidbits; updates; and corrections.

- I included endnotes for those who wish to validate my references.

And finally to nurses, historians, and readers of today and in the future I say,

> This is who we were.
> This is what we did.
> This is how Nurses of Los Angeles started everything.

Introduction: 1850

When California became a state in 1850, the treeless basin named Los Angeles had no newspapers, colleges, libraries, or public schools. The first U.S. Census of 1850 listed the population as 1,610 and the county as 3,530.[1] Residents obtained water from open canals in front of their homes that were used for bathing and dumping trash. Cows grazed in open fields. Injured people lay unattended in squalor, and orphans roamed the streets for handouts. Spanish was the dominant language, followed by English and French.

During the Mexican era, a residential home on the 300 block of North Main Street became the Capital Building. After 1847 it housed American troops from the Mexican-American War.[2] In 1850, Los Angeles County used it for its first courthouse.

Doctor Odid Macy remodeled it in 1852 as the city's first hotel: the Bella Union. He also conducted his medical practice in the hotel. That same year, the *Los Angeles Star* created the city's first newspaper using parallel columns in Spanish and English.[3]

In 1855, Thaddeus Amat, a bishop of Monterey and Los Angeles, wrote to Spain, France, and the East Coast of the United States. He asked officials for help to care for the needy residents and orphans. The Daughters of Charity of St. Vincent de Paul responded and sent six nurse nuns from Emmitsburg, Maryland: Sisters Maria Scholastica, Maria Corzina, Ana, Clara, Francisca, and Angela—three Americans and three from Spain.[4-6]

The Sisters took the railroad to Panama City and then a ship to San Francisco. From there they boarded a coastal steamer, the *Sea Bird*, and on 6 January 1856, they disembarked in San Pedro, a mere sandbar harbor at that time.[7]

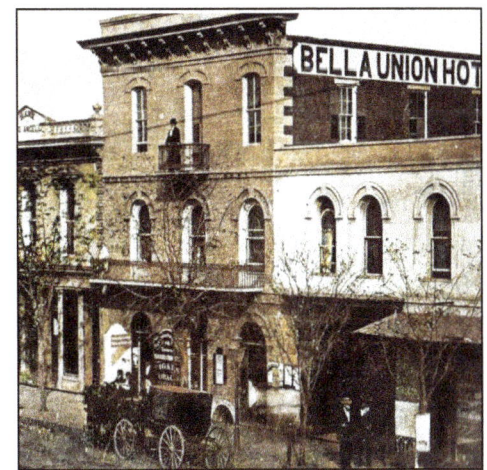

An ox cart brought them from San Pedro to Los Angeles. The cart arrived at the Bella Union Hotel, where every stagecoach stopped when it first reached the city and where every important city function occurred.[8]

Figure I.01. Bella Union Hotel, Los Angeles, c. 1871. C.

Nurses Arrive in Los Angeles: 1856-1894

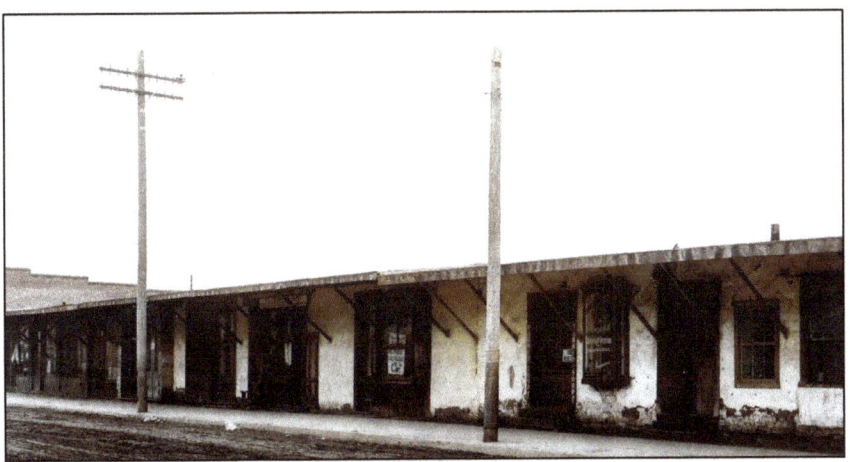

Figure 01.01. The Los Angeles Infirmary, 658-668 North Spring Street, in Don Cristobal Aguilar's adobe home, Sonora Town, 1858-1860. C. (Courtesy of Shades of L.A. Archives/Los Angeles Public Library)

The Daughters of Charity of St. Vincent de Paul organized in 1633 with a central house in Paris, France. Nursing became a vital activity. By 1650 the order contained 100 houses, and the nuns staffed many hospitals. The Sisters were in great demand as nurses in the homes of the rich. [1]

In 1856, when the Sisters of Charity arrived in Los Angeles, they opened an orphanage. A second group arrived in 1857 and created a medical dispensary for the orphanage's use. Their first infirmary began in a gardener's shed behind the orphanage when Father Raho asked them to care for a sick and dying man. The Sisters moved into the Wilson House on Alameda and Macy Streets, and the infirmary became known as Institution Caritativa. [2] Around 1858 they acquired rooms in the former home of Councilman and Mayor, Don Cristobal Aguilar, and named it the Los Angeles Infirmary.

In 1860 they bought a two-story building on Naud Street. When the County of Los Angeles decided to offer care to indigent residents, the supervisors approached the Sisters for bed space until the County could build a hospital. [3] They paid the Sisters 75 cents per patient per day. The Sisters treated fifty-two county-subsidized (charity) patients and eleven private patients the first year.

In 1870, *The Los Angeles Star* reported a private bed in the Infirmary's ward cost $1.50 per day, and a private room cost $2.50. The County paid the Sisters $1.00 per patient per day—a raise of 25 cents since they began operating. [4]

Chapter One

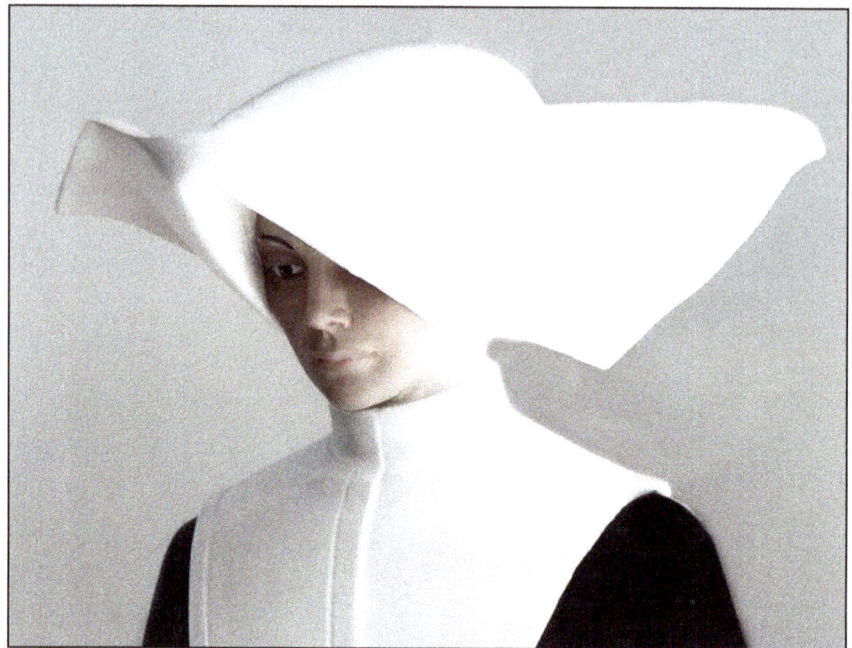

Figure 01.02. Located on the grounds of St. Vincent's Church in Los Angeles, the statue depicts an early Sister. Author photographed, 2007. C.

Elizabeth Seton founded the American Sisters of Charity in Emmitsburg, Maryland, in 1808. After she died in 1821, the nuns affiliated with the Daughters of Charity in France, founded by St. Louise de Marillac and St. Vincent de Paul.[5]

French women who lived in the area where the Daughters of Charity first started the order wore a distinctive white linen headdress. The Sisters adopted it. The famous coronet identified and protected the Sisters from harm as they attended soldiers on battlefields. The American Sisters assumed the dress style of the French Sisterhood.

Although they were nuns, the Sisters were technically not a religious order. St. Vincent de Paul would not allow them to take permanent vows; they could only promise to remain nuns for one year at a time. He advised them to adopt professional training and not obey physicians implicitly.

The Sisters of Charity did not have a cloister as other nuns did; their job was to travel everywhere. In 1853 the Sisters of Charity, in Paris, allowed Florence Nightingale to work in a hospital as a nurse for the first time. The words Sister and Daughter were used interchangeably, although St. Vincent de Paul preferred the latter.[6]

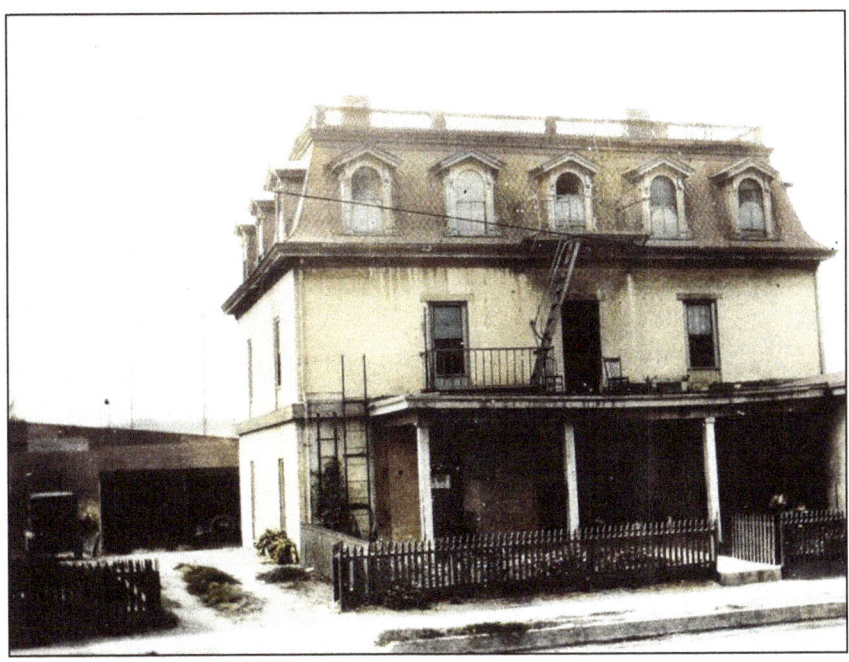

Figure 01.03. In 1860, the Sisters of Charity acquired this two-story building at 1416 Naud Street between Ann Street (named for Sister Ann) and Sotillo Street.[7] The building had three bedrooms and a kitchen. The Sisters and their helpers washed the linen in the nearby Los Angeles River.

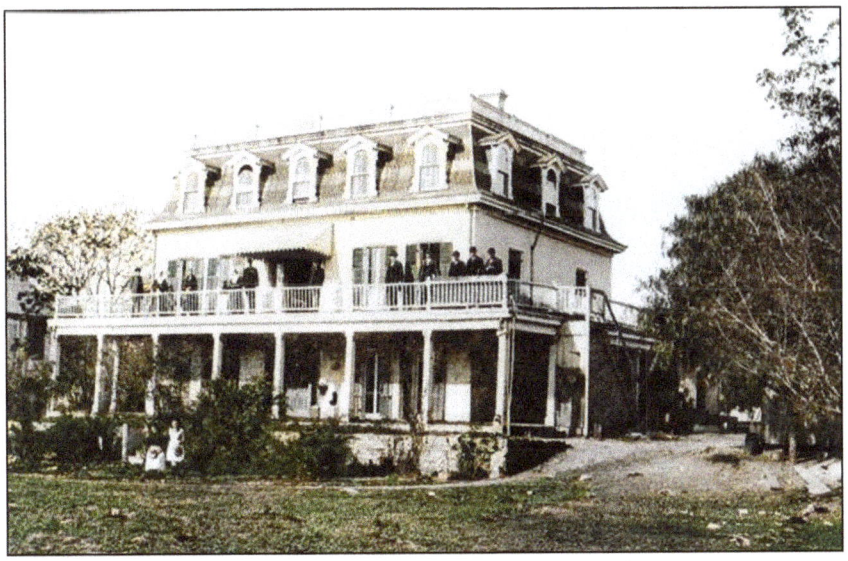

Figure 01.04. The same building after remodeling in 1904. C.

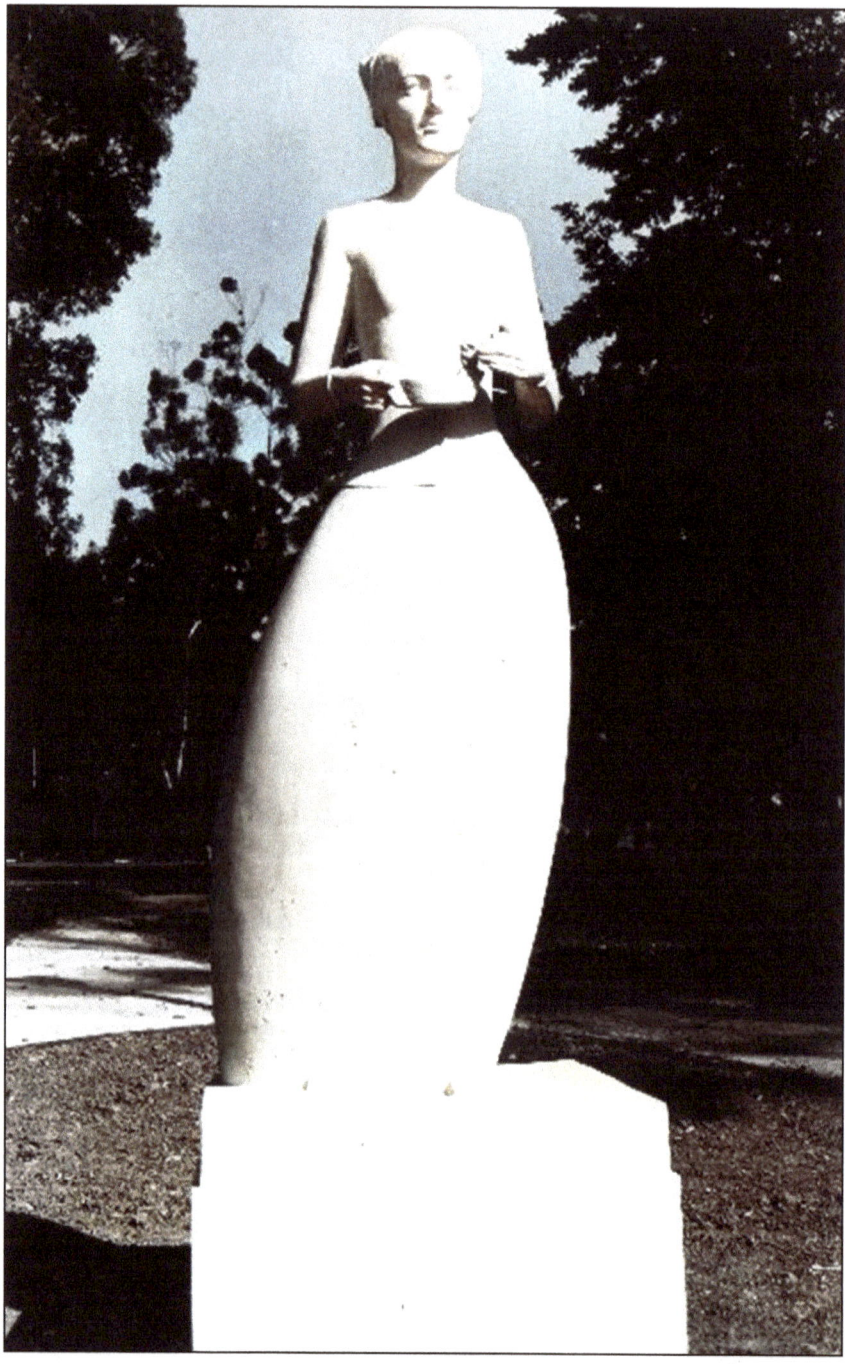

Figure 01.05. The *Florence Nightingale* sculpture at its inauguration on April 11, 1937. C. (Courtesy of Shades of L.A. /Los Angeles Public Library)

Nurses Arrive

In 1937 David Edstrom, a famous American sculptor, erected the nine-foot-high statue, *Florence Nightingale,* in Lincoln Park, Los Angeles. He used the cast stone and concrete technique Ada May Sharpless used for her 1935 *Nuestra Reina de Los Angeles/Lady of the Lake* statue at Echo Park Lake.

Nightingale trained at a hospital in Kaiserswerth, Germany, in 1851, and with the Sisters of Charity in Paris. On 21 October 1854, she led thirty-eight volunteer nurses from England to the Crimean War: ten Roman Catholic Sisters, eight Anglican Sisters of Mercy, six nurses from St. John's Institute, and fourteen from various hospitals. They reached Scutari on 4 November 1854. The barrack hospital at Scutari had no containers for water, no utensils, no soap, and no towels or clothes. [8]

When the nurses arrived, the men were lying in their uniforms, stiff with gore and covered with filth and vermin. Nightingale espoused the theory of miasma—an idea that stated poisonous vapors from decomposing matter could fill the air with noxious particles and cause disease. Germ theory was not proven until 1877, but when Nightingale scrubbed the Crimean hospital and insisted on fresh air to remove noxious particles, she inadvertently eliminated dangerous microorganisms. The death rate decreased from forty-two percent to approximately four. [9] She became a national hero in Britain.

In 1937, the Federal Arts Project erected a statue of Nightingale in Lincoln Park; the Hospital Council of Southern California sponsored it. [10] A brass plaque with an inscription was later attached to the base. Eventually, vandals defaced the statue with graffiti and broke off the arms, nose, and lamp. The city removed the plaque because they feared it would be stolen for brass.

In 1974, nurses petitioned the city to repair the statue and move it to a safer place. Conflicting groups from the County Hospital School of Nursing and California Hospital School of Nursing battled over the new location. Fifty-nine student nurses from California Hospital organized six ice cream-eating contests to raise funds for the repair. [11] The Los Angeles Municipal Arts Commission convinced the two groups to leave the statue in Lincoln Park until after the restoration. [12] However, the statue was never professionally restored or relocated. Episodes of painted-over graffiti were evident.

In 2013, Diane Harris-Hara and Joyce Jacob, from the Western Conservancy of Nursing History in Azusa, again tried to convince the city to relocate the statue for its safety: to the Azusa campus, to the County Hospital, or even to the Florence Nightingale Middle School—anywhere with a presence to protect it. [13] The City Charter declined, stating it was a gift to the entire city. In 2014 conservation artists Rosa Lowinger and Associates restored the statue, erected a barrier, and planted thorny white roses to deter vandals. A replica of the statue resides at Laguna Honda Hospital, San Francisco. [14]

Chapter One

On the facing page is one of the actual lamps Nightingale and her nurses carried during the Crimean War. The ends were made of metal, the body was paper, and a candle was burned inside. Most renderings depict her lamp as teapot-shaped. The National Army Museum stated that restricted information may have accounted for the incorrect drawings of the lamp.

English-born Nightingale is the world's most famous nurse. She started the first professional nursing school in 1860 and mentored Linda Richards—America's first trained nurse.[15-16] National Nurses Week surrounds her May 12th birthday. She wrote more than two hundred books and pamphlets. She traveled the world. She succeeded in male-dominated societies, military and medical, during a time when female role models barely existed.

The Nightingale Air Force aircraft (C-9A) was specifically designed for the movement of litter and ambulatory patients.[17] An AP-70 WWII ship, built in California, was named the USS *Florence Nightingale*.[18]

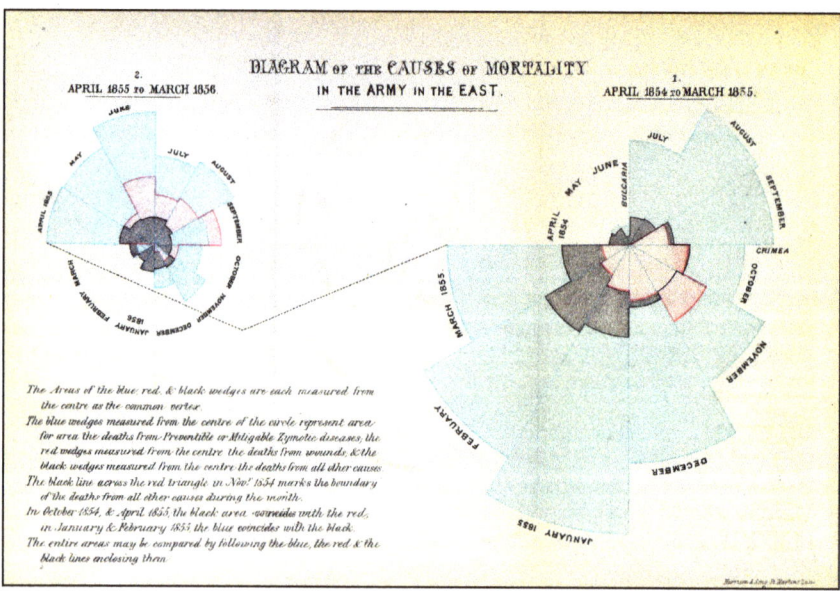

Figure 01.06. Florence Nightingale's 1858 Coxcomb Graph or Rose Diagram (a type of pie chart) she created on Crimean War mortality statistics. The inner sections of the graph illustrate that most soldiers died of contagious diseases, such as cholera and typhus, not from war wounds. (Courtesy of the Royal Collection Her Majesty Queen Elizabeth II)

Nightingale was known for her expert knowledge of mathematics and use of statistics. She created innovative charts and graphs that persuaded Queen Victoria to improve sanitary conditions in military hospitals.[19]

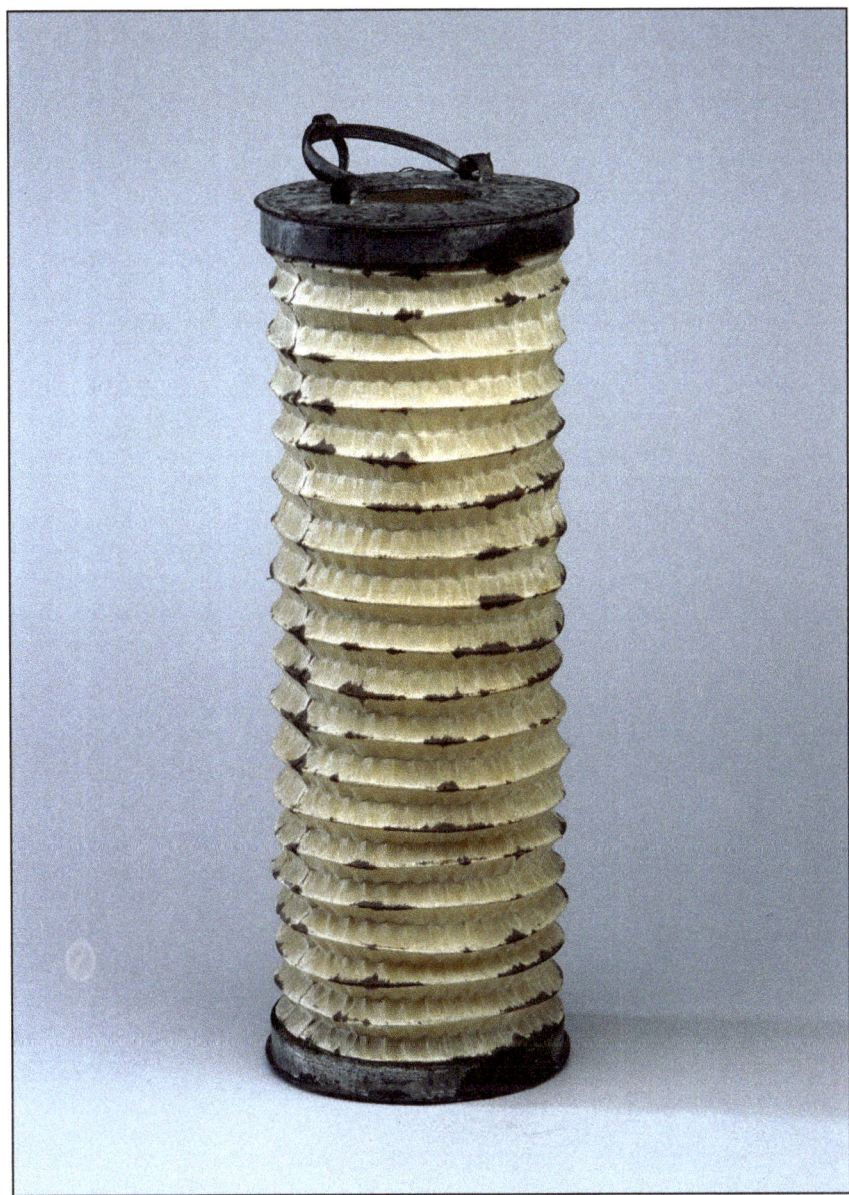

Figure 01.07. Florence Nightingale's lamp she carried in the Crimean War to conduct her nightly patient rounds, c. 1854. (Courtesy of the Council of the National Army Museum, London)

Crimean soldiers gave Nightingale the moniker "Lady with the Lamp." Sketches, paintings, and statues usually depict her holding a teapot-shaped lamp, but these renderings are incorrect. The lamp was shaped like a tube.

Chapter One

Mary Seacole's mother lived as a free Black woman in Jamaica, and her father was a Scottish soldier stationed in Kingston. Her mother, a well-known herbalist, ran a boarding house for invalid British soldiers and their family members. Seacole helped her mother care for patients with dysentery, cholera, and yellow fever. Seacole was born Mary Ann Grant; she married Edwin Horatio Seacole in 1836, but he died soon after. [20]

When Seacole heard about the Crimean War she traveled to London to volunteer as a war nurse. The War Office refused to hire her. Her second plan, to join a group of nurses headed to Crimea, did not succeed either. Rumors later spread that Nightingale refused Seacole's request to join her because of Seacole's Jamaican heritage. However, in Seacole's book she said, "Miss Nightingale had left England for Crimea, but other nurses were to follow, my plan was simply to offer myself to Mrs. H." But Mrs. H informed her "the full compliment of nurses had been secured." She wondered if "American prejudices against colour had root in England." [21] Possibly correct, but her account of this did not originate from a meeting with Nightingale.

Seacole met a friend of her late husband and they devised her third plan: they would open a hotel and store in Crimea. She used her own money to buy medicine and "home comforts" and booked a passage to Balaclava on the screw-steamer *Hollander*. They operated the British Hotel (a storehouse, a canteen, and a resting place) in the war zone from 1855-1856, selling supplies and medicine to the Army. She also cared for wounded soldiers on the battlefront. On her first trip to the front she stopped at Scutari and met Nightingale. She offered a letter of recommendation but didn't seek employment. Rather, she asked to stay the night and Nightingale accommodated her. Seacole wrote a cordial account of their meeting. [22] The French chef Alexis Soyer knew them both and reported on their friendly relations in his *A Culinary Campaign*.

In 1857, Seacole published a book about her war and travel experiences, *Wonderful Adventures of Mrs. Seacole in Many Lands*. The book became a popular and commercial success. England celebrated her accomplishments. However, when she died in 1881 she faded from memory.

In 1973, visiting Caribbean nurses discovered her London grave in Kensal Green. A Jamaican women's organization and the British Commonwealth Nurses' War Memorial restored her head stone. [23] United Kingdom schools taught her story. London erected a Seacole statue in 2003. They named two British National Health Service Awards for nurses in her honor: the Mary Seacole Leadership Award and the Mary Seacole Development Award. [24]

Artist Henry Weekes created a marble bust of Seacole circa 1859. By that time, she'd become a household name in England. In 1984 the J. Paul Getty Museum in Los Angeles secured it and placed it on permanent exhibition. [25]

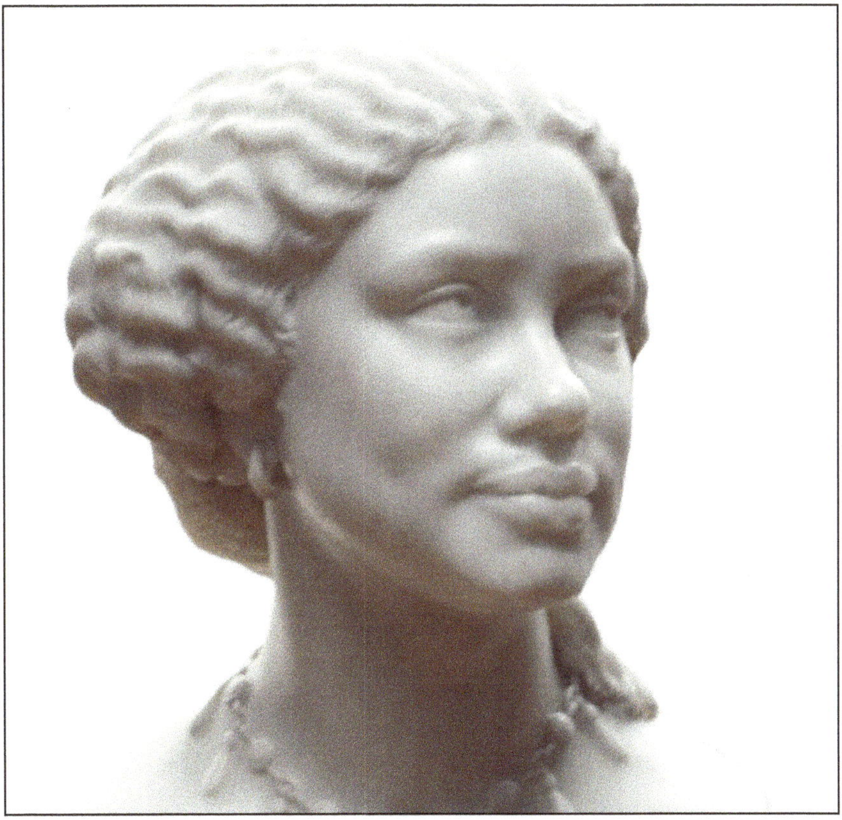

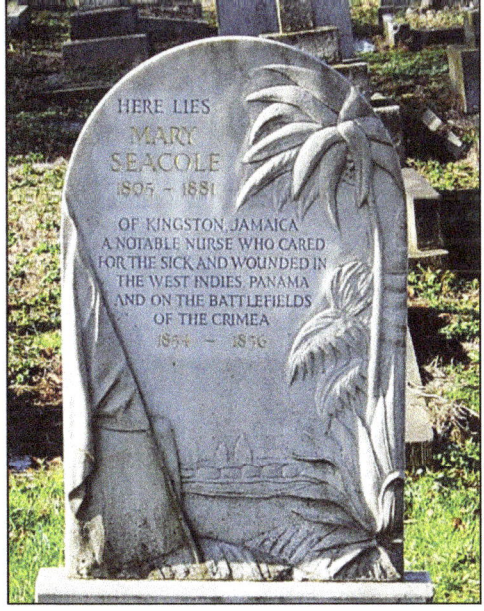

Figure 01.08. *Mary Seacole,* a marble sculpture at the Los Angeles J. Paul Getty Museum, 2009. (Courtesy of Chuck Mattick)

Figure 01.09. Mary Seacole's restored grave marker at St. Mary's Roman Catholic Cemetery in Kensal Green, 2009. (By Iain MacFarlain)

Chapter One

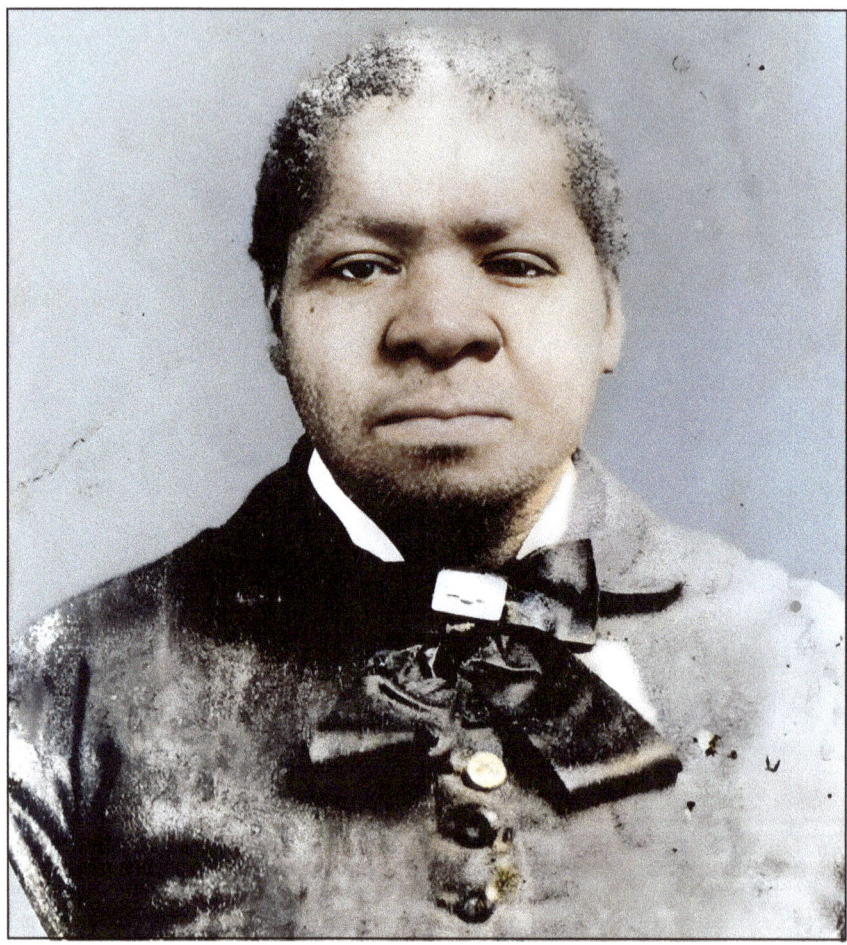

Figure 01.10. Biddy Mason in Los Angeles, date unknown. C.

Bridger "Biddy" Mason was born a slave on a Mississippi plantation. She bore three children, reportedly fathered by her plantation owner, Robert Smith.

In 1851 the family moved to San Bernardino, outside of Los Angeles. When Smith learned California was a free state that forbade slavery, he tried to relocate Mason to Texas. She refused to go. A Los Angeles sheriff intervened and helped Mason leave Smith by using the court system. She moved to Los Angeles as a free woman in 1856, at age 38, and worked as a self-taught nurse and midwife for all races and classes.

In 1866, Mason bought a plot on Spring Street for $250. She was the first Black woman in Los Angeles to own land. She purchased commercial real estate and accumulated $300,000 in holdings—a fortune at that time. [26]

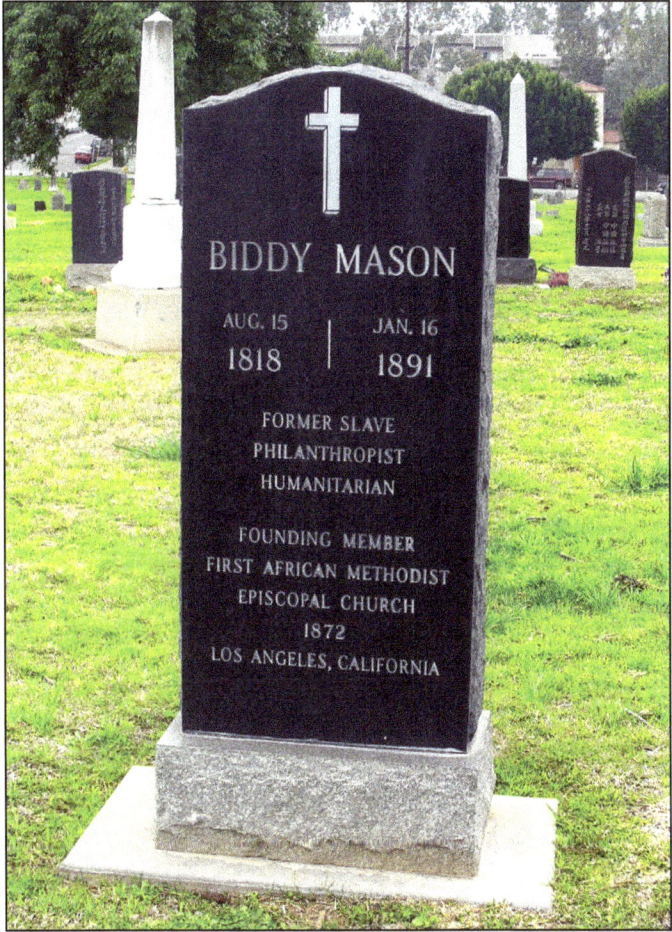

Figure 01.11. Biddy Mason's gravesite in the Evergreen Cemetery, the oldest cemetery in Los Angeles, 2009. Author photographed.

She died in 1891; however, her gravesite remained unmarked. In March 1988, the L.A. Mayor and the First African Methodist Episcopal Church (A.M.E.) erected a headstone. Mason founded the A.M.E. in 1872.[27-28]

Mason generously contributed to charities. She provided food and shelter for the poor and started an orphanage.

Her original familial dwelling was located near Broadway and Spring Streets in downtown Los Angeles. In 1989, Los Angeles proclaimed 16 November as Biddy Mason Day and erected Biddy Mason Park at 333 South Spring Street. The site contained a mural and granite wall detailing her life story. [29-30]

Chapter One

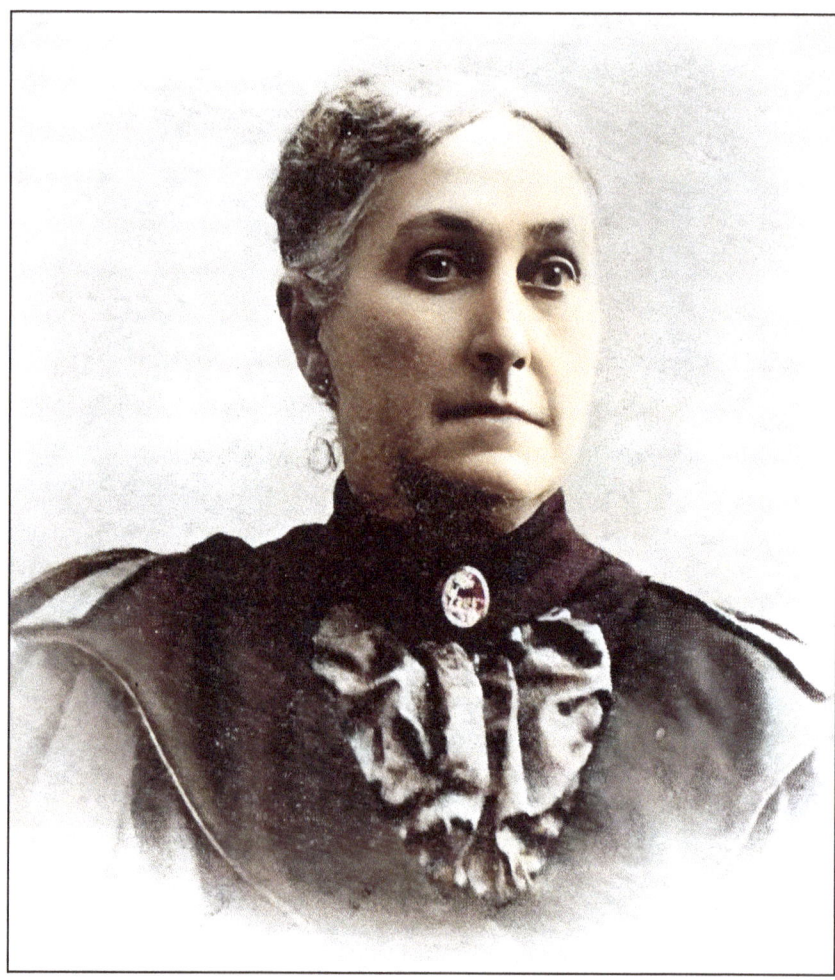

Figure 01.12. Margaret "Sister Maggie" Hayes, n.d. C.

Margaret Hayes left Chicago in August of 1863 to help the boys in blue during the Civil War. She arrived in Tennessee and was immediately assigned to Adams Hospital Number 2, in Memphis. The steamer ship, the *Sultana*, was blown up with 1900 paroled prisoners on board soon after Hayes arrived in Memphis. The emaciated, injured men were brought to her hospital; only 500 survived.

The boys in blue called her Sister Maggie. She said the boys appreciated everything she did—they gave her a valuable gold watch, which she considered "her choicest possession." She left the war in 1865 and moved to Los Angeles in 1888. She celebrated her century-old birthday in 1933 with 100 candles on a cake in her home at 1200 Forty-Fifth Street in Los Angeles. [31-32]

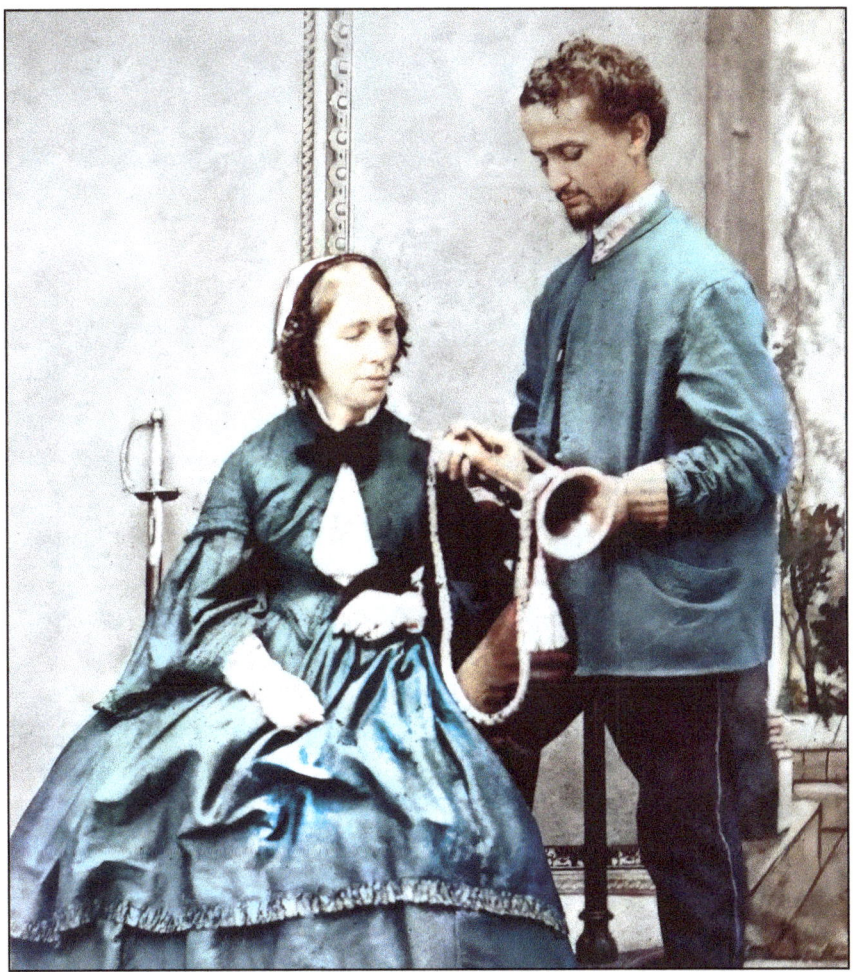

Figure 01.13. Union soldier showing Eleanor Ransom a bugle, c. 1861-1865. C. (Liljenquist Family Collection at the Library of Congress).

Soldiers and friends affectionately called Eleanor Ransom "Mother Ransom." In 1863, she was assigned to the Civil War hospital, Gayoso General, in Tennessee. Ransom said when she washed the feet of wounded soldiers, "they wept great tears of gratitude that spoke louder than words." She witnessed shipwrecks, death, and starvation. She felt so bad for the soldiers she could not function mentally or physically after returning home from the war.

She moved to Los Angeles and established several institutions that cared for the elderly and the disabled. [33] In 1904, at 90 years old, she was living in one of her institutions, the Ransom Industrial Home, when a *Los Angeles Times* reporter interviewed her for the article, "Army Nurses With Us Now." [34]

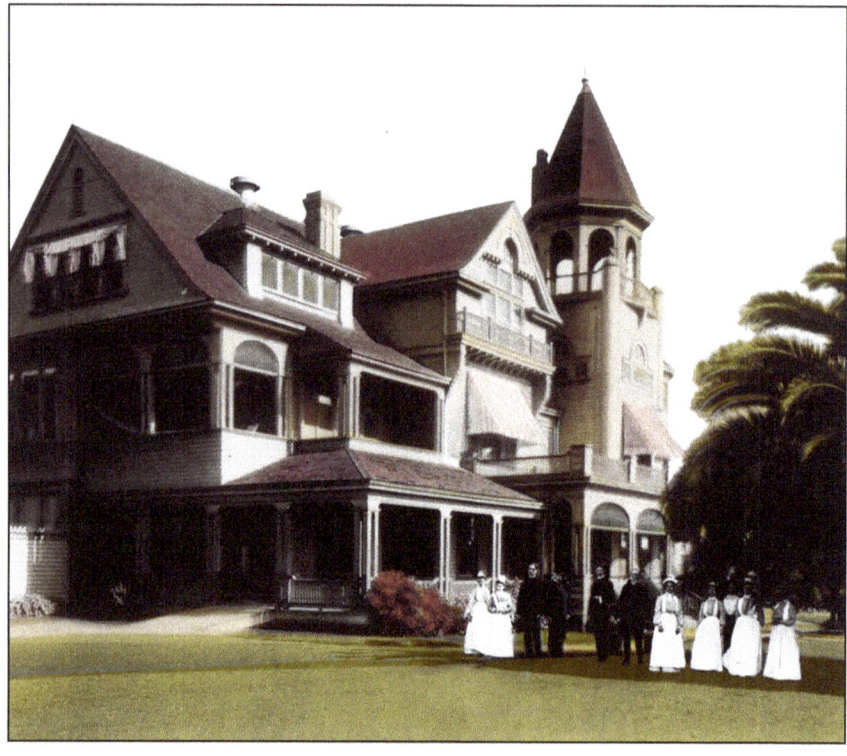

Figure 01.14. Photo postcard of nurses and doctors standing on the lawn of the Military Home Hospital, c. 1905. C.

After World War I, President Hoover combined the National Military Home and the Veterans Bureau into the Veterans Administration. Congress established the National Asylum for Disabled Civil War Volunteers in 1865.

The Asylum became known as the National Military Home or the Soldier's Home. The Pacific Branch was located in Sawtelle, a 1.82-square-mile area on the west side of Los Angeles.

A 10 September 1906 article in the *Los Angeles Times* stated immediate construction would begin for a nurses' quarter at the southwest corner of Bonsall Avenue and Sunset Boulevard—just opposite the northern extremity of the hospital. The ornate cottage would be 53 x 57 feet with many conveniences of a modern home.

The plans included a reception room with an adjoining sitting room, a room for the matron, a night nurses' sleeping room, and a bathroom with a toilet room. The west side would house a kitchen, pantry, and dining room. The second floor would consist of seven sleeping rooms and bathrooms. [35]

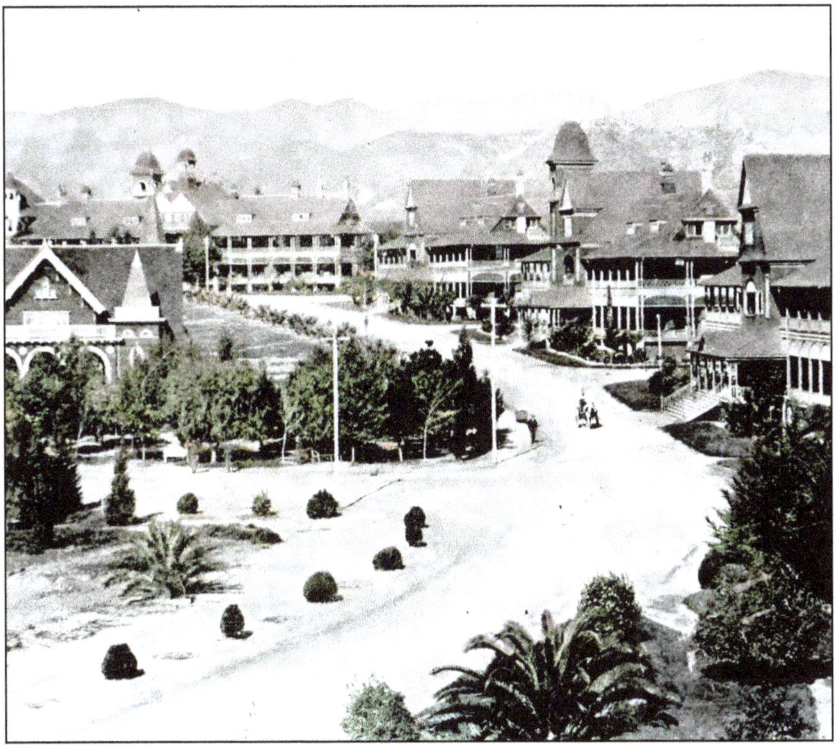

Nurses Arrive

Figure 01.15. The Soldier's Home, c. 1905. C. The 300-acre grounds contained 25 barracks with 100 men per barrack.[36]

Figure 01.16. "Ladies in the Surf" depicts nurses, who worked at the Pacific Branch of the Soldiers Home, bathing in the ocean, 1884. C. (Santa Monica Library, Connie Cramer Collection)

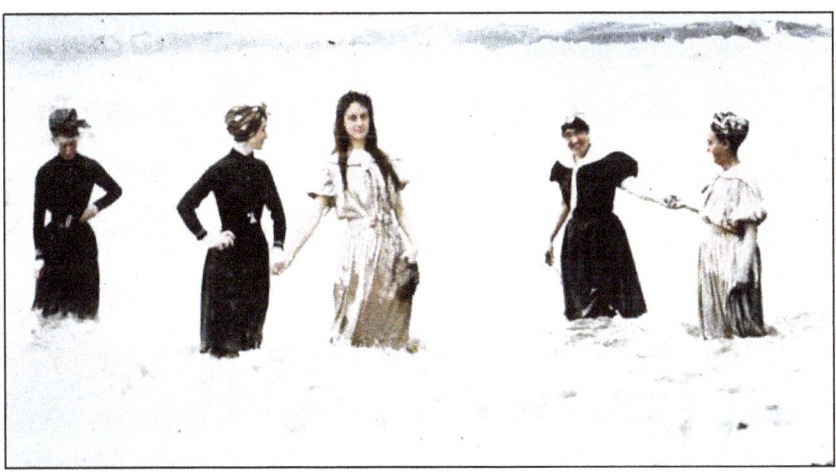

Chapter One

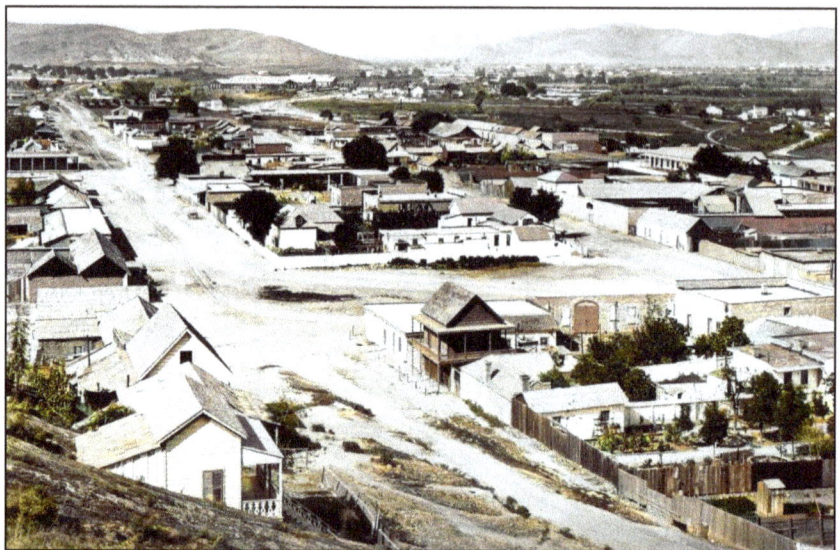

Figure 01.17. Famous photographer Carleton E. Watkins took this image of the cityscape of Los Angeles in 1880. C. The Southern Pacific Railroad facilities were visible in the distance.

The establishment of the railroad brought throngs to Los Angeles to improve chronic health conditions. Many believed in the curative effects of the perfect climate and sea breeze in Southern California. In 1880 the population of Los Angeles was 11,000; by 1890 the population had grown to 102,474, aided by the ease of railway travel. [37]

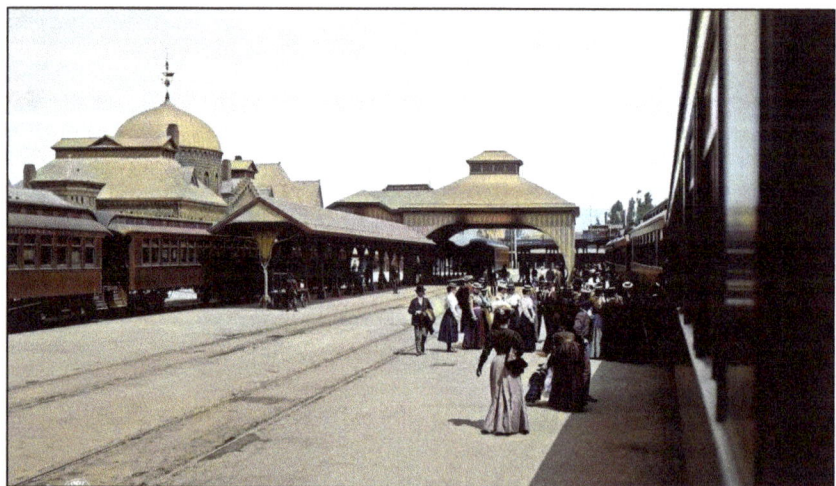

Figure 01.18. Boarding the Overland Train at La Grande Station, 1893. C.

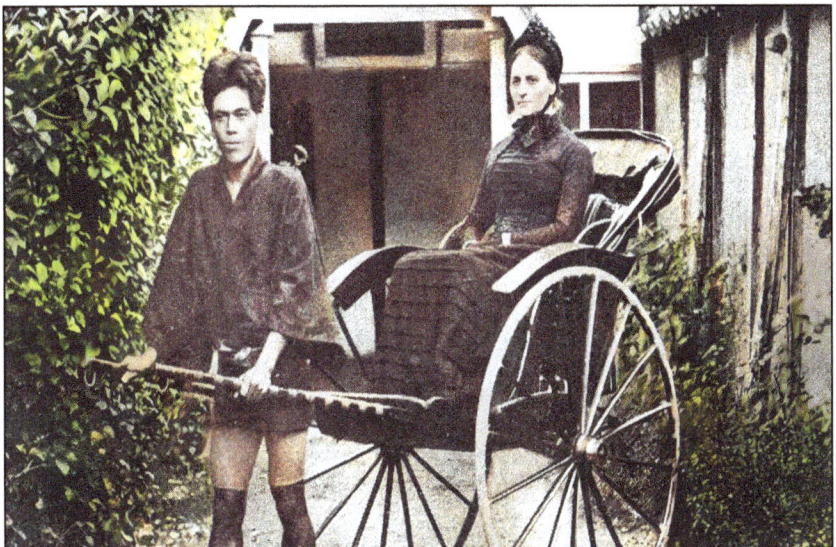

Figure 01.19. Linda Richards in a rickshaw in Kyoto, Japan, 1885. C.

Linda Richards became America's first trained nurse in 1873 when she graduated from the New England Hospital for Women and Children Nurses Training School. The pupil nurses cared for six patients from 5:30 a.m. to 9:00 p.m. They slept in small rooms between the wards. They did not wear uniforms. They had no textbooks or exams. Three young female medical interns instructed the pupils in the bedside care of patients. All medications were placed in numbered bottles as nurses were not allowed to know the names of the medications they administered to patients.

One of Richards' other four classmates, Caroline Stapfer, moved to Los Angeles and worked as a nurse-masseuse. After graduation, Richards became the superintendent for training schools in Boston, Philadelphia, New York, and in Kalamazoo Insane Asylum in Michigan. She helped improve hospitals for patients with mental illness. She is credited with conceiving the idea of charting because she kept notes on her cases. A doctor found her notes one day and said they were helpful to him. He asked her to continue to show him the notes, and this started the custom of charting.[38]

On her way to Japan, Richards spent December of 1885 in Los Angeles with Stapfer, her former classmate.[39] The American Board of Missions had hired Richards to start a training school in Kyoto, Japan; she organized Japan's first training school for nurses. She learned to speak Japanese, and although she had never sewn before, she sewed all the uniforms for her pupil nurses. The first Japanese nursing class graduated in 1888. Richards wrote a book in 1911 about her experiences: *Reminiscences of America's First Trained Nurse.*

Chapter One

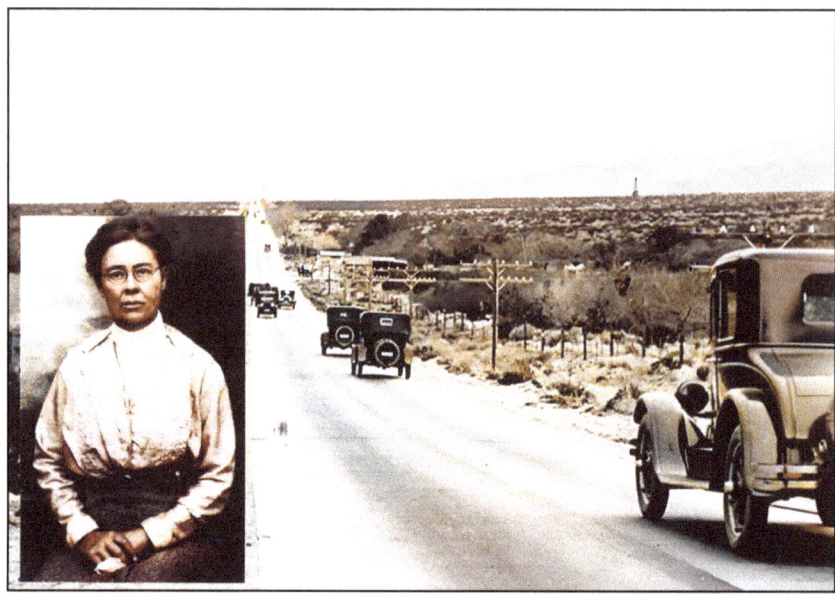

Figure 01.20. June Robertson McCarroll's photograph is set into an image of a Model T Ford driving in Coachella Valley, c.1920. A widening ridge is visible in the middle of the road. C.

June Robertson McCarroll became a nurse in Kentucky in the 1880s; she was the first Southern Pacific Railroad nurse.[40] She later became a physician in Chicago. Her husband contracted tuberculosis, so she quit her medical practice, and the couple moved to the dry climate of Los Angeles. Tuberculosis treatment during that period included sunshine and fresh air. When they arrived at the tuberculosis camp in Indio, California, she was asked to help care for patients, and her medical career started again.

Her husband did not survive his illness, but she stayed in California and became the only physician who practiced regularly in the Salton Sea to Palm Springs desert area of the Coachella Valley. She was the only physician who served the five Indian reservations for the Bureau of Indian Affairs. She traveled long hours on horseback, rode a horse and buggy, used railroad handcars, and eventually automobiles to practice medicine under primitive conditions.[41] As a doctor she witnessed the human toll from car accidents.

In 1917, McCarroll was driving her Model T Ford through Coachella Valley when an oncoming truck veered toward her car and ran her off the road. She later noticed Highway 99 had a ridge down the middle where the road had been widened; this forced cars to keep to one side and hindered them from veering into oncoming traffic. She thought a painted line down the center of the road could serve the same purpose and make driving safer.[42]

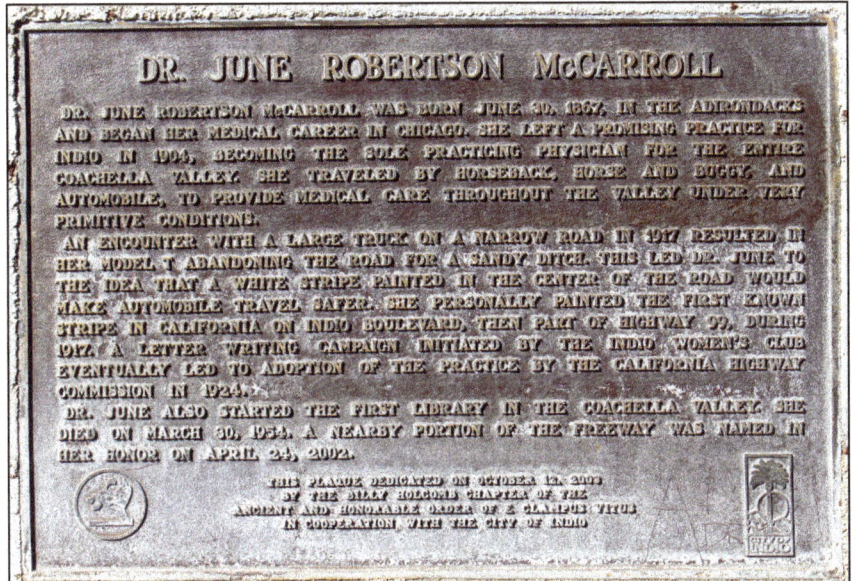

Figure 01.21. The memorial plaque, stating McCarroll's accomplishments, is located at 82921 Indio Boulevard, near the spot where the truck first ran her Model T Ford off the road.

McCarroll's incident of being run off the road spurred her idea of painting a white line down the center of the highway. She presented her idea to the Riverside County Board of Supervisors, but they were not impressed. So McCarroll hand-painted a four-inch stripe down the middle of the road, approximately a mile in length, on Highway 99 (now Indio Boulevard).

She tried to sell the idea to the board for five years without success; eventually, she asked the Indio Women's Club to assist her. They launched a statewide letter-writing campaign. After receiving the support of the county and the State Federation of Women's Clubs, she petitioned the California State Legislature to enact a resolution.

The California State Highway Commission finally adopted Robertson's idea in 1924 and, as a trial, painted 3,500 miles of lines for $163,000.

In 2002, California designated a section of Interstate 10 as the Doctor June McCarroll Memorial Freeway.[43]

McCarroll also started the first library in Coachella Valley, primarily to provide reading material for her isolated tuberculosis patients. She applied to Sacramento and was granted a state branch. The original library contained fifty to one hundred volumes.

The Great Decade: 1895-1930

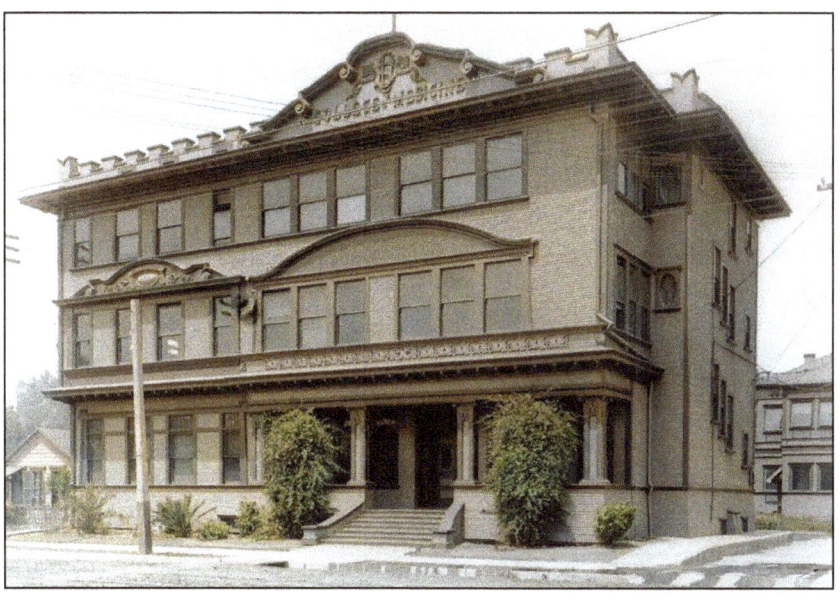

Figure 02.01. The College Training School for Nurses at the College of Medicine, University of Southern California building, 737 Buena Vista Street, Los Angeles, 1896. C. In 1905, Buena Vista became North Broadway. (Courtesy of University of Southern California Archives)

From 1890 to 1900, professional nursing education experienced a tremendous surge. Important leaders emerged, schools proliferated, and organizations were formed. The *American Journal of Nursing* distributed its inaugural issues in 1900. In 1890, only thirty-five schools existed in the United States; by 1900 there were 432.[1] Los Angeles started several schools for nurses during this great decade.

Los Angeles hospitals taught practical skills to workers to care for their patients, but none had conducted a school that taught professional nursing classes.[2] Local doctors realized the need to start a training school. The *Los Angeles Times* reported Dr. D. C. Barber went to San Francisco in 1895 to study the methods one hospital used to manage its school. Upon his return, Barber proposed County Hospital wards could be used as a training area. The progressive women in town gave their hearty cooperation to his scheme, but the County Fathers demurred at the newfangled idea. Barber represented that his plan could be secured without *any* additional expense to the county; it could hardly fail if properly managed. No expense to the county? The County Fathers agreed to his plan to use county's wards as a training site.[3]

Doctor Walter Lindley, the owner of the Sixth Street Hospital, became the president of the organization and formed a board. They incorporated faculty from the University of Southern California Medical College and started the first Los Angeles nursing school: The College Training School for Nurses.

On 10 March 1897, Miss Brennan of Bellevue Hospital in New York addressed the board of managers on training methods the New York schools employed. A few hospitals in the United States trained nurses before 1873, but they were not based on the Nightingale model.

The most important concept in the Nightingale model was that nurses would report to a superintendent nurse, not a physician. The superintendent nurse would then report to the hospital board. Most hospitals still follow a form of this model, although the word superintendent is no longer used. [4]

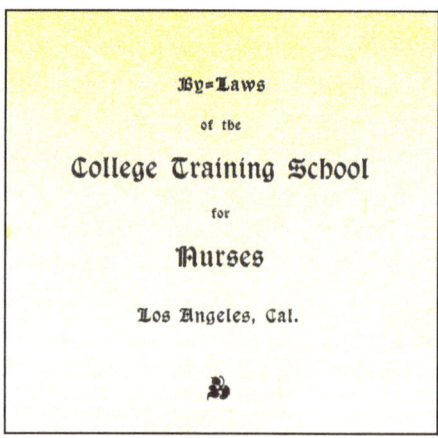

Figure 02.02. Cover of the By-Laws for the College Training School for Nurses, 1896. (Lindley Scrapbooks, Special Collections, Libraries of Claremont Colleges.)

The by-laws included voting and membership requirements, the schedule of meetings and elections, duties of the director, manager, treasurer, recording secretary, and corresponding secretary. A $50.00 contribution to the funds of the society granted a lifetime membership, $20.00 inferred an honorary membership, and a yearly payment of $1.00 as an annual member. All membership levels included the right to vote.

The *Los Angeles County Medical Center School, Looking Back a Century* book stated Lindley began the College Training School for Nurses in 1895, and it only lasted one year. [5] The book did not cite a reference. Lindley's scrapbook included items from the school dated 1896 to 1898. Yes, the idea of creating the school began in 1895 when Dr. Barber traveled to San Francisco to "learn one hospital's training methods;" [6] however, several newspapers and Lindley's records state the College Training School lasted two years.

Lindley's scrapbooks contained 1897 graduation items, including eight pupils from County Hospital and three from his hospital. [7] On 14 January 1898, the *Los Angeles Times* reported on the election of officers. Lindley remained president in 1898, but he did not own the school. [8] The college owned it.

Great Decade

The pupil's application consisted of a single page. Requirements included the applicant must have a good grammar school education, be in good health, be of good moral character, and between twenty-one and thirty- five years old.

A pupil nurse could transfer in from another hospital program. To be granted a diploma, however, she had to attend the final year at the College Training School for Nurses. The first class graduated after one year of training because the board granted one year of credit for clinical experience. After the first year, the training length became two years for every student.

Figure 02.03. A 1896 application to the school. Pupils attended thirty-four lectures in the junior and senior years.[9] (Lindley Scrapbooks, Special Collections, Libraries of Claremont Colleges.)

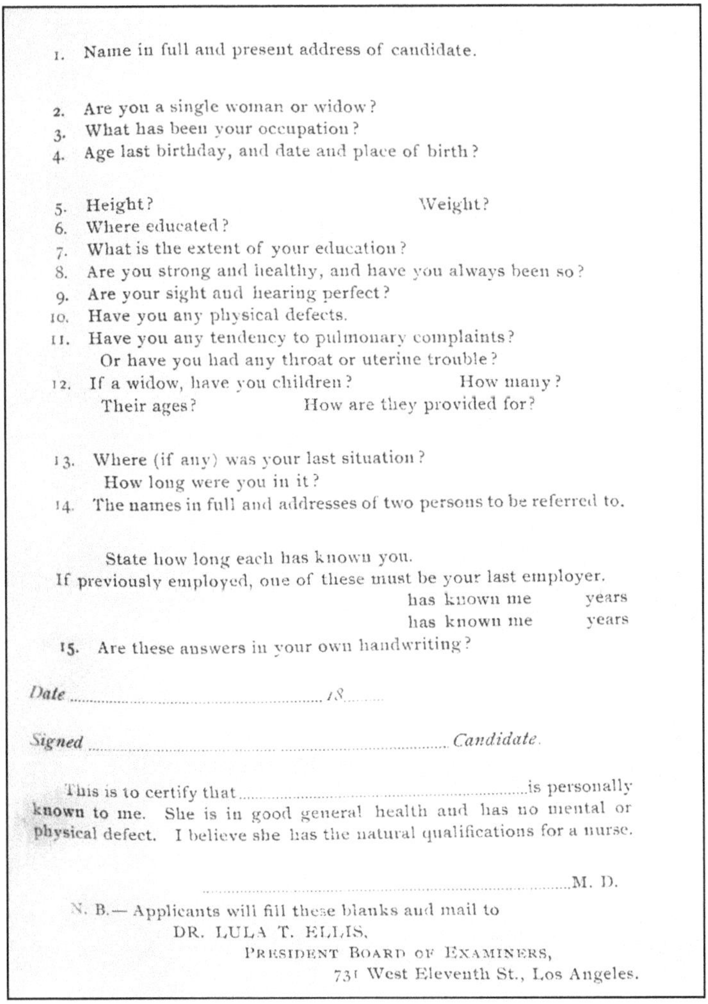

1. Name in full and present address of candidate.
2. Are you a single woman or widow?
3. What has been your occupation?
4. Age last birthday, and date and place of birth?
5. Height?   Weight?
6. Where educated?
7. What is the extent of your education?
8. Are you strong and healthy, and have you always been so?
9. Are your sight and hearing perfect?
10. Have you any physical defects.
11. Have you any tendency to pulmonary complaints?
    Or have you had any throat or uterine trouble?
12. If a widow, have you children?   How many?
    Their ages?   How are they provided for?
13. Where (if any) was your last situation?
    How long were you in it?
14. The names in full and addresses of two persons to be referred to.

    State how long each has known you.
    If previously employed, one of these must be your last employer.
                                    has known me   years
                                    has known me   years
15. Are these answers in your own handwriting?

Date _____ 18____

Signed _____ Candidate.

This is to certify that_____is personally known to me. She is in good general health and has no mental or physical defect. I believe she has the natural qualifications for a nurse.

_____M. D.

N. B.— Applicants will fill these blanks and mail to
                DR. LULA T. ELLIS,
                    PRESIDENT BOARD OF EXAMINERS,
                        731 West Eleventh St., Los Angeles.

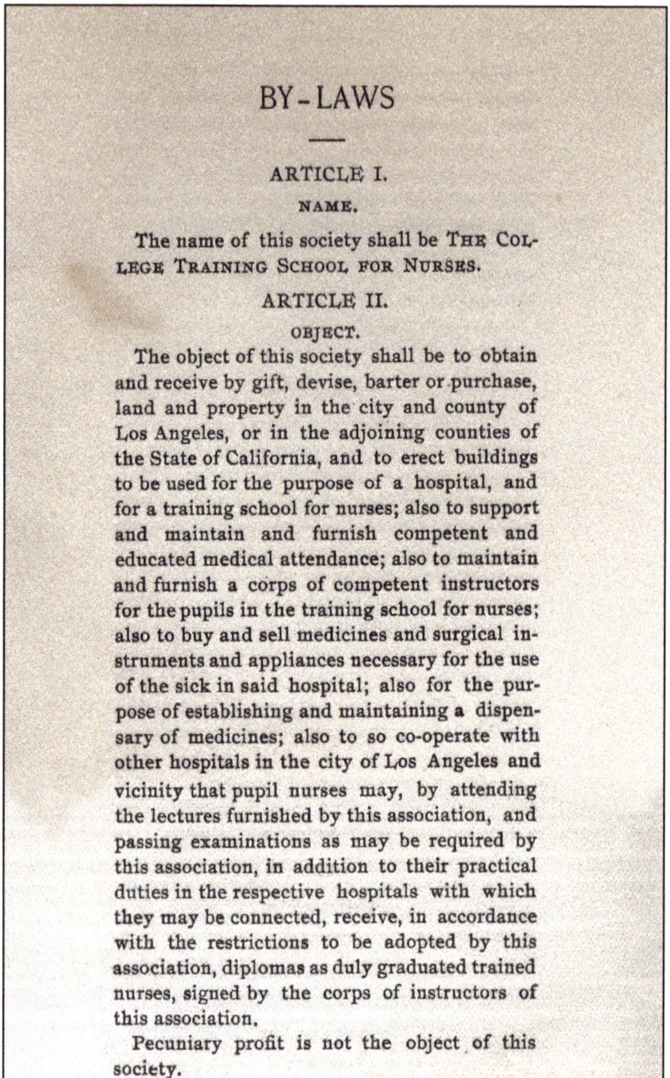

BY-LAWS

ARTICLE I.
NAME.

The name of this society shall be THE COLLEGE TRAINING SCHOOL FOR NURSES.

ARTICLE II.
OBJECT.

The object of this society shall be to obtain and receive by gift, devise, barter or purchase, land and property in the city and county of Los Angeles, or in the adjoining counties of the State of California, and to erect buildings to be used for the purpose of a hospital, and for a training school for nurses; also to support and maintain and furnish competent and educated medical attendance; also to maintain and furnish a corps of competent instructors for the pupils in the training school for nurses; also to buy and sell medicines and surgical instruments and appliances necessary for the use of the sick in said hospital; also for the purpose of establishing and maintaining a dispensary of medicines; also to so co-operate with other hospitals in the city of Los Angeles and vicinity that pupil nurses may, by attending the lectures furnished by this association, and passing examinations as may be required by this association, in addition to their practical duties in the respective hospitals with which they may be connected, receive, in accordance with the restrictions to be adopted by this association, diplomas as duly graduated trained nurses, signed by the corps of instructors of this association.

Pecuniary profit is not the object of this society.

Figure 02.04. By-Laws Article I and II, Name and Object, 1896. (Lindley Scrapbooks, Special Collections, Libraries of Claremont Colleges)

Articles I and II explained the basic ideas of the school. The pupils attended lectures at various buildings throughout the city. No documents state the exact hospitals each pupil received their clinical instructions from: they could complete a portion of training in their respective hospitals, as mentioned in the article above, or at County Hospital, as other documents state. The society did not erect a new hospital and training school as they had planned in this document.[10]

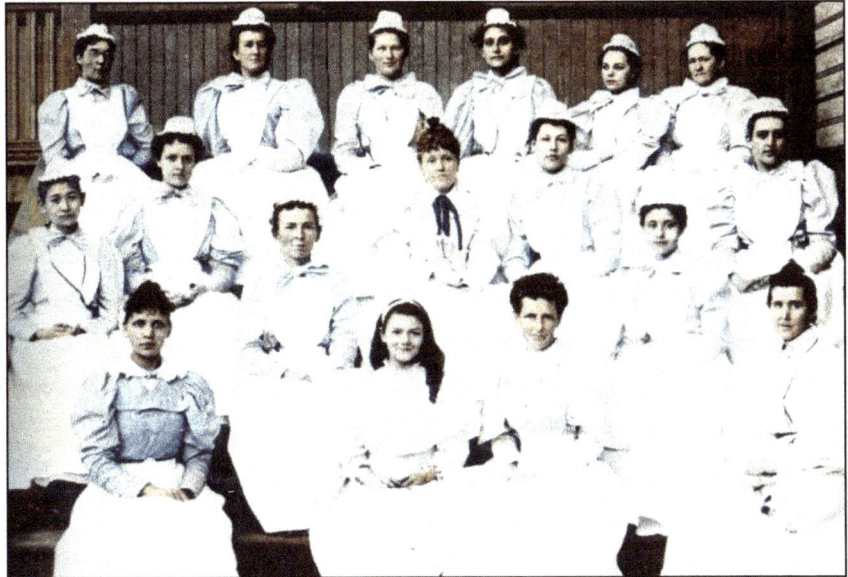

Figure 02.05. The first fourteen pupils at the College Training School for Nurses, 1896. C. Annie O'Neil, the first matron-superintendent, and her daughter are in the center front row. To her right is Elizabeth Follansbee, MD, professor of pediatrics. Their uniforms were blue and white-striped gingham with leg-o-mutton sleeves, white muslin aprons, and white caps. One woman in the front has no apron or cap but appears to wear the school's blouse and skirt; she might be a pupil with an incomplete uniform.

The *Los Angeles Times* reported the opening exercises occurred on 6 October 1896. The college extended an invitation for the public to attend. Miss Wills, the vice president, read "Duties and Responsibilities of Nurses," written for the occasion.[11]

> Thirty-four trainees sat in the center of the audience, dressed in appropriate suits that bespoke neatness, cleanliness, and good taste. The young ladies formed the center of the audience, which gathered to listen to the addresses made and papers read.[12]

Four hospitals employed the potential trainees: eighteen from County Hospital, six from the Good Samaritan Hospital, six from Lindley's Sixth Street Hospital (California), and four from the Los Angeles Sanitarium.[13]

While thirty-four trainees attended the opening ceremony, only fourteen pupils were shown in this photo. Only twelve graduated. No record could be located to explain the fate of the other twenty trainees who sat in the audience at the opening ceremony, or of the other two pupils in the photo.

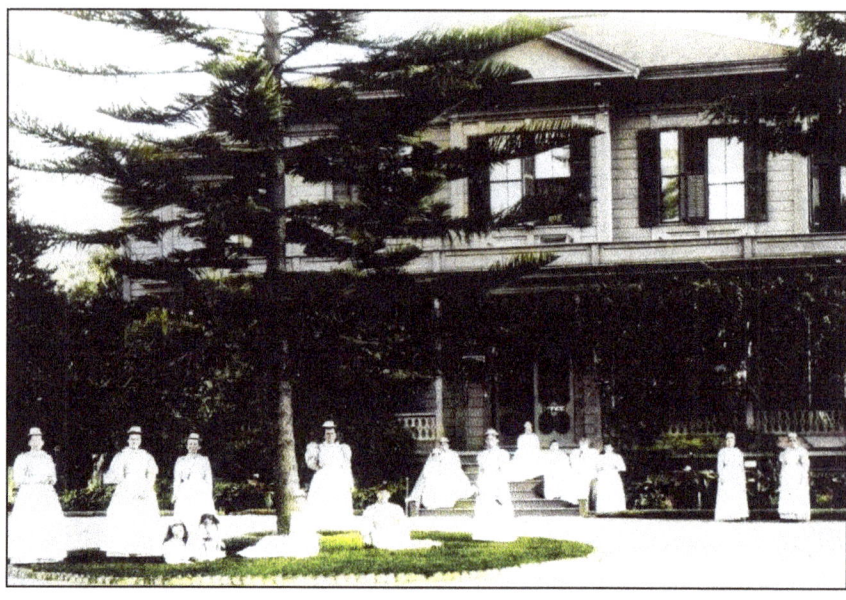

Figure 02.06. Students pose in front of the first County Hospital, 1897. C. The nursing superintendent's young daughter lies on the ground, holding her dog. The dog was dressed in white and wore a trainee's cap.

Two textbooks are listed in the brochure: *Nursing: Its Principles and Practice*, Isabel Adams Hampton, and *Essentials of Anatomy*, Chas. B. Nancrede, M.D. Hampton wrote one of the first nursing textbooks ever published—a complete week-to-week, two-year instruction manual on the training of nurses.[14]

Figure 02.07. The three textbooks used in the training school, *Nursing: Its Principles and Practice,* (Nurse Isabel Adams Hampton), *Essentials of Anatomy*, (Chas. Nancrede, MD), *Primer of Surgical Nursing*, (Frances Hayes, MD).

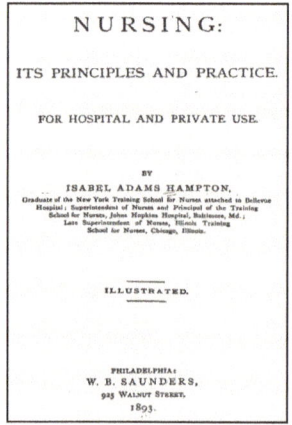 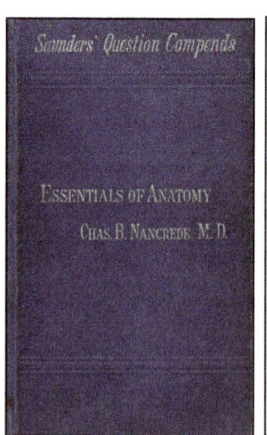 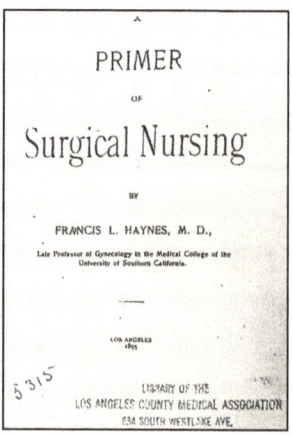

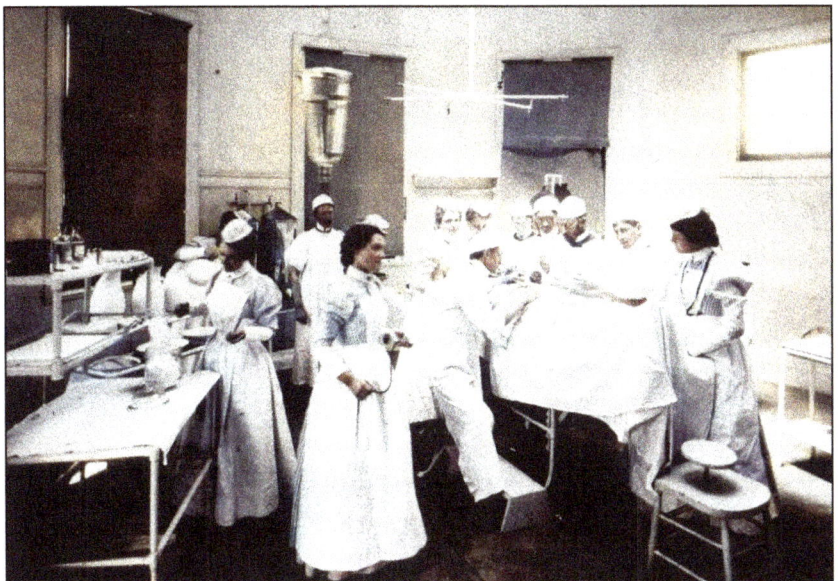

Figure 02.08. Student nurses during surgery at County Hospital. A nurse at the head of the table, wearing the same cap as the pupils, administered the anesthesia. Dr. Barber is the primary surgeon in this photograph, 1897. C.

No one wore gloves or masks. Nurses usually scrubbed their hands with disinfectant chemicals before surgery; later, they began wearing gloves to protect their hands from the caustic solutions. Joseph Lister, the father of antiseptic surgery theory, carried out the first antiseptic operation on 26 October 1877.[15] American surgeons remained skeptical of his theory. They didn't accept it until the late 1880s when an American surgeon, Dr. William Mayo, began practicing antiseptic surgery in his clinics in Rochester, Minnesota, and gradually won converts among colleagues.[16]

For surgical training, student nurses used *A Primer of Surgical Nursing* by Frances L. Hayes, MD. According to the 1899 journal, *Southern California Practitioner*, Hayes wrote a book of instructions in 1886 for nurses at Lindley's Sixth Street Hospital and printed it in 1895 for pupils at the College Training School for Nurses.

The primer contained a detailed nurses kit-list of more than 44 items: a 15x6x4 telescopic handbag (which the nurse should always carry and should be kept ready for immediate use) purgative drugs; a self-emptying bedpan; syringes; Robert's test for albumen and Haines test for sugar in a secure wooden case; a clinical and a wall thermometer; gasoline for preparing the seat of operations; and a corrosive sublimate of 7 grains mixed with 35 grains of tartaric acid put up in red powder papers and stamped "POISON."[17]

Class 1897

MISS REBECCA ALBERTS
Tehachepi, California

MISS ELIZABETH BERGHER
Hanover, Germany

MISS THERESA BABE
Los Angeles

MRS. MINNIE R. CLARK
Redlands, California

MISS ANNIE HILL
Santa Ana California

MISS MARY LAWSON
Santa Monica, California

MISS ANNIE HARPER MULLEN
Hollywood, California

MISS SARA E. NEILL
Dayton, Washington

MISS MARGARET REITZE
San Diego, California

MISS MARIETT CLARA SEXTON
Santa Barbara, California

MISS NETTIE VAUGHN
Los Angeles

MISS AMANDA ZAVITZ
Garden Grove, California

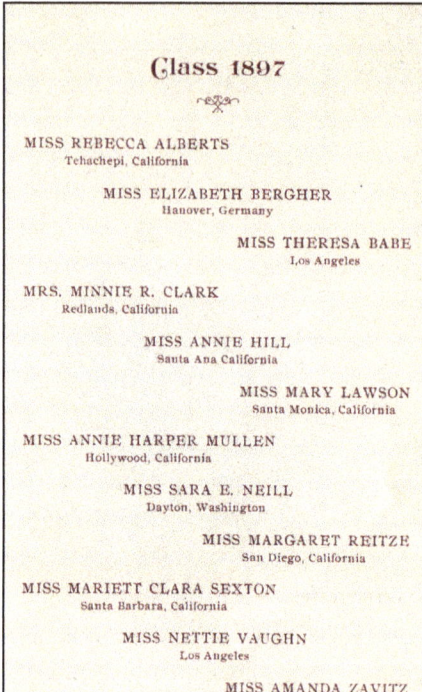

Figure 02.09. The class of 1897 graduate nurses' names.

Figure 02.10. The program cover for the first graduation exercises at the College Training School for Nurses, June 8, 1897.

Figure 02.11. Board of Directors, Faculty, and Officers Board of Managers page. (Courtesy of the Lindley Scrapbooks, Libraries of Claremont Colleges)

GRADUATING EXERCISES
TUESDAY EVENING, JUNE 8, 1897

The College Training School for Nurses

AMPHITHEATRE OF THE MEDICAL COLLEGE
737 BUENA VISTA STREET

Board of Directors and Faculty

Dr. WALTER LINDLEY	President
Dr. LEMOYNE WILLS	Vice President
Dr. W. D. BABCOCK	Secretary
Dr. GEO. L. COLE	Treasurer

JOSEPH KURTZ, M. D. — M. L. MOORE, M. D.
D. C. BARBER, M D — T. J. McCARTY, M. D.
ELIZABETH FOLLANSBEE, M. D
H. B. WING, M. D. — H. G. BRAINERD, M D.
GRANVILLE MACGOWAN, M. D.
CLAIRE W. MURPHY, M. D.
L. M. POWERS, M. D. — J. H. UTLEY, M. D.
G. W. LASHER, M. D. — H. BERT. ELLIS, M D.

Officers Board of Managers

Mrs. T. B. BROWN	President
Mrs. F. T. GRIFFITH	First Vice President
Miss M. F. WILLS	Second Vice President
Mrs. WALTER LINDLEY	Recording Secretary
Mrs E. P. JOHNSON	Corresponding Secretary
Mrs. M. L. MOORE	Treasurer

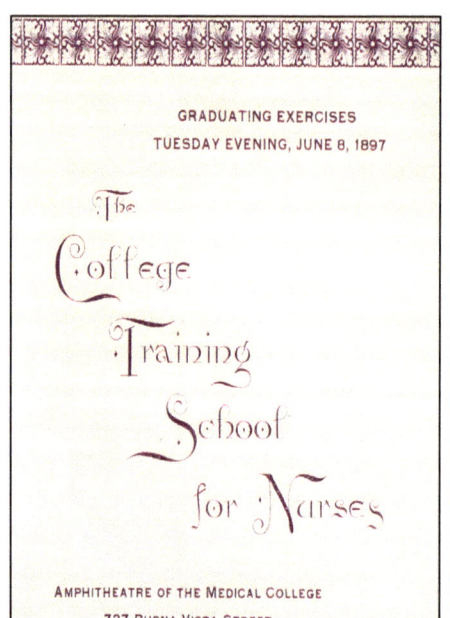

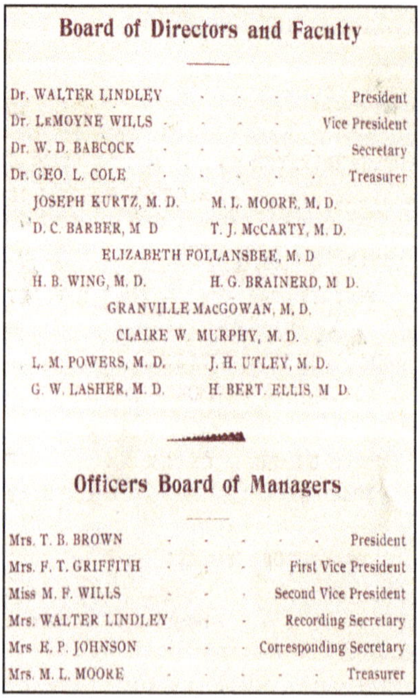

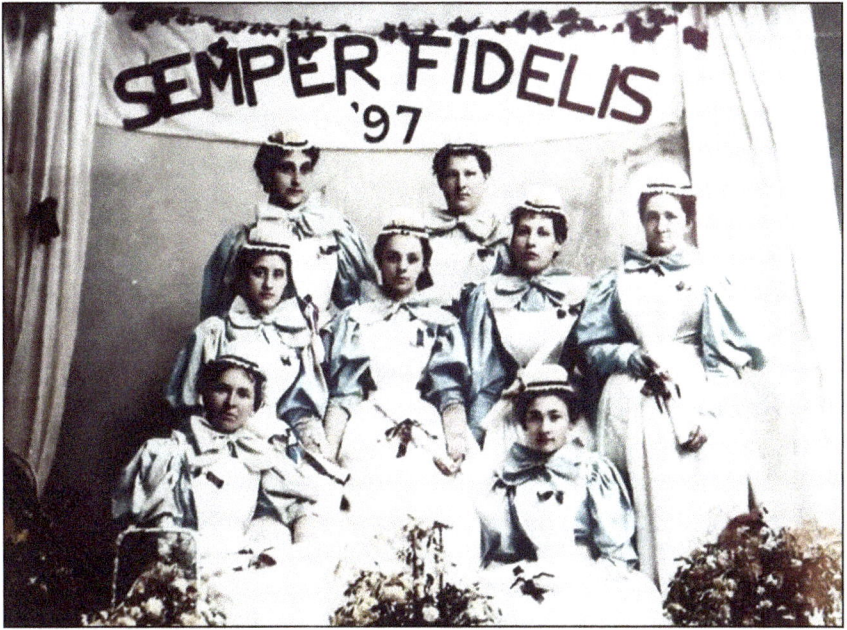

Figure 02.12. Eight of the first twelve graduates of the College Training School for Nurses, 1897. C. Los Angeles County Hospital named these eight nurses as their 1897 graduates: Teresa Babe, Elizabeth Berger, Minnie Clark, Annie Hill, Mary Lawson, Annie Mullen, Margaret Reitze, and Mariett Sexton.[18]

Four additional names appear on the graduation program, not shown in the above photograph: Bebecca Alberts, Sara E. Neill, Amanda Zavitz, and Nettie Vaugh. The first three names are listed in the 1896 *Los Angeles City Directory* as living at 315 West 6th Street (Lindley's Hospital). The other name, Nettie Vaugh, is listed in the directory as living at County Hospital.

Therefore, the first graduates of the College Training School for Nurses in 1897 included three nurses from Lindley's Sixth Street Hospital (California Hospital) and nine nurses from County Hospital. Perhaps each group returned to their hospitals for a graduation photograph. Unfortunately, a photograph of the three Sixth Street Hospital graduates could not be located.

Their graduation colors were white and gold, and their motto was "Semper Fidelis" (always faithful). Their caps had a graduates black band at the base not seen in earlier photos. According to the *Los Angeles Times*, the nurses should have received graduate medals (pins) with their diplomas, but the medals did not arrive from San Francisco in time for the ceremony.[19] The graduates have small ribbons pinned on their aprons, used in the pinning ceremony, to represent the missing graduate pins.

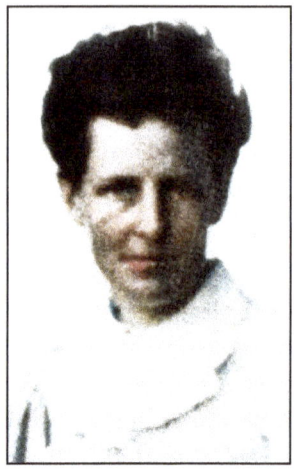

Figure 02.13. Annie O'Neil, the first matron-superintendent of the College Training School for Nurses, 1896-1897. C. O'Neil graduated from Mount Sinai Hospital, New York.

College Training School for Nurses

LOS ANGELES, CALIFORNIA.

This is to Certify, that Miss Margaret Reitz.

has completed a two years course of lectures, instruction and practice as assistant nurse, and as nurse, in the wards of the Los Angeles County and Allied Hospitals; and that she has satisfactorily passed the regular examination before the undersigned members of the Board of Examiners of the College Training School for Nurses at Los Angeles.

In Testimony whereof, the undersigned corps of instructors have affixed their signatures this Eighth day of June 1897

Executive Committee Board of Managers.

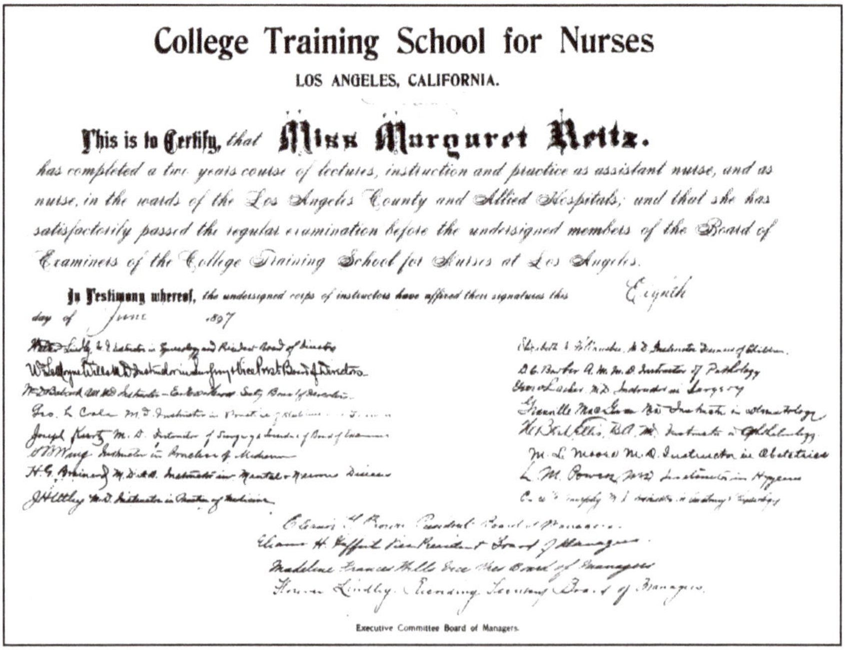

Figure 02.14. The 1897 diploma of Margaret Reitz (top row, middle of the graduation photograph, on the previous page). Her diploma included a statement of certification: "This is to certify that Miss Margaret Reitz has completed a two-year course of lectures, instruction, and practice as an assistant nurse and as a nurse, in the wards of the Los Angeles County and Allied Hospitals and that she has satisfactorily passed the regular examination before the undersigned members of the Board of Examiners of the College Training School for Nurses at Los Angeles." In 1898, she became the second matron-superintendent of the College Training School for Nurses.

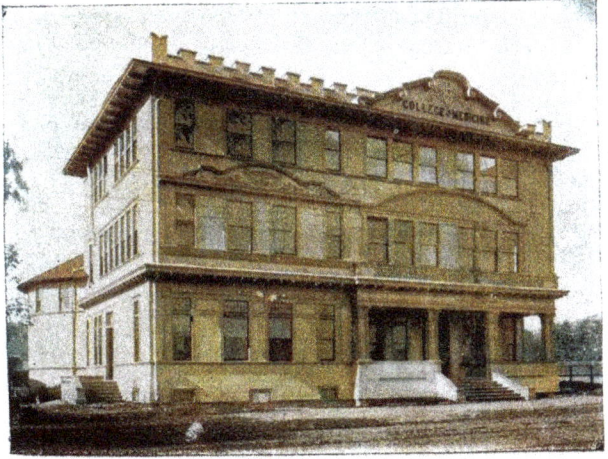

Figure 02.15. The cover of the class schedule and requirements for the second year of the College Training School for Nurses, 1897. C. A satisfactory candidate was permitted to join the school and attend lectures after a two-month trial at a recognized hospital. Candidates signed an agreement to complete the two-year course and to conform to all the rules.

The school reserved the right to terminate a pupil for any inefficiency, misconduct, general unsatisfactory record, or any reason deemed sufficient without stating the cause. (Lindley Scrapbooks, Special Collections, Libraries of Claremont Colleges)

COLLEGE TRAINING SCHOOL FOR NURSES. 5

Massage

Dr. Joseph Kurtz, 147 South Main.

Jan. 11, 18, 25, Feb. 1, 8, 15.

1. **History.** In the hands of the masseuse. In the hands of the nurse. Demonstrations on the hand and arm.
2. **Effect on Digestion.** Demonstration on chest and abdomen.
3. Demonstration on foot and leg.
4. Thigh — passive movements.
5. **Massage of Head.** Soporific effect, how obtained.
6. Demonstration on back. Back and gluteal regions. Resistive movements.
7. Sprains, dislocations, indurations, paralysis, percussion, position, use of oils.

General Medicine

Dr. H. G. Brainerd, 315 West Sixth
Dr. Geo. L. Cole, Potomac Block.

Feb. 23, March 1, 8.

1. The nervous system.
2. The heart and respiratory organs.
3. The digestive tract.

Electro-Therapeutics

Dr. W. W. Hitchcock, Byrne Block.

March 15, 22.

Practical application of electricity.

Insanity

Dr. H. G. Brainerd, 315 West Sixth.

March 29, April 5, 12.

1. The care of the nervous and insane.
2. What to do for special forms of insanity.
3. Occupation for the invalid and convalescent.

Diseases of the Skin

Dr. Granville MacGowan, Bradbury Block.

April 19, 26.

1. Anatomy and care of the skin.
2. Nursing in diseases of the skin.

Figure 02.16. Page five of the pupils' busy schedule. (Lindley Scrapbooks, Special Collections, Libraries of Claremont Colleges)

The schedule shows they traveled to many downtown locations for lectures. They attended Tuesday eight o'clock evening lectures on obstetrics, children, contagion, massage, general medicine, electo-therapeutics, insanity, diseases of the skin, and dietetics—after they had worked a long shift in the hospital. Friday evening included anatomy and physiology, bacteriology and pathology, hygiene (at the City Hall), medical lectures, surgical lectures, and gynecology. Much of the content in the schedule is listed exactly as Isabel Adams Hampton wrote in her nursing textbook.

Massage became an important component of worldwide nursing education until it gradually declined in the late 1920s. The details of the class schedule demonstrated the importance of massage in 1897. Massage disappeared from nursing curricula by the 1950s, except for the custom of a nighttime back rub for patients on bed rest. Nurses also studied treatments using devices that administered mild electrical currents.[20] They employed three forms of electricity: galvanic, faradic currents, and static electricity.

Rest, massage, and electrical currents were the treatments for patients diagnosed with nervous or insane disorders. They recommended complete isolation as the first step in the treatment: little or no reading or writing and bed rest for four to ten weeks to further inhibit the patients' movements.[21]

Hysteria, epilepsy, and insomnia were the diagnoses described in Hampton's book. Although they used the word patient, they frequently substituted "she," revealing the gender they most often confined for an insanity diagnosis.[22]

TRAINED NURSES GRADUATE.

Interesting Exercises Held at the Medical College.

The Medical College, Buena Vista street, was the scene last evening of the graduating exercises of the College Training School for Nurses. The room was very prettily decorated in pink and green, the class colors, adn the nurses looked very neat and cool in their blue and white-striped gighams, with snowy muslin aprons and dainty white caps. There were five graduates from the class of 1898, Miss Ethel H. McFarland of Mentone, Miss Etta Mae Prosise of Long Beach, Miss E. Alberta Speer of Covin, Miss R. Louise Walling of Garden Grove, and Miss Ginerva Inmann of Norwalk.

Figure 02.17. This announcement appeared in the *Los Angeles Times* on June 4, 1898—the second class of five graduates from the College Training School for Nurses. The *City Directory* lists these five graduate nurses as living at the County Hospital. By this date, the nurses at Lindley's Sixth Street Hospital had begun to train at his new facility, California Hospital. This was the final graduation class of the College Training School for Nurses. Many Los Angeles hospitals subsequently began their own training programs.

Chapter Two

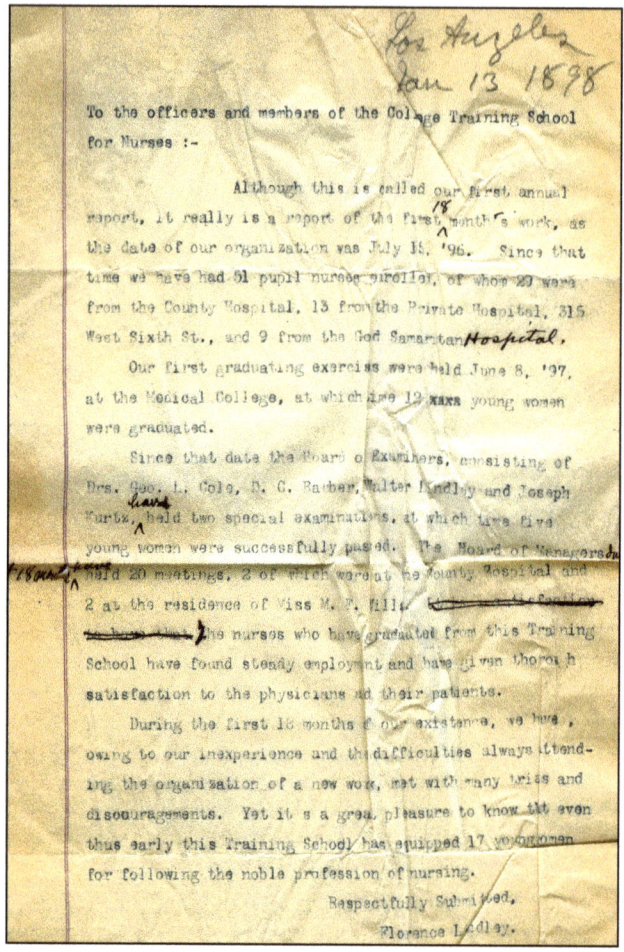

Figure 02.18. Letter to the Board of the College Training School for Nurses, January 13, 1898. (Lindley Scrapbooks, Libraries of Claremont Colleges)

The recording secretary wrote the above letter to the board. The letter stated the college had enrolled fifty-one pupil nurses in the first eighteen months: twenty-nine from County Hospital, thirteen from Lindley's Private Hospital; and nine from the Good Samaritan Hospital (although Good Samaritan had their own school, they probably attended the College Training School's lectures). She further stated, "It is a great pleasure to know that even thus early in this Training School we have equipped seventeen young women for following the noble profession of nursing." She does not specify the seventeen names; however, twelve graduates from the first class and five from the second equal seventeen. She did not mention the status of the other thirty-four enrolled pupil nurses. The secretary's letter also stated the Board of Examiners held two examinations, and five (unnamed) nurses passed.

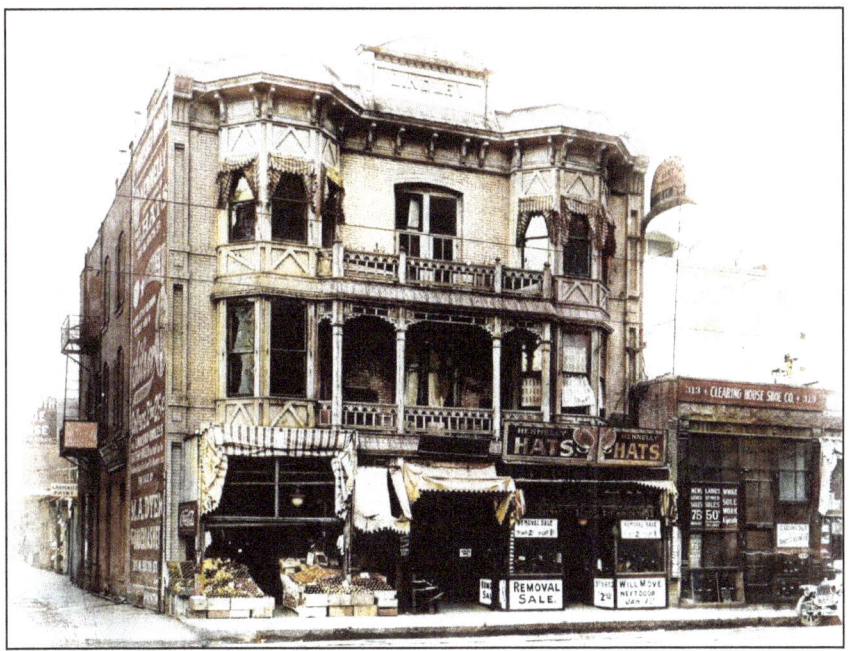

Figure 02.19. Doctor Walter Lindley's Sixth Street Hospital, 315 West Sixth Street, c. 1900. C. The top of the building is stamped 1887 Lindley. Hennley's Hats occupies the first floor, right side. The grocery store, on the left, advertised rooms for 50 cents. (Special Collections Division, Louise M. Darling Biomedical Library, University of California, Los Angeles.)

Lindley opened the three-story Sixth Street downtown building in 1887. Physicians used the first and second floors. Although the building had no elevators, the third floor contained six to eight beds. They called it the Private Hospital, Sixth Street Hospital, or Lindley's Hospital. Some references refer to it as the first California Hospital building because Lindley later founded California Hospital.

Nurses Sara Neill, Bebecca Alberts, and Amanda Zavitz were listed in the 1896 *Los Angeles City Directory* as nurses who lived and worked at Sixth Street Hospital. All three graduated from the first class of the College Training School for Nurses in 1897.

The California Training School for Nurses opened on 11 June 1898; four nurses graduated on 10 June 1899. The 1899 city directory listed one of the nurses, Althea Clark, as living at Sixth Street Hospital; Lindley might have continued operating a business there. Lillian Simpson and Susan Purdam lived at 1414 South Hope—the address of the new building of California Hospital. Mary Sergeant lived at 406 West 28th Street.

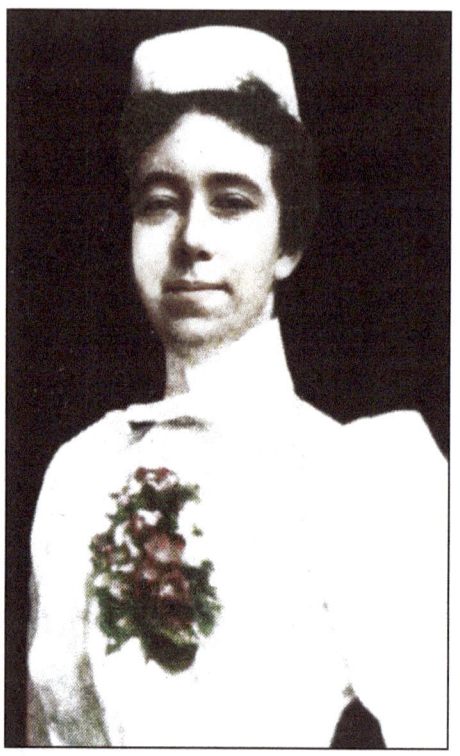

Figure 02.20 Sara E. Neill, a graduate of the 1897 College Training School. C. She became the first superintendent of the California Hospital Training School for Nurses in 1898. Her responsibilities included selecting all training students. She served as nursing superintendent from 1898 to 1924.

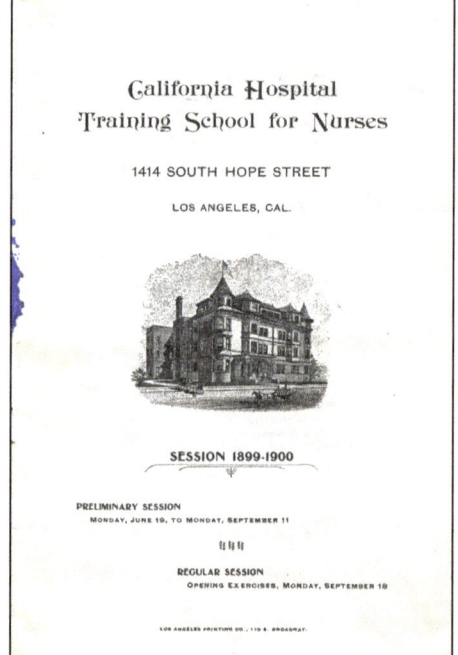

Figure 02.21. The schedule for the first session of classes in the new building on Hope Street at California Hospital, 1898. (Lindley Scrapbooks, Libraries of Claremont Colleges)

Great Decade

> *The President and Incorporators*
>
> *of the*
>
> *Training School for Nurses of the*
>
> *California Hospital*
>
> *cordially invite you to attend the*
>
> *First Annual Commencement*
>
> *Ebell Hall, 724 S. Broadway,*
>
> *Los Angeles, Cal.*
>
> *at eight p. m. on Thursday, June twenty-ninth,*
>
> *Eighteen hundred and ninety-nine.*

Figure 02.22. The invitation for the first commencement exercises of the Training School for Nurses, California Hospital, June 29, 1899. (Lindley Scrapbooks, Libraries of Claremont Colleges)

Graduates....

✢

Miss Althea F. Clark, Los Angeles

Miss Lillian Simpson, Los Angeles

Miss Susan A. Purdam, Los Angeles

Miss Mary Sergeant, Los Angeles

Figure 02.23. The names of the graduating nurses: Miss Althea F. Clark, Los Angeles; Miss Lillian Simpson, Los Angeles; Miss Susan A. Purdam, Los Angeles; and Miss Mary Sergeant, Los Angeles, 1899.

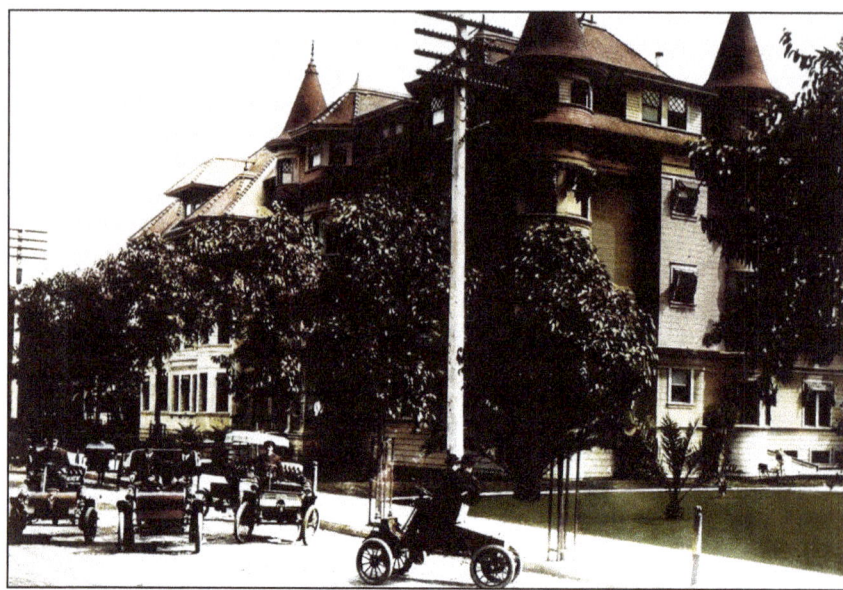

Figure 02.24. California Hospital with small cars in front owned and driven by hospital doctors, c. 1900. C. Walter Lindley and twenty-two physicians from the Private Hospital purchased a site in a quiet area at 15th and Hope streets. They opened California Hospital on 1 June 1898.

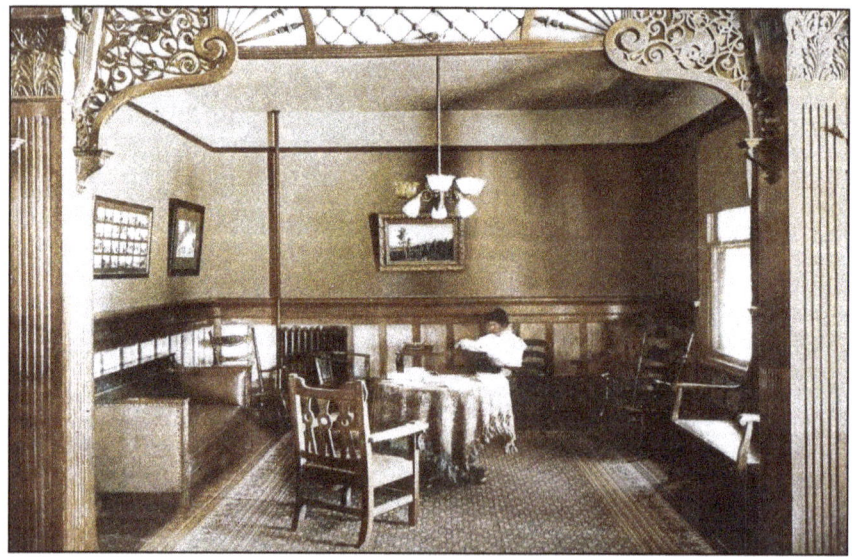

Figure 02.25. A nurse reads in the parlor at the nurses' home, 1898. C. Buelah Wright, dean of the College of Oratory, gave the nurses a course in reading and use of the voice in conversation to add culture to the nurses repertoire. [23]

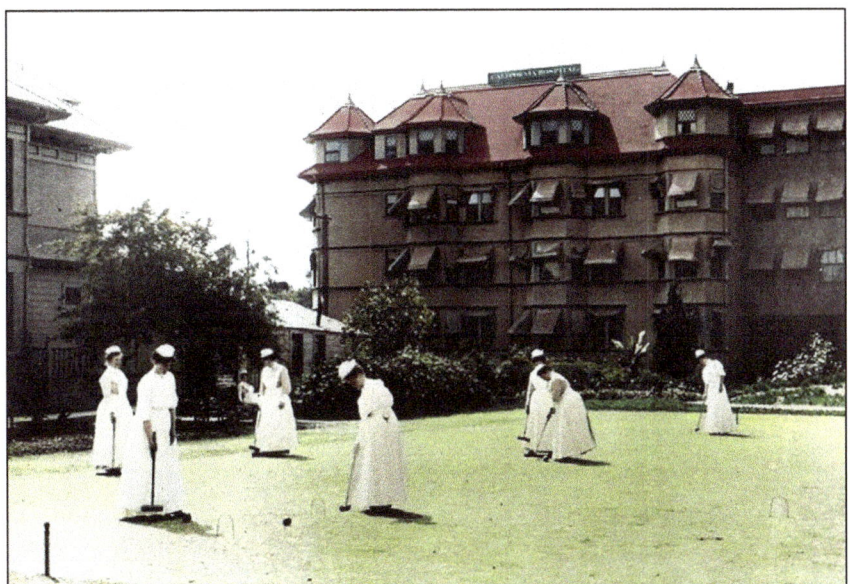

Figure 02.26. Nurses play a croquet game on the lawn of the California Hospital. The hospital prepared a daily paper to read to the nurses during lunch. The superintendent said the paper educated them and gave them subjects for conversation—a respite from thoughts of disease and gossip.[24]

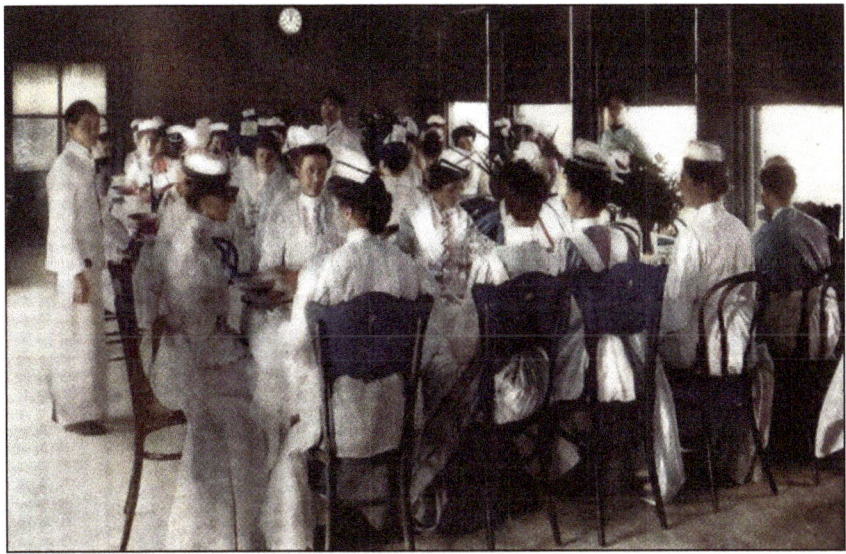

Figure 02.27. This image is titled, "Twelve O'clock," c. 1900. C. A graphophone allowed nurses to choose two music selections during evening meals. (Lindley Scrapbooks, Libraries of Claremont Colleges)

Chapter Two

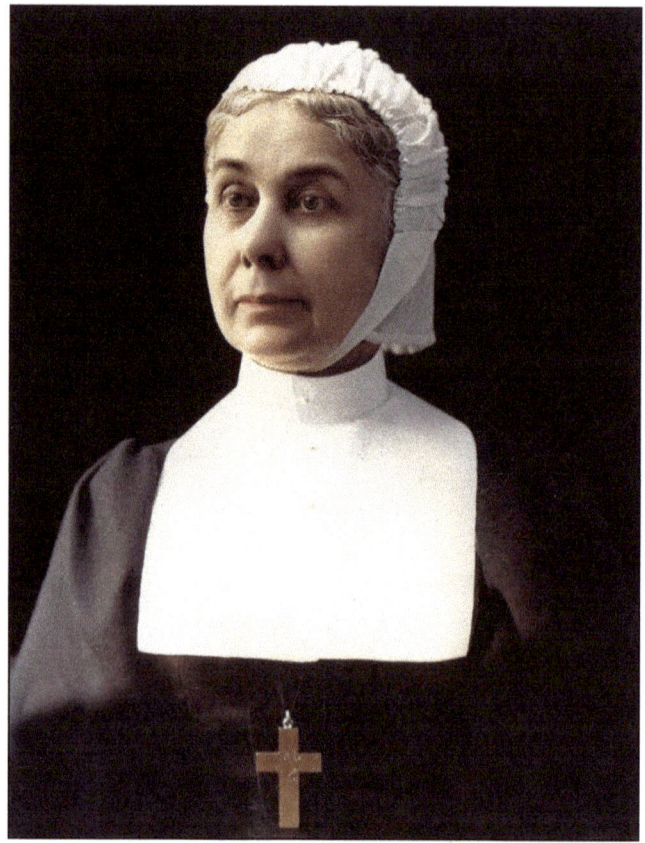

Figure 02.28. Sister Mary Wood, n.d. C. (Good Samaritan Hospital Archives)

In the 1880s, the California Diocese of the Episcopal Church asked Sister Mary Wood, a member of the small order of the Good Shepherd in San Francisco, to travel to Los Angeles as a missionary. [25]

She witnessed the needs of the frail who had traveled west to find health and prosperity. Using her own money, she rented a cottage at 215 Olive Street and opened a nine-bed hospital in 1885. The first year she was the business manager and chief nurse. She cared for ninety-two patients but had to turn away many more.

Her abilities impressed St. Paul's Protestant Episcopal Church, and in 1886 they assumed funding; they named it the Los Angeles Hospital and Home for Invalids and appointed Sister Wood as matron-superintendent. Later, a private citizen made a sizable contribution. The hospital constructed a larger building at 924 West Seventh Street in 1896, and they changed the name to the Hospital of the Good Samaritan. [26]

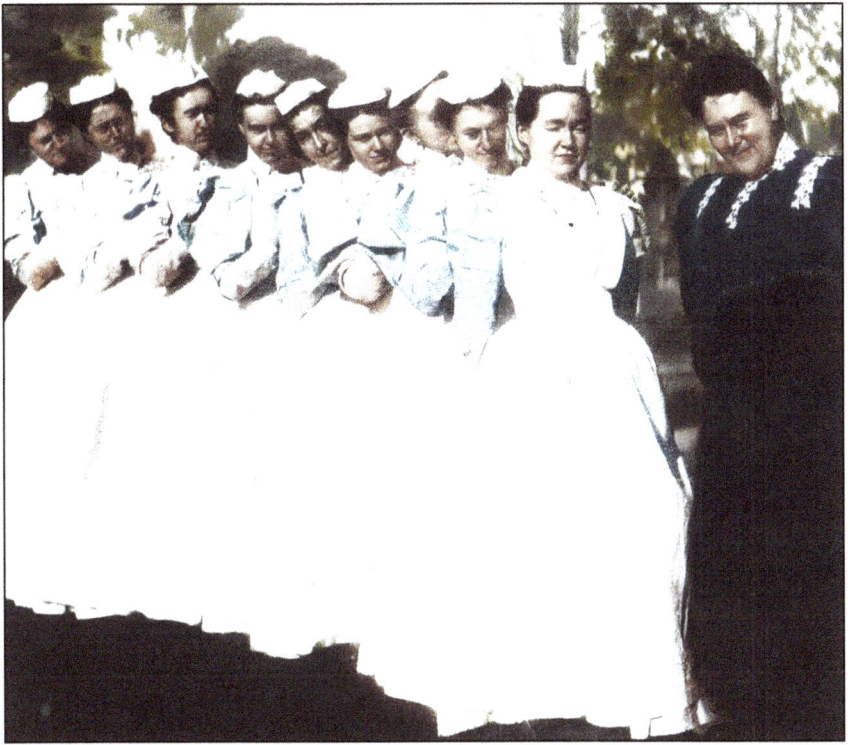

Figure 02.29. The class of 1898 and 1899, at the Training School for Nurses of the Hospital of the Good Samaritan: Era Burton, Catherine Caldwell, Alice Thorn, Josephine Meyer, Emma Bolman, Evangeline Post, and Bertha Swisher. C. The woman dressed in black is the first superintendent of nurses from 1897 to 1898, Harriet Pahl.[27] (Good Samaritan Hospital Archives)

In 1898 Pahl demanded an increase in salary to $75.00 per month. The hospital fired her. The subsequent superintendent could not manage the budget, so the hospital asked Pahl to return. She remained superintendent from 1900 to 1911.

In 1904, the school changed from a two-year to a three-year program. The junior pupils received only room and board for the first two months of the probationary period. During probation, Pahl observed the pupils carefully for their physical strength, education, endurance, tact, adaptability to work, and powers of observation and judgment. If accepted into the school, the pupils signed an agreement to comply with regulations.[28]

Pupils received $5.00 per month the first year, $7.50 for the middle year, and $10.00 in the senior year. The school stated the money was for books and laundry, not a salary. The instruction was considered full pay for services.[29]

Chapter Two

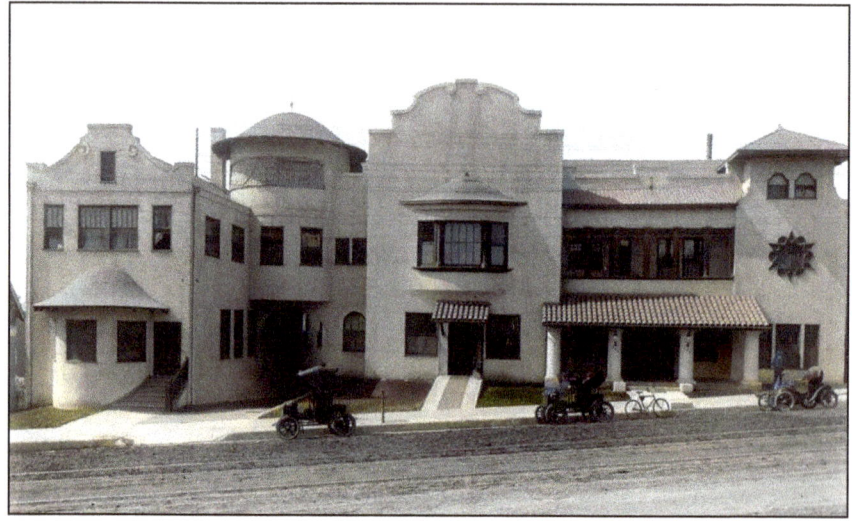

Figure 02.30. A photo postcard of the Good Samaritan Hospital located at 924-934 West Seventh Street, 1907. The writing on the back, from a nurse, indicated the nurses' home was the building to the far right that she called the dormitory—a later addition to the original building. In 1911 the hospital moved to its final location in a residential area on Orange Street, now called Wilshire Blvd.

Figure 02.31. Foot surgery at California Hospital. Note the open window. Most are not wearing masks and only the surgeon is using gloves, n.d. C.

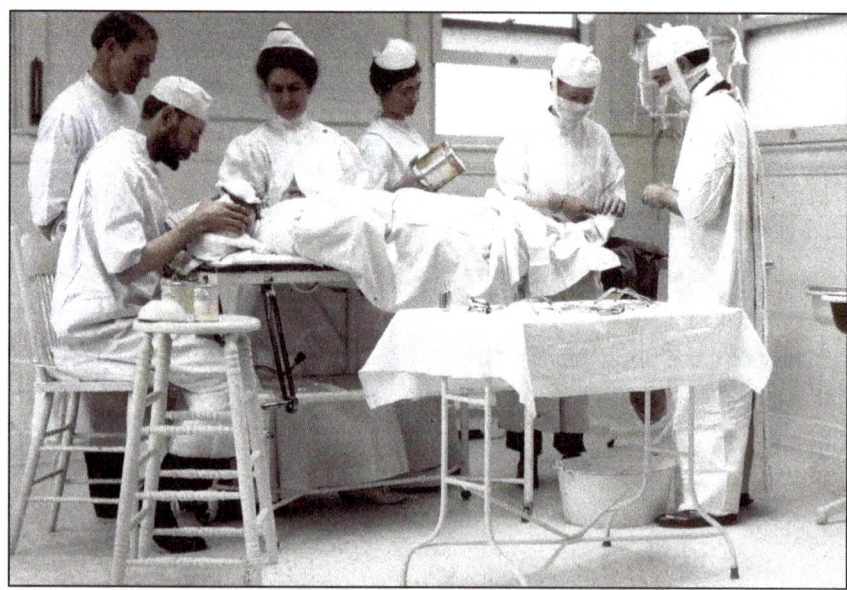

Great Decade

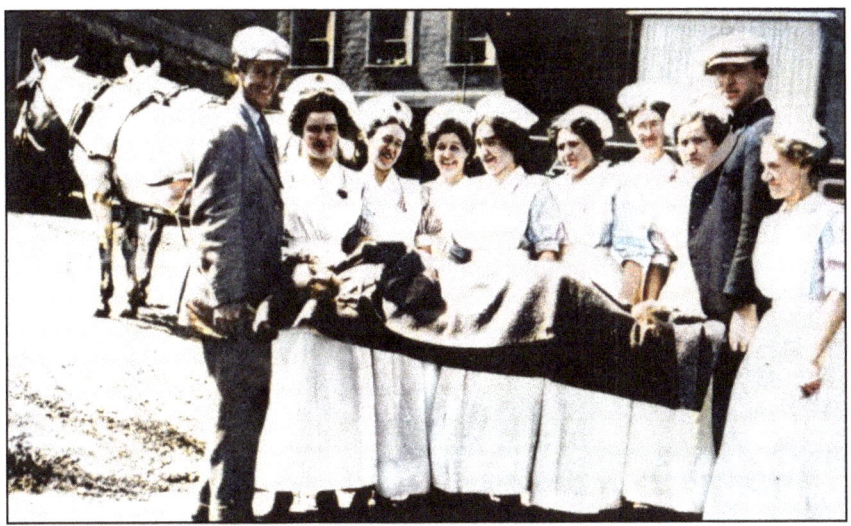

Figure 02.32. Student nurses from County Hospital posed with J.H. Goodhew in front of his first ambulance, 1905. C.

Figure 02.33. When Dr. Barber realized the College Training School for Nurses was destined to close, he asked County Hospital if he could transfer it there.[30] These eleven nurses graduated in 1899—the year the location and name changed from the College Training School for Nurses to Los Angeles County Hospital Training School for Nurses at County Hospital. The County Board of Supervisors did not approve the school until 1901.[31]

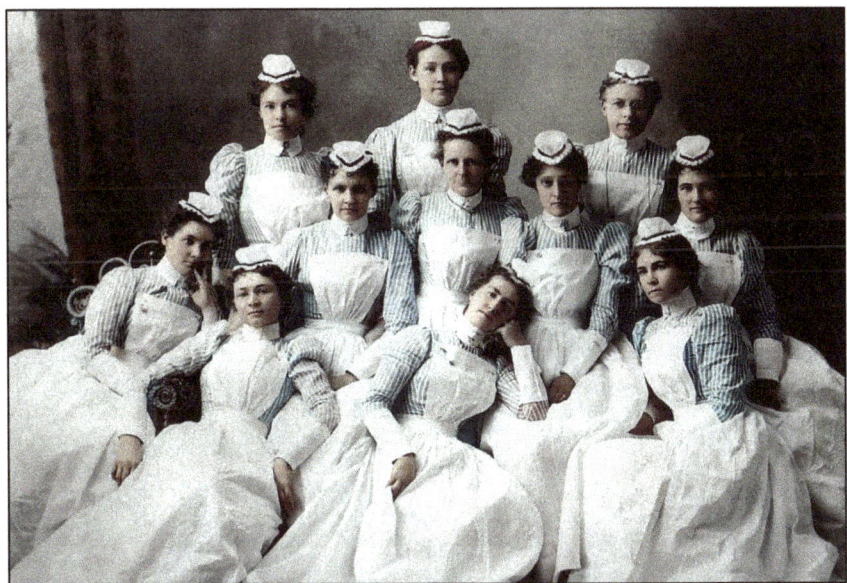

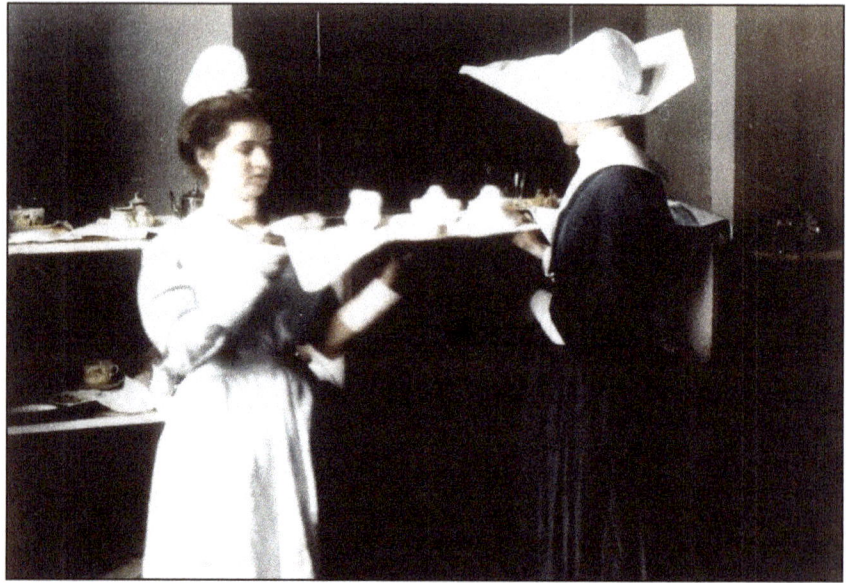

Figure 02.34. A Daughter of Charity, at the Los Angeles Infirmary Training School for Nurses, teaches a student nurse how to serve a patient, n.d. C. The school began training nurses in 1899, graduated its first class in 1901, and its last class in 1974. [32]

Figure 02.35. Nurses and doctors in surgery at Los Angeles Infirmary, c. 1908. The hospital was known by several names: Institucion Caritativa, Sister's Hospital, Los Angeles Infirmary, St. Vincent's Hospital, and finally St. Vincent's Medical Center. Los Angeles' oldest hospital closed in 2020.[33]

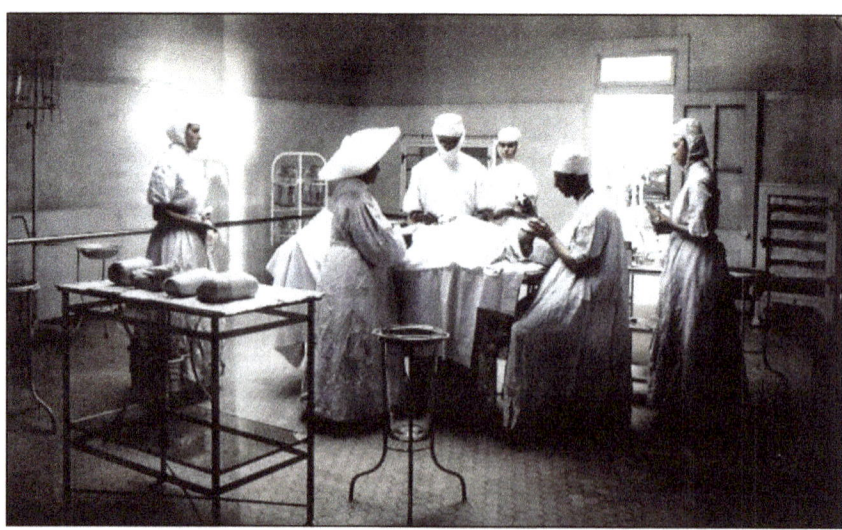

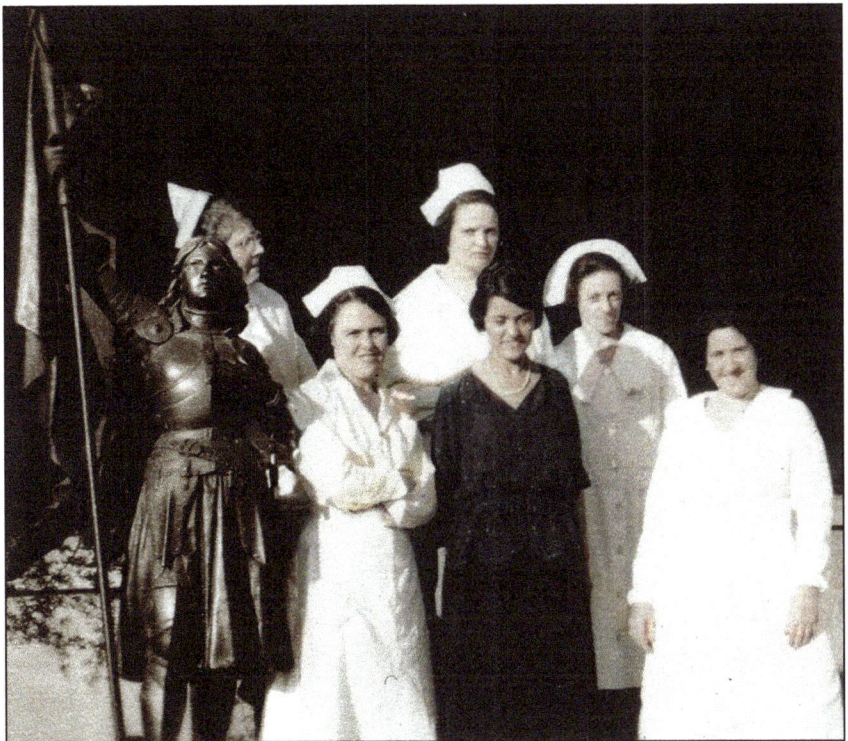

Figure 02.36. French Hospital nurses standing next to the *Jeanne d'Arc* (Joan of Arc) bronze statue, n.d. C. (Private Collection)

Some say no one knows who placed the statue; it just appeared one day. Others say the French Benevolent Society erected it in 1964—they owned the land underneath it. The hospital was located at College and Castelar (later Hill) Streets in the Los Angeles area called Chinatown.

The French Hospital opened in 1870. Initially, a couple performed both housekeeping and nursing duties. In April 1903, they received their first four apprentice nurses. The nurses were paid $7.00 per month for the first year and $14.00 the second year, including laundry.

In 1904 Yvonne Clos, a graduate nurse from Paris, France, became matron-superintendent. She worked at French Hospital until she retired. Clos was a highly respected person in the community. [34]

The *Jeanne d'Arc* statue stood in front of French Hospital, eventually called Pacific Alliance Medical Center, until it closed in 2017. The French Benevolent Society rescued the statue and donated it to Childrens Hospital. Childrens did not make immediate plans for *Jeanne d'Arc*. [35]

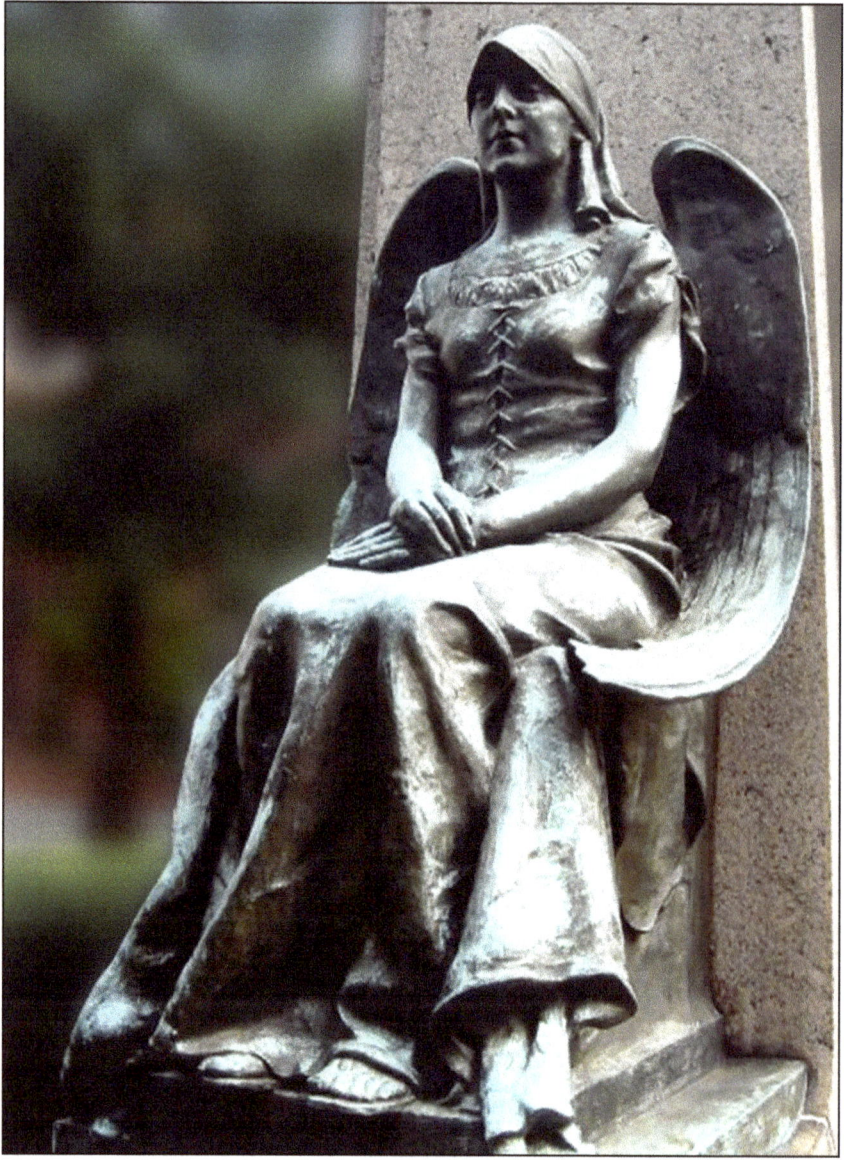

Figure 02.37. Jerome Connor sculpted this Civil War Nurses Monument in 1924, located at M Street & Rhode Island Ave., Washington, D.C., n.d.

In 1861, Dorothea Dix, Superintendent of Women in the Civil War, advertised for nurses over the age of 30 who agreed to wear only brown or black dresses, without bows, curls, or jewelry. Nurses were paid 40 cents and one ration per day. The Sisters of Charity and the Sisters of Mercy also worked in military hospitals and close to the fighting front.

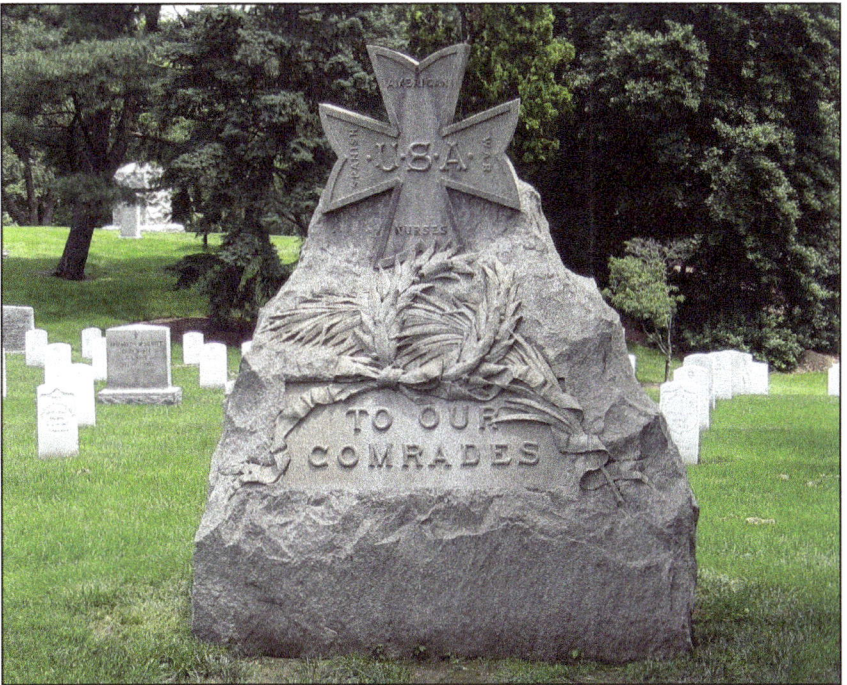

Figure 02.38. Veterans erected the Spanish-American War Nurse Memorial in Arlington National Cemetery in 1902.

Carlie G. Patterson served as a nurse in Cuba during the Spanish-American War, in 1898, and later as superintendent of nurses at California Hospital in Los Angeles.[36] She graduated from the Methodist Episcopal Hospital School of Nursing, New York, in 1893.

The U.S. government had advertised for nurses to join the Spanish-American War in April 1898. Hundreds of untrained women applied. The National Society of the Daughters of the American Revolution (DAR) organized an examining board to separate the trained from the untrained. Nurses were required to have graduated from a training school and have an endorsement from a nursing superintendent. Female physicians could also apply as nurses. The first appointed were those immune to yellow fever.

The Sisters of Charity sent two hundred nuns from their order. The National Red Cross organized nurses, furnished money for transportation, and paid a $28.00 stipend for nurses serving at Army Hospitals. In August 1898, the Surgeon General's Office established the Army Nurse Corps Division with 1,200 nurses. They stationed nurses at hospitals and camps in the United States, Puerto Rico, Cuba, Honolulu, the Philippine Islands, and on a hospital ship named the *Relief*. The war ended in December of 1898.

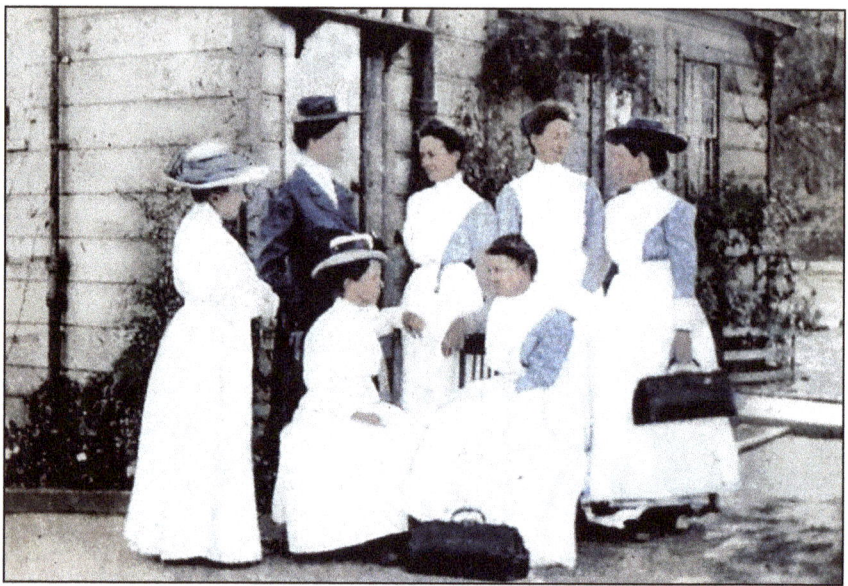

Figure 02.39. Maude Foster Weston (the dark uniform) with public health nurses at the College Settlement call station, n.d. C. (Los Angeles County Department of Public Health)

The concept of nurses living in a settlement house began in New York when Lillian Wald started Henry Street in 1893. Settlement nurses would move into a house in a depressed area of the city (often populated by new immigrants) and care for community health needs. They were first called district nurses and later visiting nurses.

The first Los Angeles house, the College Settlement, opened in December 1895 in an old adobe at the corner of Ord and Castelar streets. In 1897 Maude Foster Weston, president of the Los Angeles College Settlement Association (LACSA), petitioned the County to pay a district nurse a salary. Weston was an educated socialist, not a nurse. Help from her twin, Nancy Foster, and their inherited wealth allowed Weston to engage in public health reforms. The city agreed with her idea: on 22 November 1897, Los Angeles became the first city in the U.S. to pay for the services of a district nurse. [37]

In February 1898, the settlement moved to 428 Alpine Street, and one trained nurse moved in. Public Health Nurses cared for 21,749 patients and made 102,446 home visits during the sixteen years of the LACSA's existence. They attended to colds, sores, and minor infections. Febrile and zymotic diseases were the second most common reasons for visits.[38] Zymotic was the term used for diseases that were contagious, contracted from putrid matter, and transmitted through the air. [39]

LOS ANGELES
Board of Health, School Nursing Department.

Established in 1903.

Number of nurses: Four.

Salary: $75 per month.

Hours: 8:30 a. m. to 5 p. m.

Plan of Work: In May, 1903, school nursing was started experimentally by one of the College Settlement nurses, under the supervision of the health officer. In 1904 a special school nurse was appointed by the city to take up the work systematically. There are now four on the staff, one of whom inspects the children in the day nurseries, children's hospitals, etc.

Figure 02.40. School Nurse data. Figure 02.41. District Nurse information. Images from *Visiting Nurses in the United States*, Yssabella Waters, 1906.

Instructive District Nursing for the City of Los Angeles, College Settlement, 428 Alpine Street.

Established in March, 1898.

Number of nurses: Five.

Salary: $75 per month and carfare.

Hours: 8 a. m. to 5 p. m. Sundays and evenings are free. One half day off duty twice a month.

Classes of cases cared for: Surgical, medical, obstetrical, and tuberculous.

History and Plan of Work: In December, 1897, the College Settlement appealed to the city council to appropriate a monthly allowance of $50 for the salary of a district nurse. The request was granted, and Los Angeles became the first city in America to establish municipal visiting nursing. A monthly allowance of $50 was made, which was in 1903 increased to $75. The city now supports five district nurses, all of whom work under the supervision of the College Settlement.

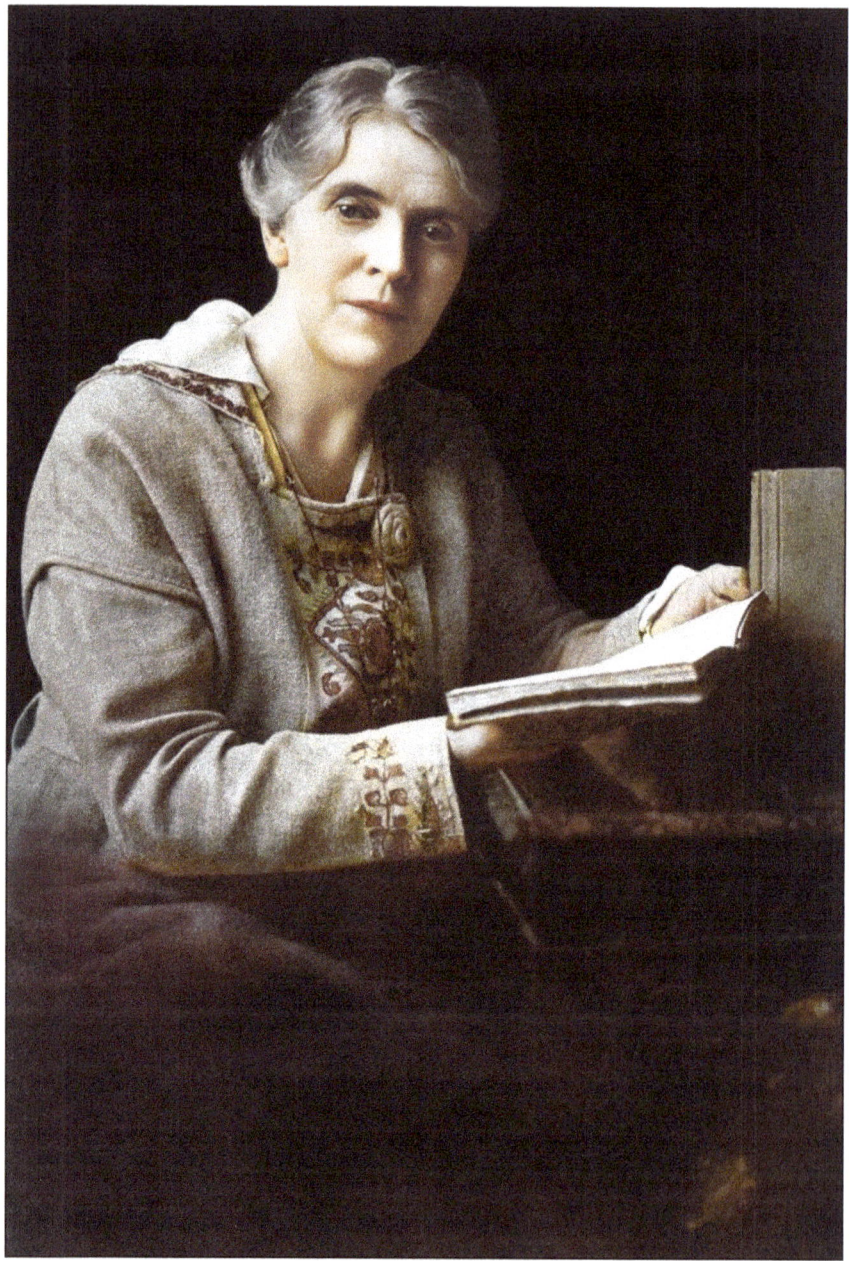

Figure 02.42. Margaret Elliot Frances Sirch in Los Angeles, 1938. C. Sirch established *The Trained Nurse*—the first permanent monthly magazine for nurses in the United States—just one year after she graduated from nurses's training. Sirch published her first issue of *The Trained Nurse* in August 1888. The name later changed to *The Trained Nurse and Hospital Review*.

Great Decade

"We had twelve-hour duty and often worked extra and for night emergencies," Sirch told Antonia Potemkina, a Pasadena nurse who interviewed Sirch in 1938. "The floors were of stone. The wards were chronically crowded, so the beds had to be placed down the center. There were no elevators. But we had excellent men orderlies who helped with the lifting."

The hospital sent senior students outside for private cases to add to the hospital finances. During the last six months of Sirch's training, she served as acting superintendent. Following her 1887 graduation from Buffalo General Hospital, the trustees appointed her to the position permanently. "I doubt I would have accepted the position with such meager preparations, but I was young then, and I did not know my own limitations." [40]

She worried that nurses had no post-graduate educational opportunities and said they often felt "scientific isolation" if they worked in private homes or small facilities. She discussed this with a publisher, Alfred Rose, and he proposed a magazine. She started *The Trained Nurse*. Catherine Dunlop, of Los Angeles, was one of the first subscribers to *The Trained Nurse*.

In 1903 she moved to Los Angeles. The City Health Department hired her as a staff nurse in 1910, however, only after California revoked the law prohibiting married women from working in government positions.

She became chief nurse for the Bureau of Municipal Nursing in 1913. The bureau absorbed the College Settlement, including visits to tuberculosis patients, maternity supervision, the teaching of home nursing in infectious diseases, and inspection of boarding houses. She established and supervised Baby Milk Stations that evaluated infants' health and provided free milk.

She took charge of the State Board of Charities and Corrections (later called the State Department of Social Welfare), which included all territories south of the Tehachapi. A Division for Blind Aid and a Division of Adoption were added to her lengthy list. The Retirement Act of 1937 forced her to retire at the age of seventy. Many considered Sirch to be the founder and builder of the Welfare and Health Departments. [41]

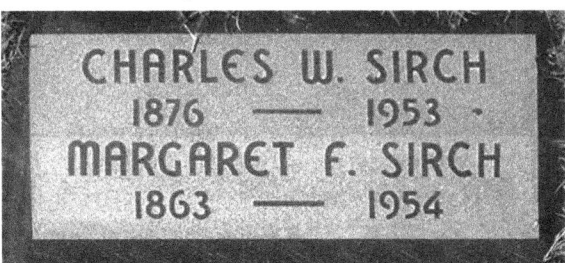

Figure 02.43. The Sirch's gravestone in Rosedale Cemetery, Los Angeles.

Chapter Two

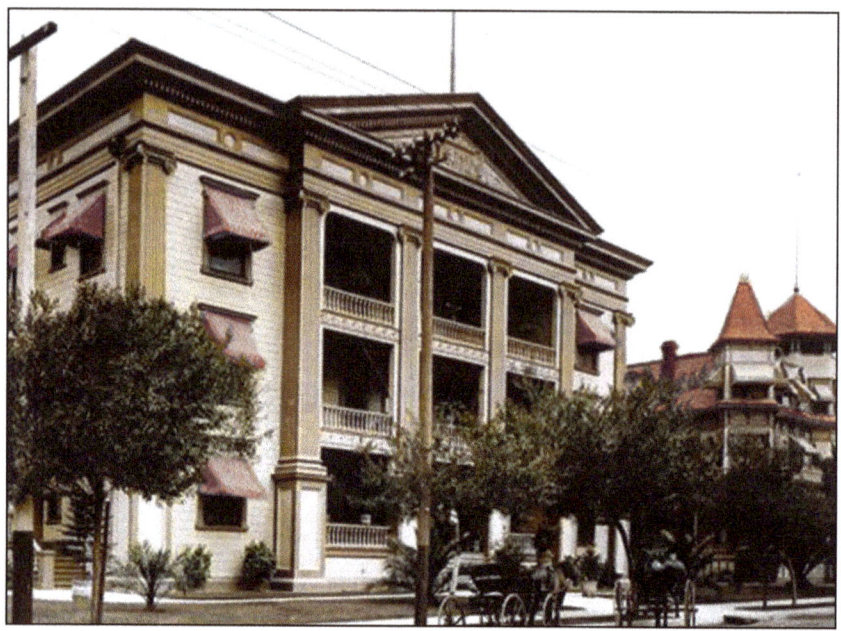

Figure 02.44. The Pacific Hospital, 1902. C. The original building was in the back. The new surgery building was in front. (Courtesy of USC Archives)

The *Los Angeles Herald* announced the Pacific Hospital opened at 1319 Grand Ave on 22 December 1899.[42] On 9 September 1902, the new building opened—only surgical cases were admitted there. The building looked like a handsome private home rather than a hospital. The floor had inlaid wood; the rooms were furnished with brass beds, bird's-eye maple, mahogany, polished oak, and walnut. The seventy-five unique rooms had suites and private baths. A nurses' lecture room touted reclining chairs, couches, and game tables.[43]

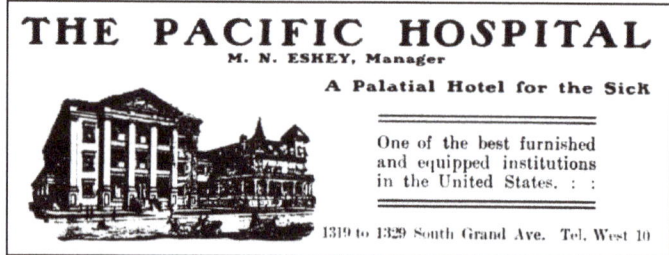

Figure 02.45. A Pacific Hospital advertisement in the *Los Angeles City Directory*, 1903. The 1901 & 1903 directories listed the address as 1319 to 1329 S. Grand Ave. The Pacific Coast Architecture Database stated it operated there from 1901 until 1905. In 1918, the Naturopathic Institute and Sanitarium of California was listed at the same address with no mention of who occupied the building between 1905 and 1918.[44]

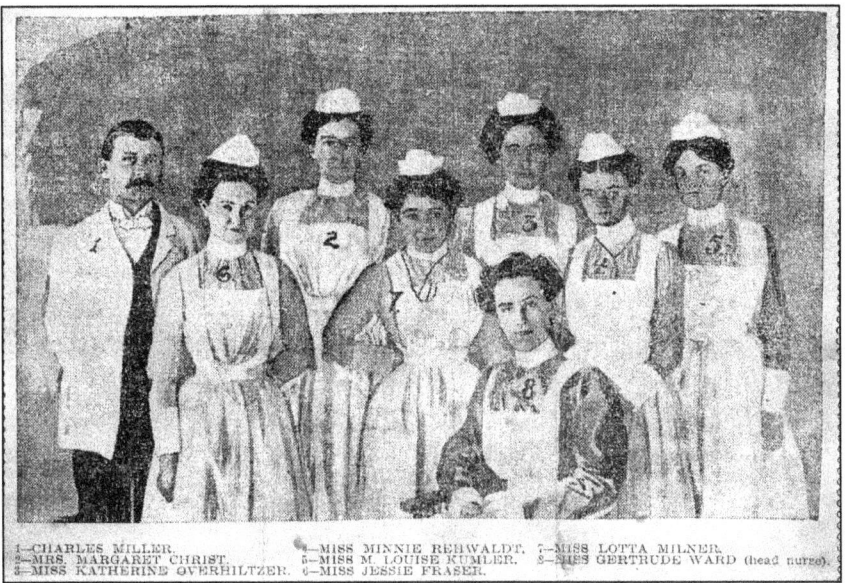

Figure 02.46. The first graduation class of seven nurses at The Pacific Hospital Training School, December 16, 1901. Charles Miller, Minne Rehwaldt, Lotta Milner, Margaret Christ, Louise Kumler, Katherine Overhiltzer, Jessier Fraser. The head nurse, Gertrude Ward, is sitting in front. (Lindley Scrapbooks, Special Collections, Libraries of Claremont Colleges)

Very few records exist regarding The Pacific Hospital Training School. The *Los Angeles Herald* reported graduate that Katherine Overhiltzer accepted a position as head nurse in Williams, Arizona; Margaret Christ took charge of a hospital in Hawaii; and Lotta Milner stayed on as head nurse.

Figure 02.47. This 1903 newspaper advertisement for Pacific Hospital asked only for lady applicants, even though the inaugural class listed the first man to graduate from a nurses' training school in Los Angeles: Charles Miller in 1901.

In Lillian Balding's graduation program, she was listed as the first 1908 graduate and the only nurse from Los Angeles. The other graduates traveled from Colorado, Ontario, Illinois, and Iowa to attend this desirable training school.

> **TRAINING SCHOOL FOR YOUNG LADIES.**
>
> **Los Angeles Can Boast of Having One of the Best Furnished and Equipped Hospitals in the World.**
>
> The class of the training school for 1903 will graduate the latter part of May. From May 8th to May 24th a limited number of young ladies of education and refinement will be admitted to the training school. The applicant must be in good health, and between the ages of 22 and 35, and have the best of references.
>
> This school has the standard course of three years, and all of the advantages of the eastern schools.
>
> Young ladies desirous of entering the school will please write for catalogue and application blanks, addressing or calling at THE PACIFIC HOSPITAL, 1329 South Grand avenue, Los Angeles, California.

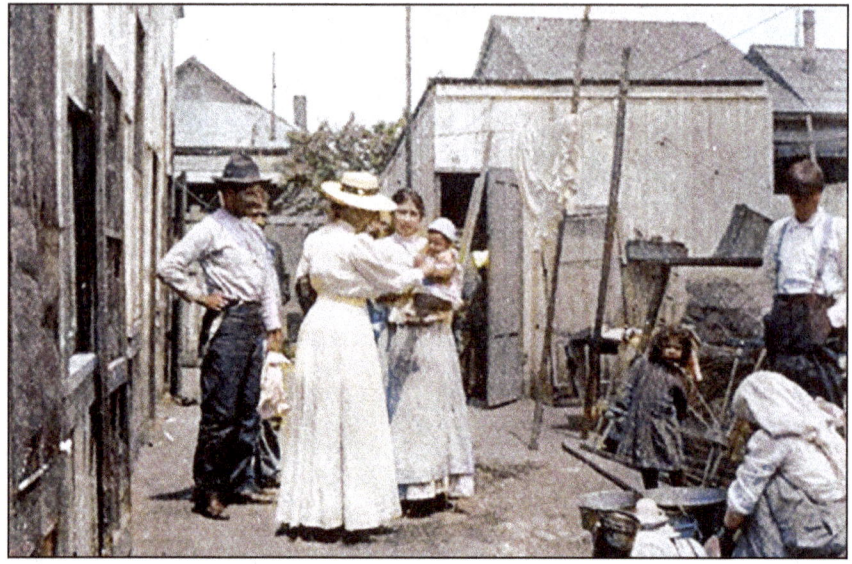

Figure 02.48. Nurse Johanna Von Wagner inspecting the house courts, Los Angeles, c. 1908. C.

When Los Angeles initiated the College Settlement scheme, public health nurses began to assess housing conditions in living areas called house courts. The house courts, later called "slum areas," consisted of poorly constructed, single-story row houses with one to three rooms. They shared common sewage and water facilities, which was a recipe for the spread of diseases. This experience transformed public health nurses into knowledgeable house inspectors during the normal course of patient visits.

Public health nurses developed an interest in environmental housing reforms with regard to lack of ventilation, absence of light, and overcrowding—the 621 house courts contained 3,671 dwellings of 9,877 people. [45-46]

In 1908, Los Angeles hired a graduate nurse and leading New York housing inspector, Johanna Von Wagner, to be the Los Angeles Housing Inspector—the first woman and first nurse in that position. Von Wagner had lectured on the subject locally, to the State Board of Massachusetts, and the International Women's Congress. She claimed working knowledge of six languages, which helped with the four thousand Russian immigrants of the house courts. During one of her assessments, she said the "wretched habitation of some immigrants has made it possible for them to pursue their opium habit." [47]

Von Wagner remained the most prominent inspector until she resigned in 1912. Reformers continued to refine the environmental factors of house courts, but the living conditions in the areas remained lacking.

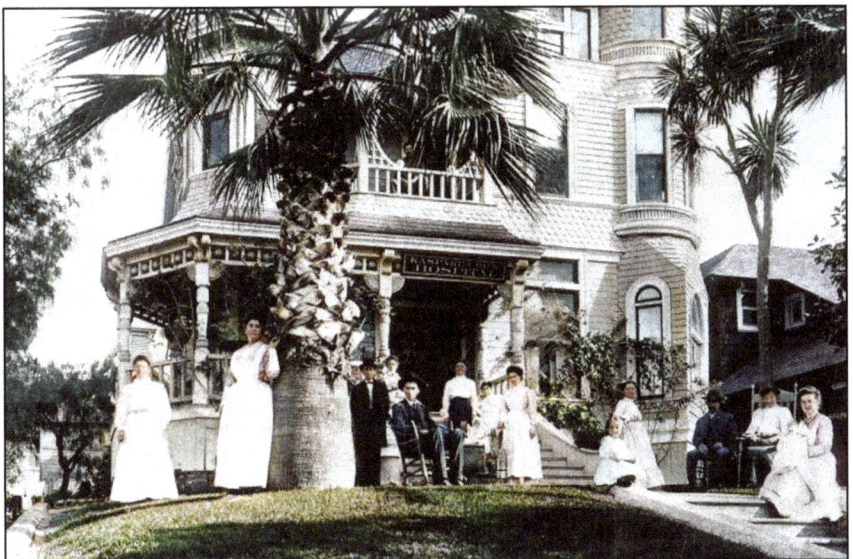

Figure 02.49. Nurses and doctors standing in front of Kaspare Cohn Hospital in the early 1900s. C. (University of Southern California Archives)

Mae Comport joined Kaspare Cohn Hospital as one of its first nurses hired when it opened in September 1902. When the hospital promoted her in June 1903, Comport became the youngest superintendent nurse in the United States at twenty-two years old. [48]

She graduated from Sister's Hospital Training Program (St. Vincent's Hospital). Although she was not Jewish, she spoke Polish, Russian, and Hebrew. May Gray was the assistant superintendent. Comport and Gray are probably pictured above in this early 1900 photograph; the exact names of the nurses are not known. The hospital boasted they admitted one hundred "inmates" in its first year and only six deaths (from tuberculosis). [49]

Kaspare Cohn, a two-story, fifteen-bed hospital, was located at 1443 North Carroll Street. The building was first a private residence and then became Wooly Sanitarium. In 1902, the Jewish Benevolent Society decided to endow a hospital for the Jewish indigent. One of the best-known Jewish pioneers of Los Angeles, Kaspare Cohn, donated the building as a memorial to his son, Samuel Cohn, who had died in Los Angeles. [50]

The building still stands in the famous section of Los Angeles known for its Victorian-era home; however, it's no longer a hospital. Kaspare Cohn moved its location, and in 1930 it became Cedars of Lebanon Hospital, named after the religiously significant Lebanese cedar tree. In 1961 it merged with Mount Sinai Hospital to form Cedars-Sinai Medical Center.

Chapter Two

> **BREVITIES.**
>
> The first annual meeting of the Los Angeles County Nurses' Association will be held at the parish house, St. Paul's Pro-Cathedral, Olive st., at 2:30 o'clock on the afternoon of Oct. 4, 1904. There will be an election of councilors, following which Dr. Walter Lindley, dean of the medical dept. of the University of Southern California, will address the nurses upon the value of organization, and the benefits to be derived from State registration All grauduate nurses are cordially invited to be present.

Figure 02.50 The *Los Angeles Times* announcement for the first annual meeting of the Los Angeles County Nurses Association—the beginning of the law that required all nurses to register, October 4, 1904.

Before 1905, the State of California did not require the registration of nurses. Correspondence training schools advertised in newspapers. Anyone could use the title of nurse. This practice confused the hiring public, who could not tell which nurses had received formal training and those who had not. In response to this issue, a movement began to register nurses to protect the public and establish professional cohesion. After the 1905 law passed, it became a misdemeanor for anyone to call themselves a registered nurse without certification.[51]

> *The people of the State of California, represented in senate and assembly, do enact as follows:*
>
> SECTION 1. Commencing in the month of July, 1905, and at least semi-annually thereafter, the board of regents of the University of California shall hold, or cause to be held, such examination or examinations as they may deem proper to test the qualifications and fitness of applicants for certification and registration as registered nurses within the State of California. Such examinations shall be practical in character, and a reasonable notice designating the time and place thereof must be given by publication in at least two daily papers published within the State of California.
>
> SEC. 2. All applicants for examination must furnish satisfactory evidence of good moral character and of having complied with the provisions of this act relative to qualifications; and any examiner may inquire of any applicant for examination concerning his or her character, qualifications or experience, and may take testimony in regard thereto, under oath, which he is hereby empowered to administer.
>
> SEC. 3. All persons satisfactorily passing such examinations shall be granted by the board of regents of the University of California a certificate stating that he or she is a registered nurse within the State of California, and shall thereafter be known and styled as a registered nurse. The secretary of the said board of regents shall keep in his office a book showing the names of all persons to whom certificates as registered nurses have been granted. Graduates of all training schools for nurses which shall have been approved by the said board of regents may be certified as registered nurses, without examination, at any time within three years after the passage of this act, upon payment of the fee prescribed in section four hereof.

Figure 02.51. The law requiring nurses in California to take an examination, pay a fee, and register, 1905. (Lindley Scrapbooks)

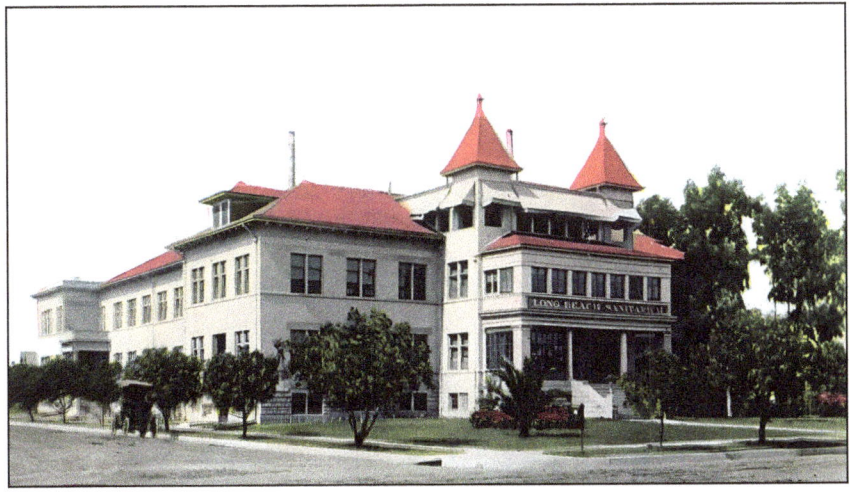

Figure 02.52. Long Beach Sanitarium photo postcard, Long Beach, 1910.

In 1876, the Los Angeles Chamber of Commerce launched a publicity campaign to attract businesses. They advertised the health benefits of the perfect climate and fresh sea air in Southern California. Doctors built sanitariums, and people traveled to Los Angeles for health vacations.[52]

The patients also traveled to Los Angeles hoping to heal incurable illnesses. A large influx of patients with tuberculosis (referred to as consumption at that time) arrived to be cured. No cure existed. Some of the patients had sufficient funds to live in luxurious sanitariums and sanatoriums; few people had enough funds to support themselves through the lengthy tuberculosis recovery process. Patients who had no money were sent to the County Hospital pneumonia and fever wards. Those with mild symptoms often recovered after months of rest. Serious cases did not survive.[53]

The advertisement on the back of this postcard bragged they did not have a nurses training school—they hired only graduate nurses. The Kellogg brothers coined the term sanitarium, (a health retreat) for their premiere facility in Battle Creek, Michigan.[54] The brothers developed corn flakes and used the brand name Sanitas for their first corn flake cereal.[55] Sanitas meant healthy in Latin.

Sanitariums were the forerunners of spas: they served residents quality meals in beautiful dining rooms and provided therapeutic treatments. Hospitals used the term sanatorium—especially for facilities that housed tuberculosis patients—but some hospitals used the word sanitarium to lessen the fear of staying in a tuberculosis-occupied facility. Because of this confusing naming practice, both sick and health-seekers occupied the same buildings.

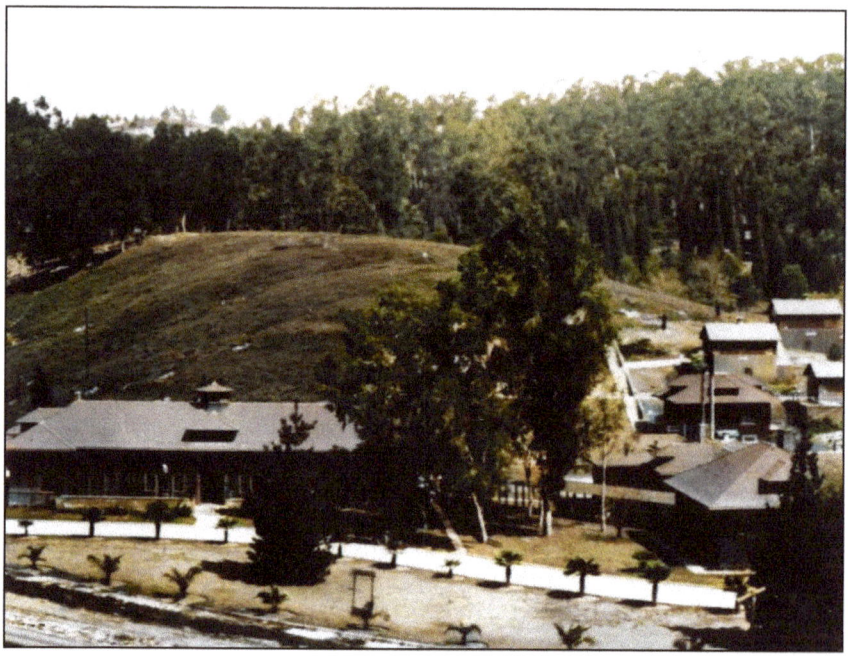

Figure 02.53. Barlow Sanatorium's infirmary, with a covered walkway to the cottages, 1902. C. (Courtesy of Barlow Respiratory Hospital)

Walter Barlow moved to Los Angeles to recover from a mild case of tuberculosis and opened a sanatorium. To ensure privacy and fresh air, he bought a twenty-five-acre site in Chavez Ravine, next to Elysian Park, from J. B. Lankershim for $7,000. [56-57]

He constructed groups of cottages and opened Barlow Sanatorium. Fresh air, sunshine, and bed rest were the only treatments available for tuberculosis in the early 1900s. Because of the infectious nature of the disease, some Barlow residents were nurses and doctors who had contracted the disease while caring for infected patients at other hospitals. [58]

Patients moved from the infirmary to the cottages when their bacilli counts decreased. Each cottage had a donor's nameplate on its side. The cottage on the facing page is the Al Malaikah Mystic Shrine Cottage. [59] Some members of the early Al Malaikah order are listed as Knights Templar.

Porches were required for the sun cure (known as heliotherapy). Rest, however, was the main treatment. Bed rest was strict—patients' feet were not allowed to touch the floor for years. Nurses pulled the beds outside, with the patients in them, to maintain their bed rest. When patients' health improved, they had to learn to walk again due to muscle atrophy from inactivity.

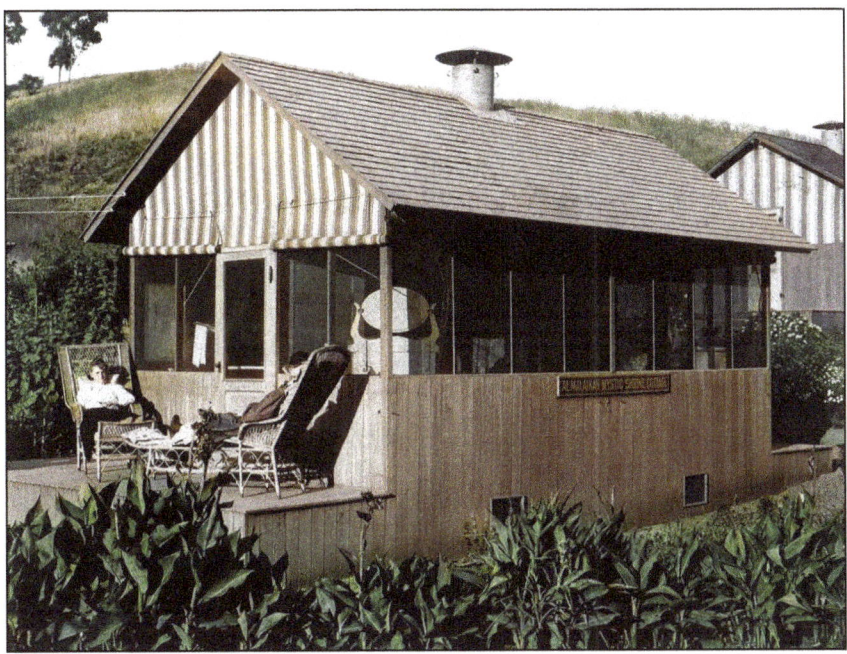

Figure 02.54. Two patients on the porch of an original Barlow Sanatorium cottage, 1907. C. (Courtesy of Barlow Respiratory Hospital)

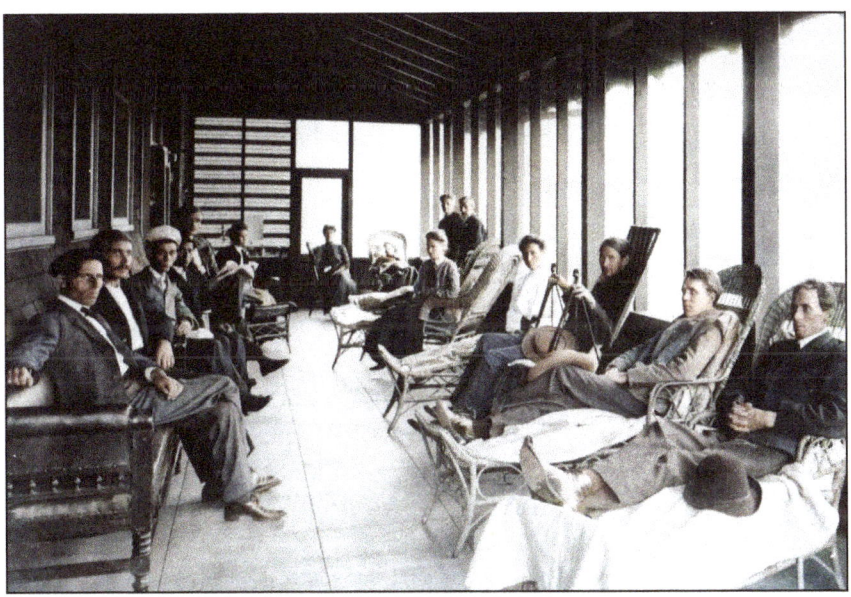

Figure 02.55. Men and women sitting on the infirmary porch taking heliotherapy, the therapeutic use of sunlight, 1902. C. (Barlow Respiratory)

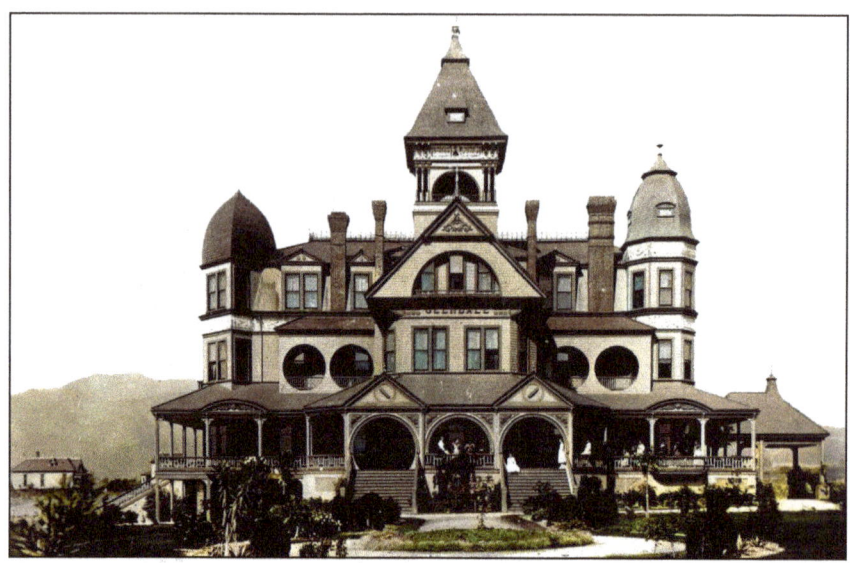

Figure 02.56. Glendale Sanitarium, early 1900s, before they added the sanitarium sign. C. (Courtesy of Glendale Adventist Medical Center)

The Glendale Hotel was built in 1880 on East Broadway between Jackson and Isabel Streets. The population of Glendale was fewer than 500. The houses were built far apart; the hotel felt as if it were in a rural area. It became St. Hidla's Hall (a girls' school) in 1887 and later Glendale High School. In 1905, the Battle Creek Sanitarium in Michigan bought the property for $12,000. They converted the building to The Glendale Sanitarium—a surgical hospital for the sick and a sanitarium for tourists.[60]

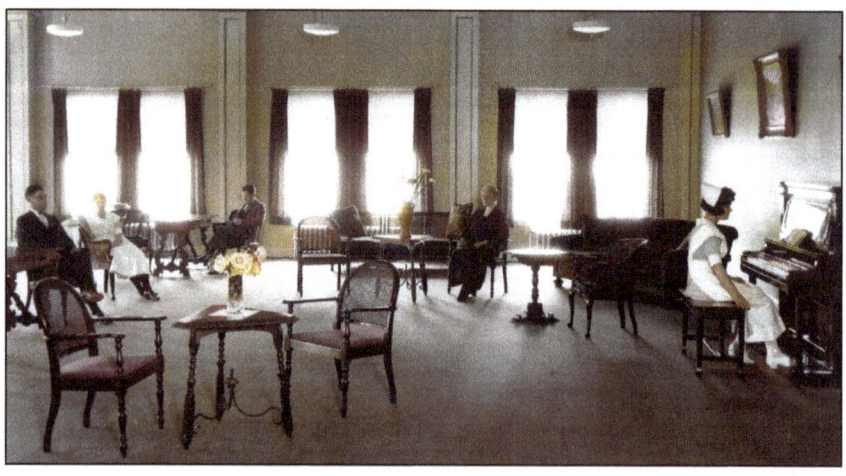

Figure 02.57. Nurses and patients relax in the Glendale Sanitarium parlor.

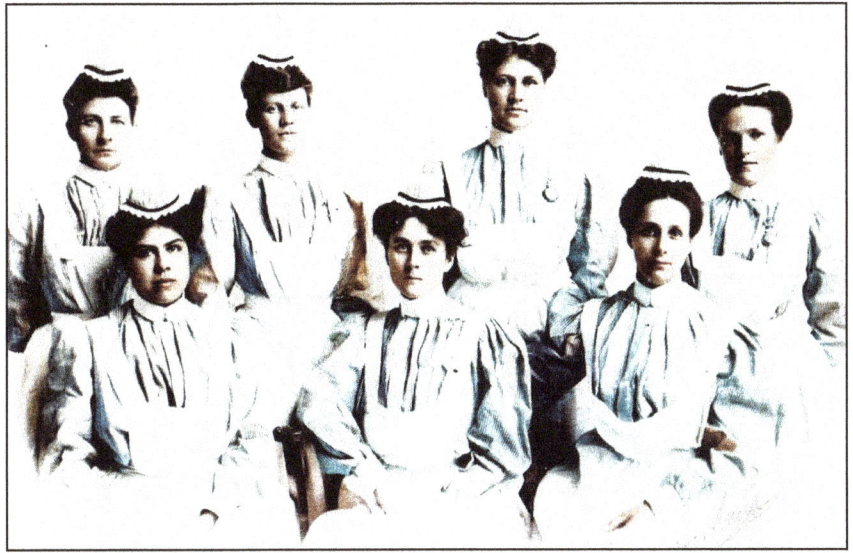

Figure 02.58. The first graduating class of the Glendale Sanitarium Training School for Missionary Nurses, 1906. C. Christine Meyers, Nellie Ray, and Edith Stevens, L to R. Standing are Barbara Chapman, Edwina Wager, Amanda Buckley, and Helen Henton. (Glendale Adventist Medical Center)

They opened a nurses training school in 1905. The entrance requirements included completion of nine grades. No fees were charged. The program consisted of two years of training, after a three-month probation. Glendale awarded the inaugural class a one-year credit because the pupils had worked in the Los Angeles Sanitarium prior to the start of training.

They wore blue cambric dresses, white aprons, and ruffled caps. Long sleeves, high-bishop collars, ankle-length skirts, and high-top black shoes were required. Short hairstyles and corsets were forbidden.

The pupils worked twelve to twenty-four hours every day. They provided all of the chamber work and special duty. They worked in the laundry, set up tables in the patients' dining room, and waited tables three times a day. They cared for all the patients. The probics had no days off; they were usually allowed one half-day off on the Sabbath.

Boxes were nailed together and painted white as supply cupboards; they converted two of the bedrooms into operating rooms. Before each surgery, pupils washed every inch of the walls and floors of the room with bichloride of mercury 1:1. Then, they sealed the doors and windows and fumigated with formaldehyde for eight hours. The hospital employed only three graduate nurses: a head nurse, a surgery supervisor, and a night supervisor.

Chapter Two

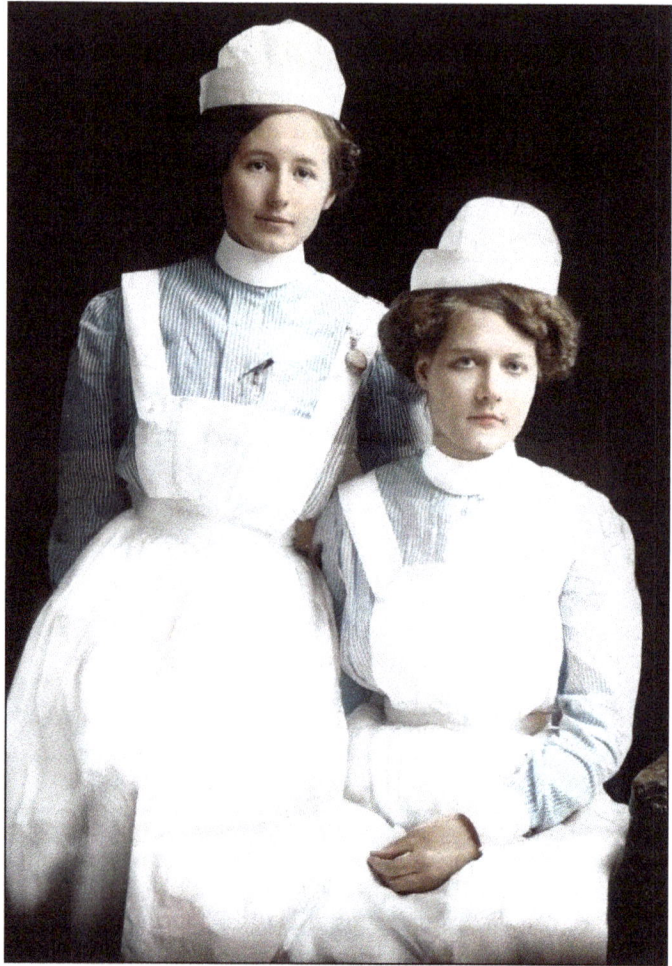

Figure 02.59. Lenora Lacey, standing, Glendale Sanitarium's first nursing supervisor, a 1901 St. Helena Sanitarium Training School graduate. Lacey said this about her training:

> We did not have a single classroom in which to meet; classes were held in the dining room under the store and laundry, in a shed-like laboratory building up on the hill above the sanitarium, when it wasn't being used as a morgue. During the first year, there were two or three female nurses, one male nurse, and one practical nurse.
>
> There were no nurses on duty at night, no night clerk, and no call service. If a patient rang the bell at night, the head nurse would peer over the balcony from her room on the second floor. If the patient rang twice, the nurse would go down and attend to the call. [61]

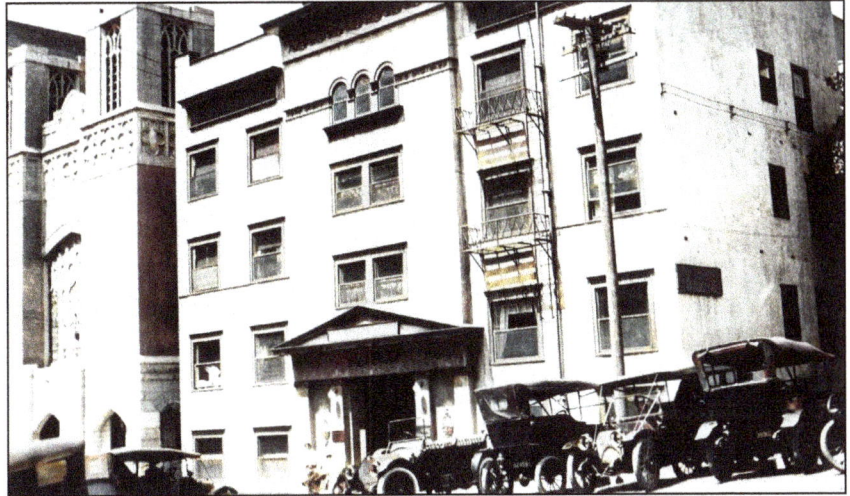

Figure 02.60. The German Methodist Deaconess Hospital on 447 South Olive Street. (Special Collections, Louise M. Darling Biomedical Library)

In February 1904 the *Los Angeles Times* reported the opening of the new German Methodist hospital: eighteen nurses from the German Methodist Mother House in Cincinnati moved to Los Angeles to staff it. Ella Sheila was appointed as the matron.

One novel feature of the hospital, advertised to the public, was the eight disinfecting baths for the nurses. The patients rooms were thus arranged: when a nurse went on duty or retired from duty, it was absolutely necessary for the nurse to pass through the disinfecting spray baths. [62]

German Methodist physicians practiced eclectic medicine. By 1915, eight accredited schools existed, and 2,000 Eclectic Physicians practiced in the U.S. The Eclectics used botanicals, which they deemed safer; however, they also performed surgery. California Eclectic Medical College was formed in Los Angeles in 1907 on Hill Street between 3rd and 4th. The college closed in 1915. Eclectic schools faded or fell victim to unscrupulous management. The last one closed in 1939.

In June 1904, reports began to circulate in the *Los Angeles Times* that the German Eclectic Hospital would be sold. The hospital denied the rumors: they said the hospital was running at full capacity. Twenty-five nurses were on staff; they had requested more from Cincinnati, and they had formed classes for a training school for nurses. Eleven pupils had already applied. [63]

Despite their denials, by 1905 the Germans had moved out, and Clara Barton Hospital had moved in—the second location of the Clara Barton Hospital.

Chapter Two

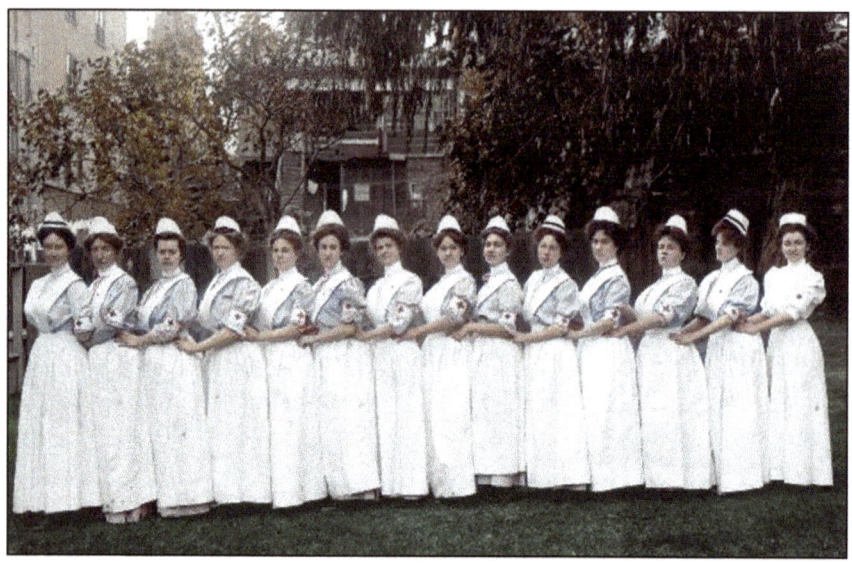

Figure 02.61. The Clara Barton Training School for Nurses trainees in front of the nurses home, 1908. C. The first class graduated in 1905.

The original 1903 thirteen-bed Clara Barton Hospital was located at the corner of Pico and Hope Streets. The hospital moved to a sixty-bed building on 447 South Olive Street in 1905.

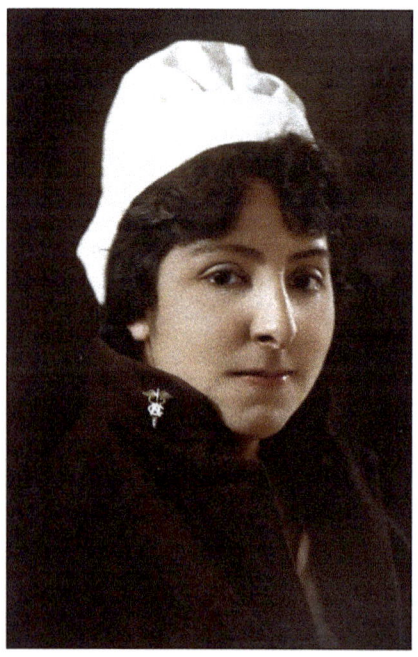

Figure 02.62. Marie Moreno, a 1917 graduate of the school, wore her Army Nurse Corps cape and pin on her collar, n.d. C. (History & Special Collections Division, Louise Darling Biomedical Library, UCLA)

In 1991 Moreno updated the Clara Barton Alumni Association minutes. "I'm lucky to keep as well as I do at 96. Do all my own housework. Sometimes I use someone for heavy work. Did a great deal of canning fruits and also found a 14-day pickle recipe that my mother had, so I did that too. The kids will get a surprise for Christmas. I bought only toys for the little ones. The doctor said that germs are afraid of me. Love, Marie" [64]

Great Decade

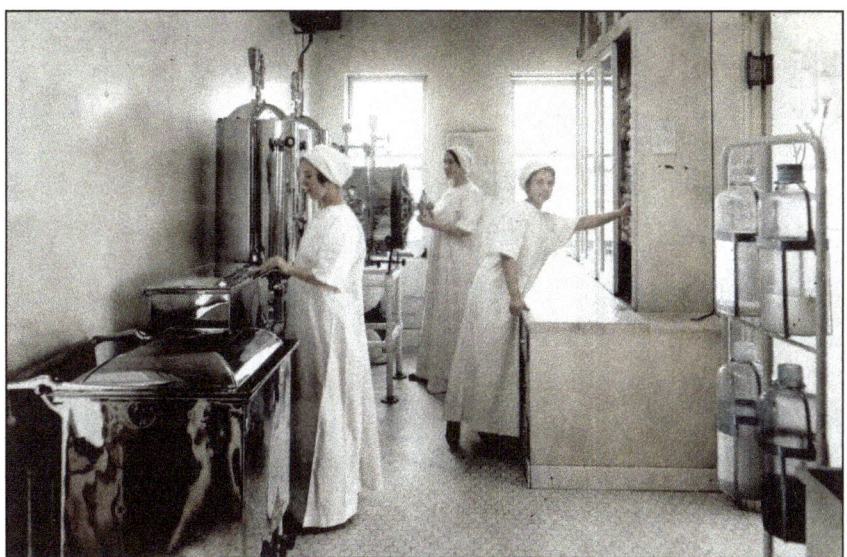

Figure 02.63. Nurses sterilizing items at Clara Barton Hospital, c. 1905. C. Self-taught nurse Clara Barton founded the Red Cross in 1881. Her nephew, H.P. Barton, named the hospital in her honor, not because Barton was his aunt. He named it because she dedicated her life to philanthropic work.

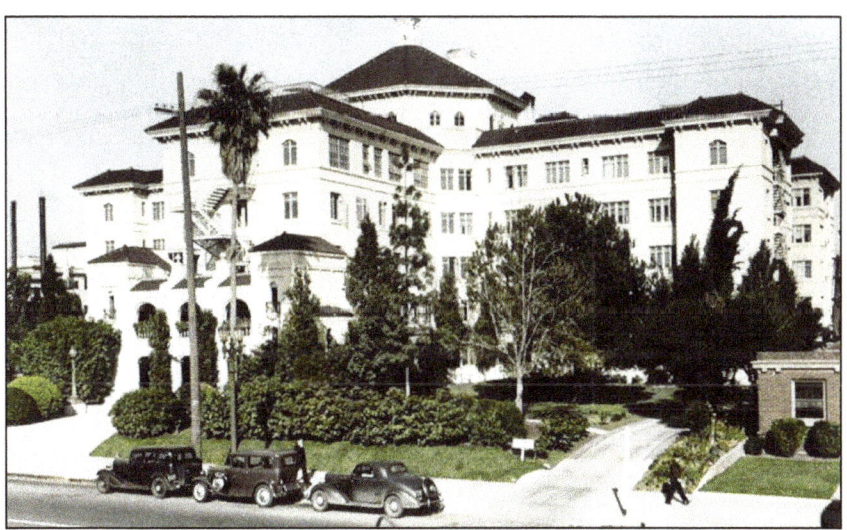

Figure 02.64. Hollywood Clara Barton Memorial Hospital, c. 1928. C. In 1926, the hospital moved to and merged with Hollywood Hospital, on Vermont, to become Hollywood Clara Barton Memorial Hospital. In 1944, Hollywood Presbyterian Hospital moved in. Queen of Angels merged with them in 1989. They became Queen of Angels-Hollywood Presbyterian.[65]

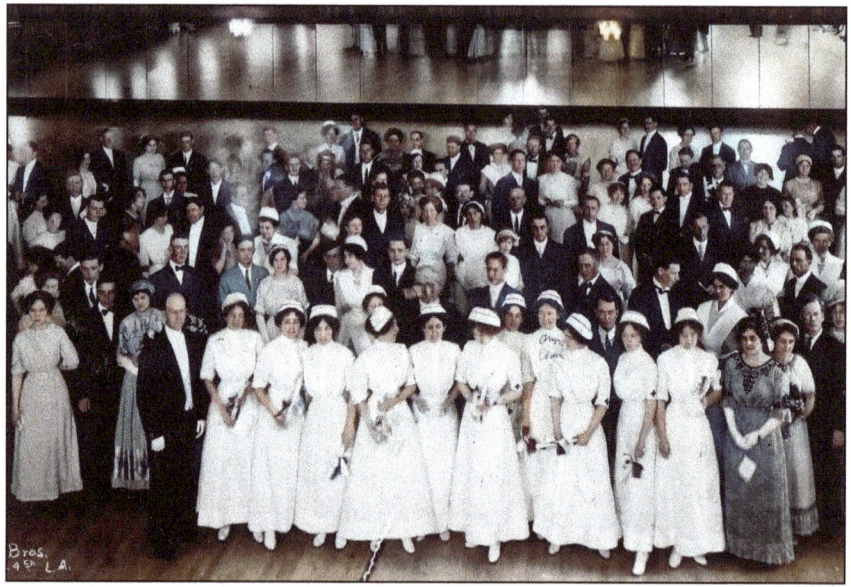

Figure 02.65. Clara Barton Training School graduation ceremony, 1913. C.

Figure 02.66. Sixty-five alumni attended this homecoming dinner of the Hollywood Clara Barton School of Nursing, 1938. C. (History & Special Collections Division, Louise M. Darling, Biomedical Library, UCLA)

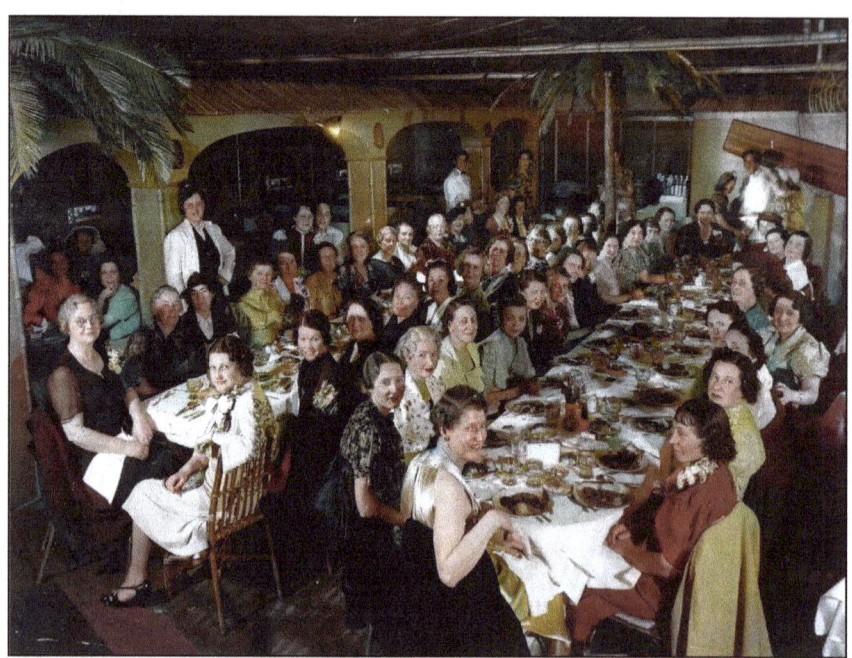

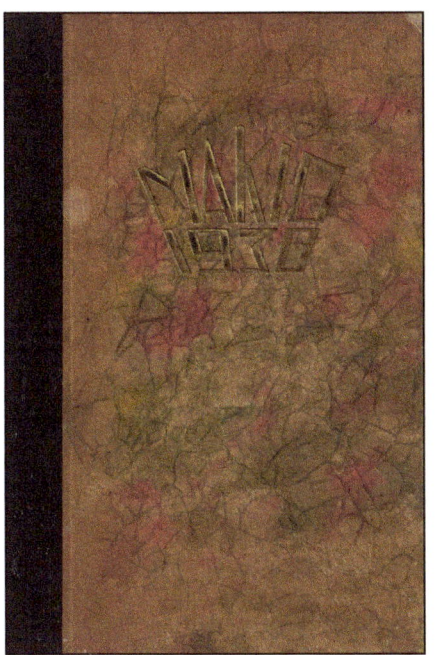

Figure 02.67. The 1930 *Makio*.

Supervisors Last Words to Probies

Is the flower room all straightened?
Did you fill the well with ink?
Did you wash the dirty dishes?
That were left in the kitchen sink?
Did you do your charting proper?
Did you see the telephones were in?
Did you give the patients water?
If you didn't, it's a sin.
You'll have to hurry up a bit!
I think you're awfully slow!
You must do you work quite proper
And then I'll let you go.

Figure 02.68. Barbaretta Taylor Jackson's Hollywood Clara Barton School of Nursing yearbook photo, 1930. C.

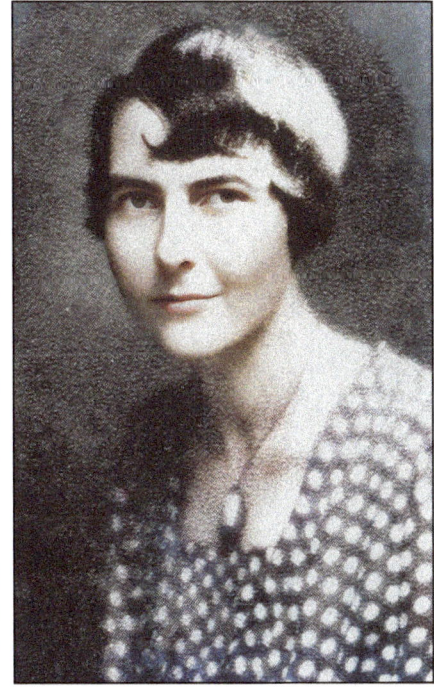

Jackson was listed in the 1930 *Makio* as Secretary of the School Alumnae Association. Sixty-one years later she was still listed as the secretary.

In the May 1991 Alumni Minutes, she informed the group, "Our treasury is empty and the bank account is closed."[66]

Jackson had saved many school items: the original secretary's book, photographs, pamphlets, yearbooks, tickets, and sheets of newspaper clippings about the school.

In 1993, she gathered the items and donated her entire school collection to the University of California, Los Angeles Archives.

Chapter Two

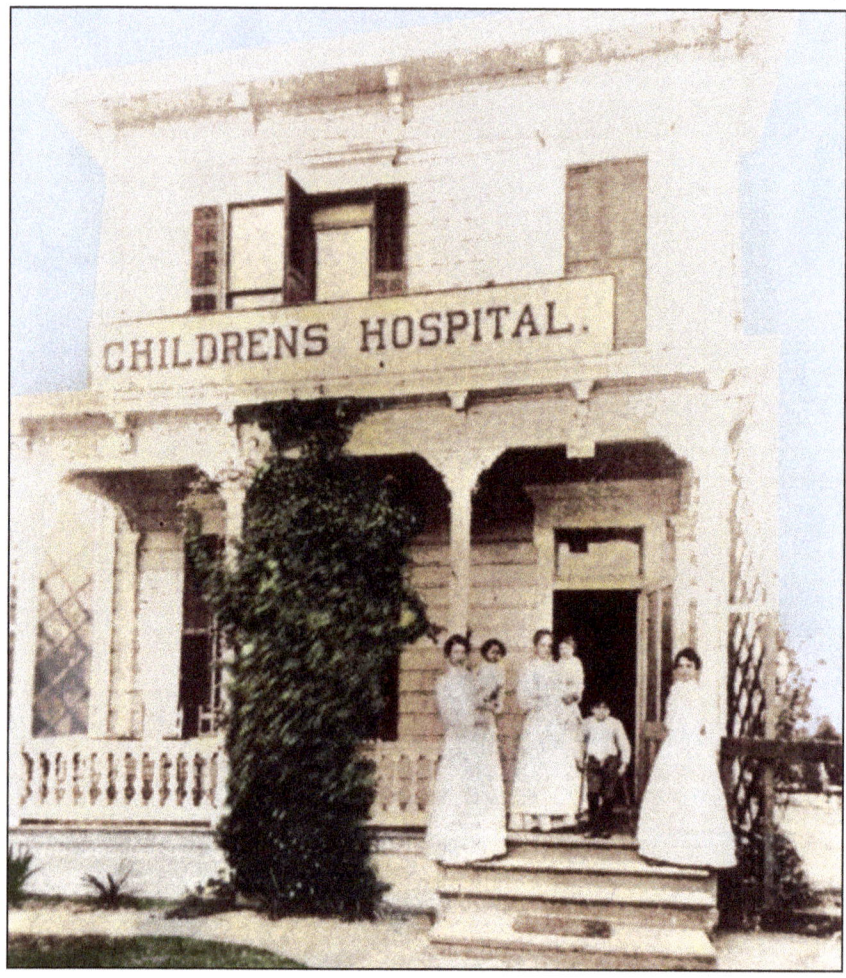

Figure 02.69. The first Childrens Hospital on Castelar Street, c. 1902. C. In 1912 they constructed a new building at Sunset and Vermont. [67]

Childrens Hospital began with four beds in a leased Victorian house on the corner of Castelar (later Hill) and Alpine Streets in 1901. The first floor contained an office, a reception room, a dining room, and a kitchen. The matron's (head nurse) quarters, a bathroom, and a sick room with four little white beds were located on the second floor. [68]

Businesses donated the four pediatric beds, a kitchen table, a dresser, a bureau, ten pillows, an iron bed, a mattress, silver and chinaware, twelve oak chairs, a roll-top desk, two wicker chairs, a library table, five dollars worth of paint, ten dollars for labor, and monetary deposits of $3,816. Hundreds of men and women attended the grand opening on 22 January 1902.

Great Decade

A non-dated letter from the secretary and manager of California Hospital to Mrs. William Johnston (president at Childrens 1904–1907) stated they had made arrangements so that four to six student nurses from California Hospital would work at Childrens for three months.[69]

Childrens would directly pay California Hospital student nurses the same stipend California paid them: eight dollars per month for a first-year student, twelve dollars for a second-year student, fifteen dollars for a third-year student, and car fare to go back and forth to lectures at California Hospital. Since Childrens had yet to start their own school and had no regular supply of student nurses, they needed nurses to care for patients.

The beginning of the nursing school at Childrens is not well documented, but Helena Barnard wrote a letter concerning the school in 1915 to the *American Journal of Nursing*. Barnard, a graduate of Johns Hopkins Training School for Nurses, had been a former president of the California State Nurses Association and a former member of the board of managers at Childrens.[70]

Bernard said Superintendent Marian Vinnier, also a graduate of Johns Hopkins, had organized the Childrens Hospital Nursing School in 1914. She said the school was the first nurses training program in California to establish instruction on a tuition basis.[71]

Grace Watson, a graduate of Teachers College, Columbia University, was hired as the first instructor. Twenty students were in the first class: half had studied one to three years in college, and one had a college degree. They affiliated with California State Normal School, a teachers' college downtown on 5th and Grand, for chemistry, dietetics, and other courses.

In May 1915, the management made an abrupt decision to hire a business woman, not a nurse, as superintendent. With that, Vinnier resigned as she felt she could no longer maintain the ideals of the school. Students were disappointed and unwilling to accept inferior education; they expected the higher ideals and training would be maintained. Bernard endorsed them.[72]

On 5 February 1915, the *Los Angeles Times* reported, "Didn't Like it So They Left: Young Mutiny Among Student Nurses at Childrens Hospital." Good Samaritan Hospital and Pasadena Hospital rushed a corps of student nurses to fill the vacancy. None of the graduate nurses at Childrens walked out.

Students on rotation, and some staff nurses, lived in the nurses home. In 1927, they added a new building and a new nurses' residence.[73] The custom of student nurses on a clinical rotation at Childrens continued. Modern nursing students, however, rotated to learn, not to assist with patient care. No records were located to indicate Childrens restarted the nurses training school.

Chapter Two

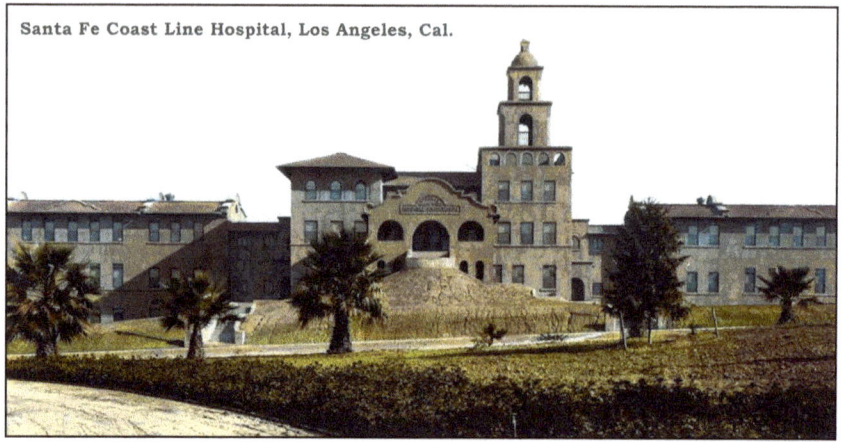

Figure 02.70. Santa Fe Coast Line Hospital photo postcard, 1907. C. The Santa Fe association purchased four acres for $5,500, in 1890, on the east side of Hollenbeck Park. The Southern California Railway used the land to build a hospital for its employees in 1905. The building included a well-appointed operating room, nurses quarters, beautiful recreation rooms, and a dining room. A separate section of the building was devoted to Mexican patients who "received the same care as their English-speaking coworkers."

Heated and lighted tents were located outside the building to house tuberculosis patients. Jersey cows and flocks of chickens roamed the grounds. Workers tended the garden to assure patients had fresh milk, butter, eggs, poultry, and vegetables. The association collected dues from the Southern California Railway employees to run the hospital: fifty cents from employees who received a salary of less than $100.00 per month, and one dollar for employees who received $100 or more.[74] In 1915 the patient census was 941.

SHE WOULD BE GOOD OLD MAID.
NURSE WEDS BUT SAYS NIX ON MARRIED LIFE

J. D. De Haven went to the Sana Fe Hospital as a nurse. Amoung the women nurses was Miss Agusta Relgleman, sweet and dainty. She was devoted to her work, but by persistent wooing, covering six weeks, Mr. De Haven gained her consent to marry him. They went December 31, 1911, to Santa Ana, and return to this city a happy married couple; this is, the groom was happy.

His joy turned to gloom when, as testifed in his divorce suit before Judge Myers yesterday, the bride clamly informed him she was going on night duty. The following morning she told the head nurse, Lena Matthews, she did not love her husband.

"I don't care for any man," she plaintively sighed.

"Why did you marry him, then?"

"I don't know."

She stole away to her home in Pennsylvania. She still used her maiden name, refusing to be known as Mrs. De Haven.

Judge Myers granted the decree on the ground of desertion.

Figure 02.71. An October 12, 1914 article in the *Los Angeles Times* told the saga of the marriage and divorce of a pair of nurses who worked at Santa Fe Coast Line Hospital.

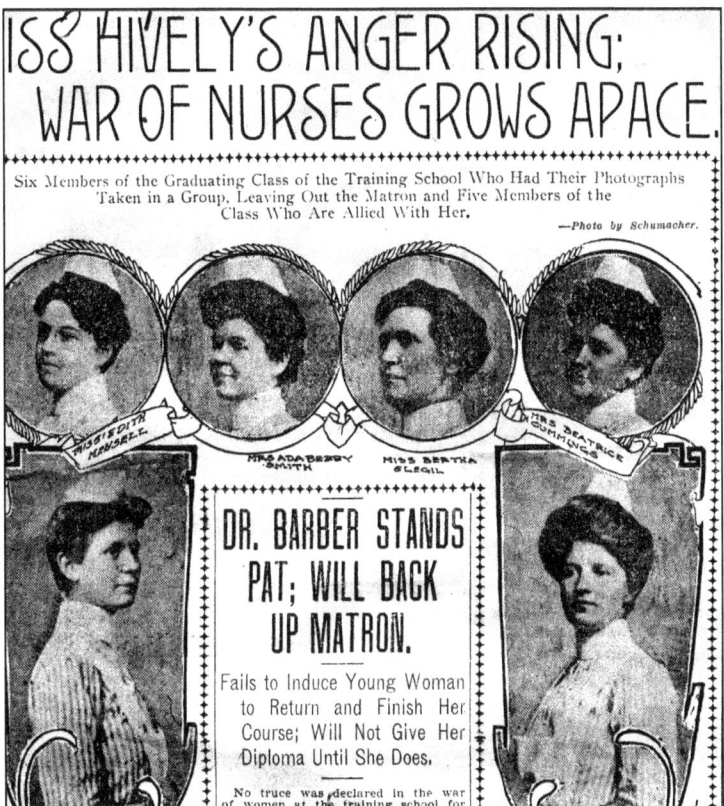

Figure 02.72. Student Nurse Hively is shown in the lower right side, 1905. *The Examiner* printed an article about an argument between a student nurse and the superintendent of County Hospital in September 1905. Student Bessie Hivley stated she was overworked and discriminated against. She claimed other students had been given a diploma before finishing the two-year program. She wanted to leave, and she wanted her diploma.

Dr. D.C. Barber told Hivley she needed four more months of training for the diploma—they would not bend the rules. Barber said, "It is like this with these girls. They are young and come here unused to hard work. They have all sorts of whims and they run up against the matron. Now the matron must have discipline, or there would not be any training school. When she sets her foot down, then the girls get mad."

In a follow-up article, the Matron Estelle Woods claimed, "Hively would not rise in the morning at the hour prescribed for a nurse of her rank and file." Hively left the hospital and finished her training at a school in San Bernardino.[75] (Lindley Scrapbooks, Special Collections, Libraries of Claremont Colleges)

Chapter Two

Angelus Hospital, Los Angeles, Cal.

Figure 02.73. The Angelus Hospital at the corner of Washington and Trinity Streets in the year of its completion, 1906. C. The bone room, a pathological room, a dissecting room, and an anatomical room were located on the third floor. The *Los Angeles Herald* touted the building as the first fireproof hospital and lauded its Grecian design and accoutrements. [76-78]

The patient rooms had no sharp corners, angles, door castings, moldings, mop boards, or chair railings. The thirty-six rooms contained a bathtub and vented air expelled to the outside by a fan in the basement. The four-tiled operating rooms had adjacent washrooms, dressing rooms, and two large etherizing (anesthesia) rooms. Gardens covered a sun parlor on the roof.

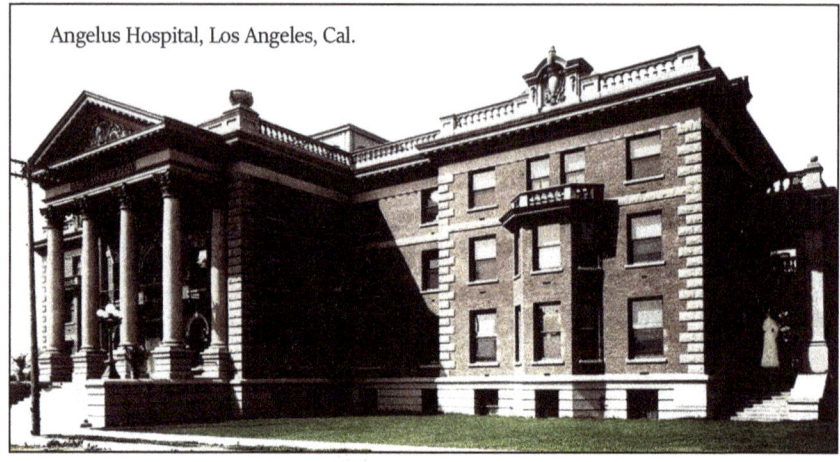

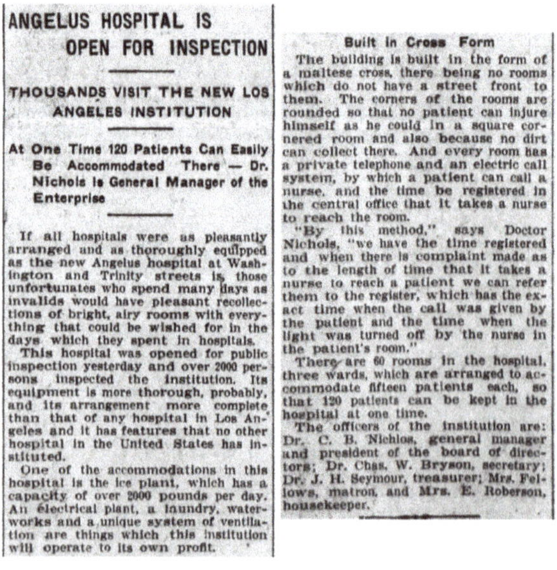

Figure 02.74. A 1906 article extolled the multiple features and beauty of the new Angelus Hospital.

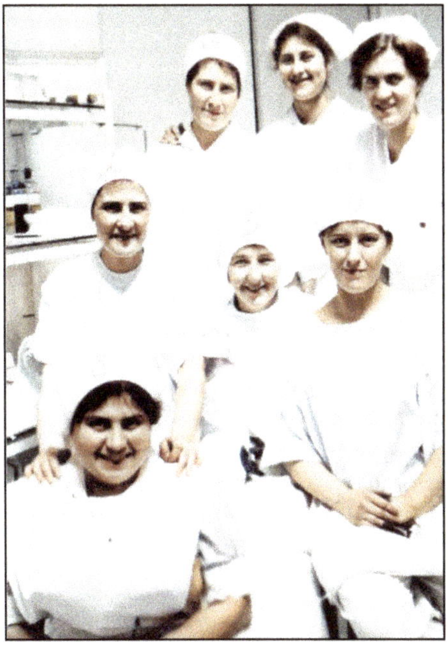

Figure 02.75. Angelus Hospital Training School student nurses with graduate nurses, n.d. C. (Whittier Public Library)

The Angelus Hospital Training School for Nurses graduated its first class of five graduates on 28 June 1908: Mary Dolan, Edith Johnson, Emma Johnston, Antionette Piago, and Sophia Voeltzel. The colors were blue and gold. They decorated the lecture hall with American flags and their class motto was "Semper Paratus."

When the nurses received their graduation pins, the speaker told the attendees the pins were "beautiful enough for a princess, and yet a princess could not wear them." [79]

Figure 02.76. Harriet Waugh Pahl, 1913. C. Pahl was the superintendent of nurses at Good Samaritan from 1897 to 1911 and then the superintendent at Angelus Hospital.

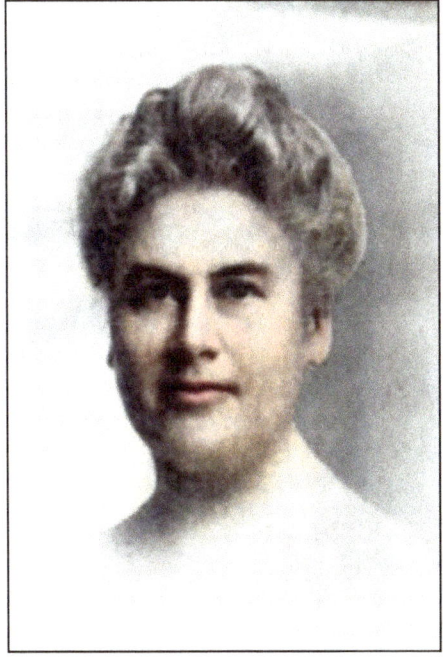

In 1904, she was elected the first president of the Los Angeles County Nurses Association. The nurses began the organization to fight for a standard of recognition.

Only nurses with scientific training and recognized abilities could join. LACNA planned to take their cause to the legislature to request the passage of a bill to elevate nurses to the same standard occupied by physicians.

Pahl graduated from the Illinois Training School for Nurses in Chicago, Illinois, in 1893. She married Peter C. H. Pahl, a well-known Los Angeles surgeon. [80]

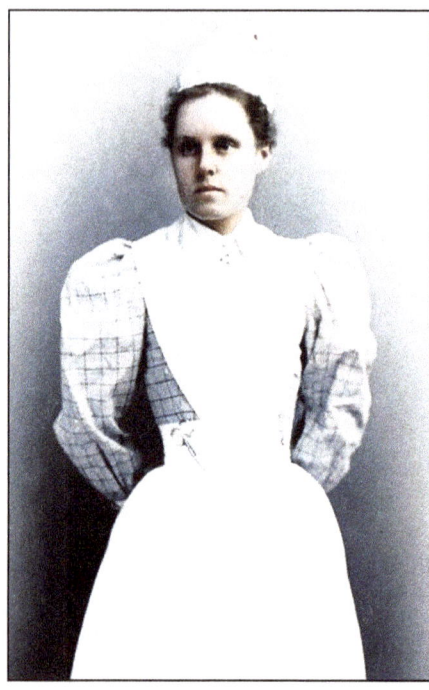

Figure 02.77. Anne Williamson's graduation photograph at New York Hospital School of Nursing (Cornell University), 1896. C.

After graduation, she cared for Rudyard Kipling in his home when he had pneumonia. She said nurses often worked for twenty-four hours without a break—people thought they were superior beings who could work without rest.

When the Spanish-American War began, Williamson wrote to her mother's friend, Clara Barton, and joined the Red Cross in Cuba. A yellow fever epidemic among soldiers forced her reassignment to Sternberg Hospital, which was filled with 2,000 typhoid patients.

When Williamson attended school, no one used gloves or masks in surgery—they scrubbed their forearms with a stiff brush and poured solutions over their hands. Many surgeries were performed at the patient's home on a kitchen table. During her first home surgery with a well-known Los Angeles surgeon, she went to the patient's home the day before, rolled up the rugs, and scrubbed the house. She used a wad of cotton in a cone of newspapers to deliver ether or chloroform anesthetic. She said despite the primitive methods, patients usually made a wonderful recovery. [81]

In 1908, Williamson became the director of nurses at California Hospital School of Nursing. She worked there for forty years. She once led a successful protest when a major studio produced an unflattering movie, *War Nurse*, because she had lived the truth and the movie did not show it. She detailed her many accomplishments in her book, *50 Years in Starch*, yet she always insisted, "She was just another nurse." [82]

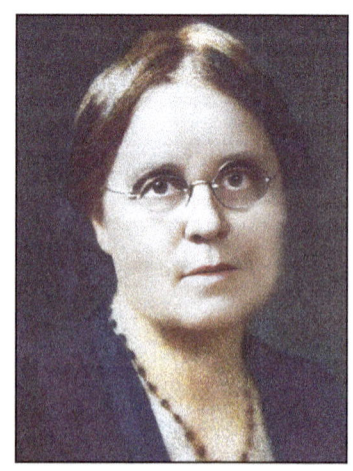

Figure 02.78. Madame President of the California State Nurses Association, Anne Williamson, 1927. C.

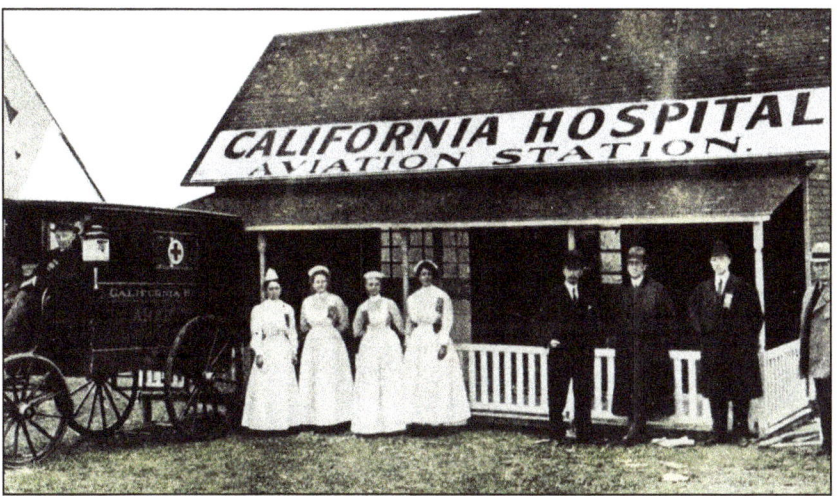

Figure 02.79. Anne Williamson, left, with unidentified nurses, ambulance drivers, and doctors at the Los Angeles International Aviation Meet, Dominguez Field, 1910. C.

Organizers contracted California Hospital to set up a camp hospital for the Los Angeles International Aviation Meet in 1910. A portable house company assembled Cottage No. 2, which included a room with windows, a small kitchen, and folding stairs to reach the supply room on the second floor.

Pacific Surgical Instrument Company installed an operating table, an instrument table, and stands for irrigation and washing. A circulating water wagon supplied water. The Los Angeles Ambulance Company was stationed near the hospital to transport injured flyers from the field. Anne Williamson took charge of the field hospital.

Lacerations from propellers and other minor incidents kept the hospital busy and women breastfed babies in the hospital for privacy. On the fourth day a famous aviator, Arch Hoxie, crashed his plane and died instantly. The ambulance rushed him to the hospital, but they couldn't save his life. [83]

Figure 02.80. A clipping from the *Los Angeles Herald*, January 23, 1910.

GIVEN AVIATION MEDAL

Miss Anne A. Williamson, superintendent of nurses of the California hosptial, was presented with a medal, a duplicate of those given to the aviators, by a representative of the aviation committee of the Merchants' and Manufacturers' assoiciation yesterday. The medal was given to Miss Williamson in recognition of her services in the hospital on the avaiation field.

Chapter Two

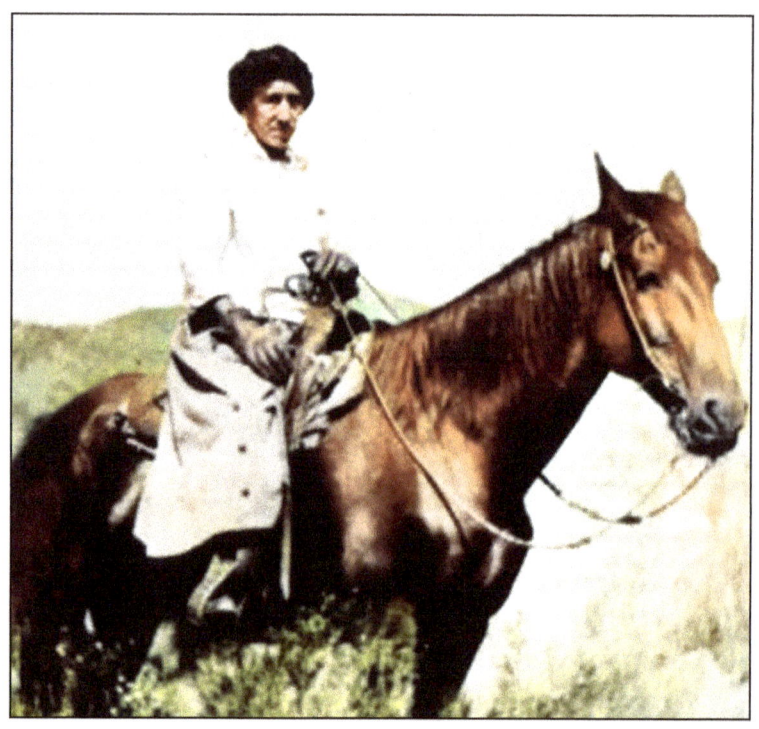

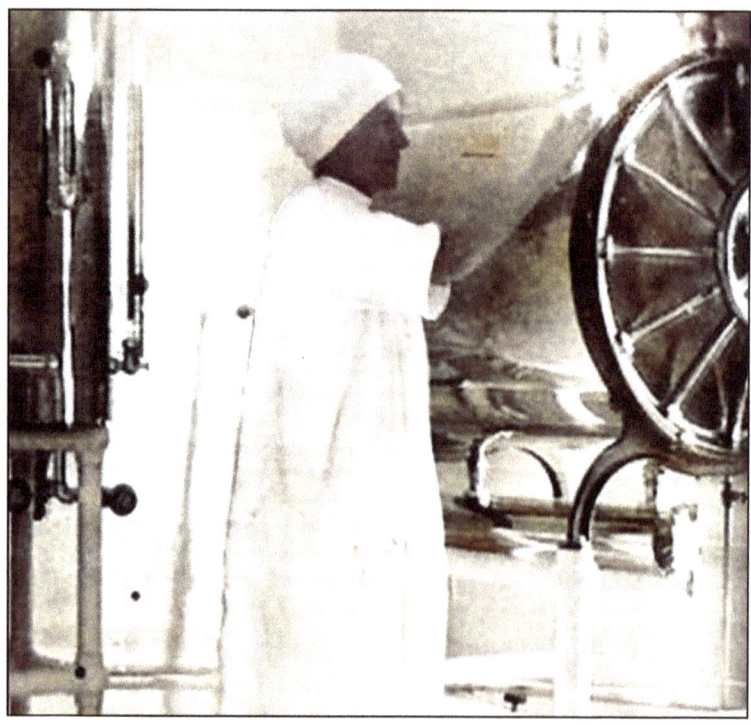

Elizabeth Cuddeback followed her grandmother on her rounds delivering babies. She liked to listen to her grandmother tell stories about the time she worked with Florence Nightingale during the Crimean War. Her grandmother had trained in Germany.

Her father was a blacksmith. Her mother had twelve children; only three survived. Because of her mother's asthma, Cuddeback assumed most of the responsibilities in the home, and her family had to move frequently because of her mother's health.

When she was seventeen, Cuddeback read a newspaper ad from a Texas hospital that operated a school for training nurses. She wanted financial independence; she wanted out from under her parents' rule. She had only recently completed the eighth grade; she applied, and the hospital accepted her. She graduated in 1907 after four years of training, twelve hours a day.

When she neared graduation, a woman from the Panama Canal came to her training school to recruit nurses. She wanted to work in the Panama Canal as a nurse, but her mother would not sign the permission form.

In 1908 Cuddeback moved to Los Angeles to work as a special nurse (private duty) for patients with typhoid. She worked with Native Americans in the Tehachapi Mountains and also attended ambulance calls: she set broken bones, delivered babies, and "fixed hobos with mangled arms who arrived on the Southern Pacific Railroad." [84]

Figure 02.81. Elizabeth Cuddeback on her nursing rounds to Native American patients in the Tehachapi Mountains, north of Los Angeles. C.

Figure 02.82. Elizabeth Cuddeback used a sheet steamer that stretched the wrinkles, n.d. C. (Courtesy of Sherna Berger Gluck/Feminist History Research Project at California State University, Long Beach)

Figure 02.83. Elizabeth Cuddeback, later in life, n.d. C.

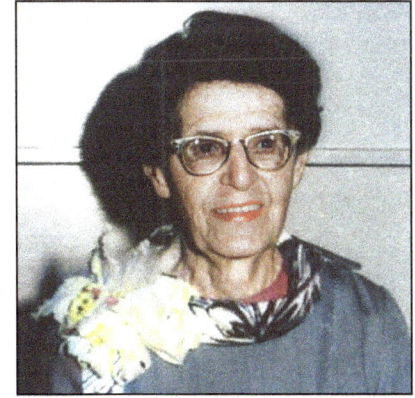

Chapter Two

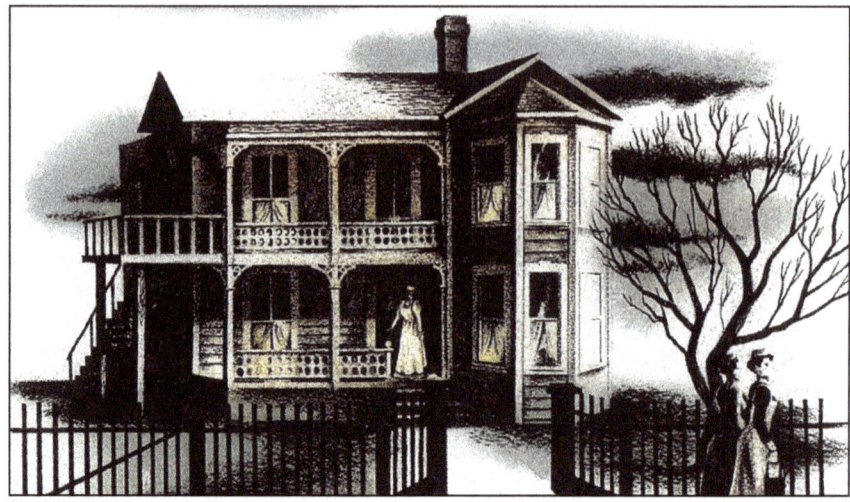

Figure 02.84. The first Methodist Hospital of Southern California, 1903. C.

In 1903, Methodist Hospital began with five beds in a two-story building downtown on Hewitt Street. The first patient was a Chinese woman. In 1915, they remodeled the mayor's residence, at 2826 S. Hope, into a 100-bed hospital and later expanded to 225.[85] Their operating rooms were the first in Los Angeles with air conditioning.[86] In 1953 they opened the first post-operative recovery room in the city.

In 1925, they built a nurse's residence across the street that housed 150 graduates and students—an underground tunnel connected the nurse's residence to the hospital. The hospital and school moved to Arcadia in 1957. The last nursing class graduated in 1958.[87]

Figure 02.85. The first graduate nurses of the Methodist Hospital School of Nursing: Meryle Dunham, Grace Wilson, and Minnie Wilson, 1915. C. Charlotte Armstrong, right, was the first Superintendent of Nurses.

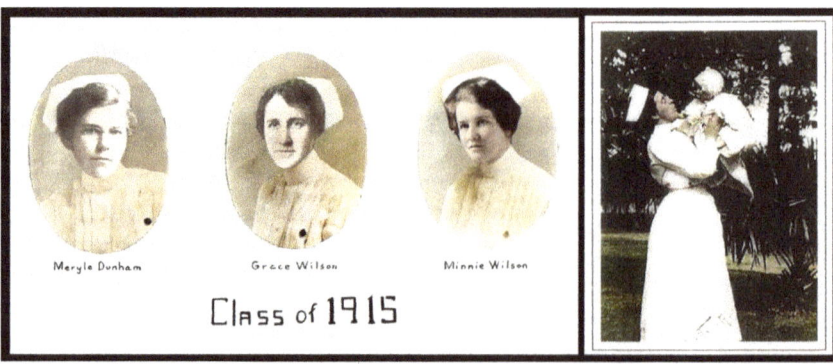

Great Decade

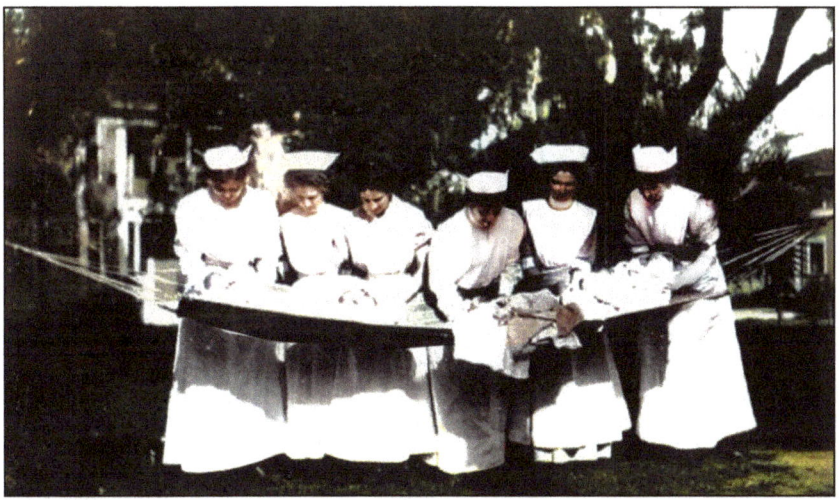

Figure 02.86. Nurses arranged babies in a long sling outside of Methodist Hospital, n.d. C. The original hospital building (1903 to 1915) is in the background. (Courtesy of Methodist Hospital)

Figure 02.87. Methodist Hospital nurses at the first Nurse's Alumni banquet at Christopher's Café, June 1919. C. World War I had recently ended, and the banquet displayed a patriotic flag. The popular Christopher's Cafe, located at 241 South Spring Street, specialized in frozen dainties. They advertised their ice cream was made from the highest grade of pasteurized cream tested at 120 degrees for safety. They delivered. 88

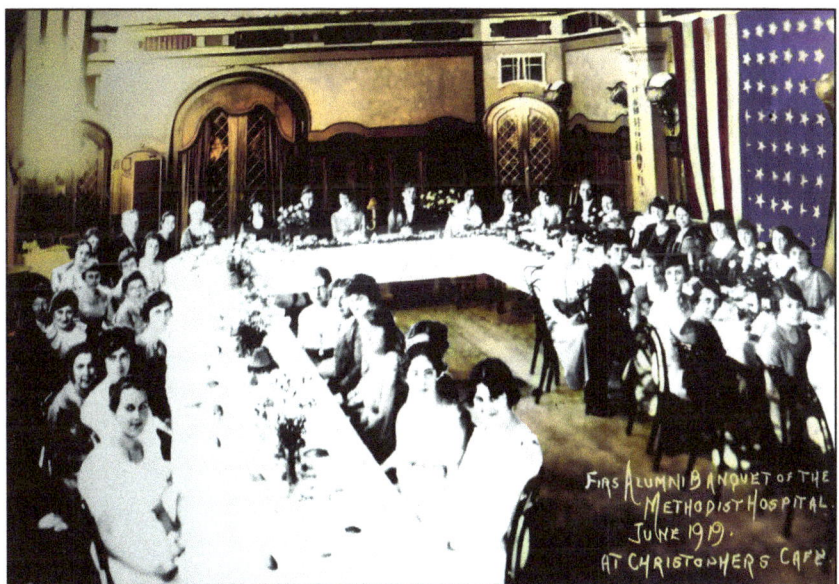

Chapter Two

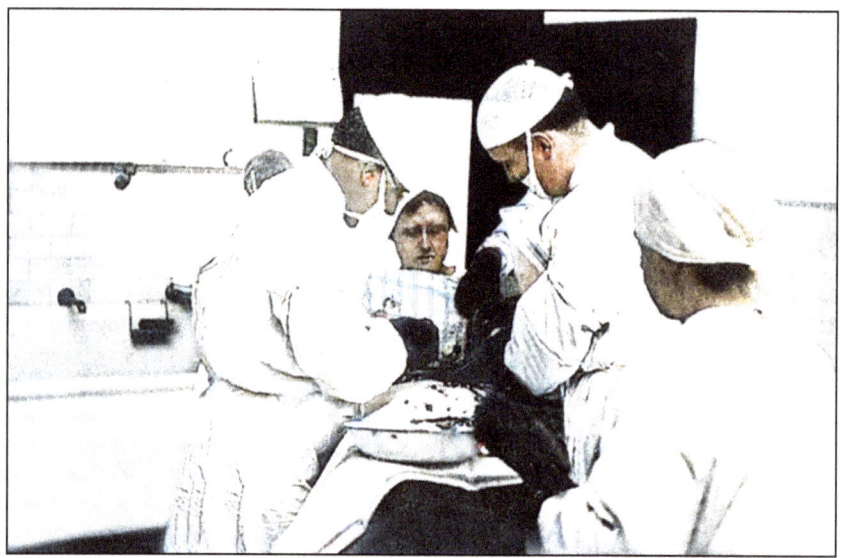

Figure 02.88. Surgeon Charles H. Mayo operating; Florence Henderson is seated at the head of the table, an unknown surgeon is on the right, and Mary Doyle Marceau is the surgical nurse at the end of the table, c. 1913. C. (Courtesy of Mayo Historical Unit, Mayo Clinic, Rochester, Minnesota)

In the early days of surgery, any available person administered the anesthetic: doctors' wives, nurses, or even secretaries. In 1904, doctors at the Mayo Clinic (then called St. Mary's Hospital) realized trained nurses provided excellent anesthesia care and decided to hire them specifically for the job. Franc Florence Henderson, Alice Magaw, and Mary Hines were the first three nurses they hired. Magaw had already been administering anesthesia at St. Mary's for several years. [89]

When Henderson graduated from Bishop Clarkson's Training School for Nurses in 1900, William and Charles Mayo heard about her nursing abilities and offered her a job. Until that time, Magaw and one doctor administered all the anesthetics. In 1904 the doctor left for a trip, and Henderson permanently took his place. Magaw, often called the Mother of Anesthesia, had already mastered this skill and was respected for her ability. She taught Henderson. The nurses administered ether using the open-drop method—placing drops of an anesthetic on a cloth over the patient's nose and mouth. They had no machines to monitor the patients; they relied on observation of skin color, vital signs, and the patients' movements.

Henderson excelled in anesthesia and trained other nurses and physicians; she helped define the early profession of nurse anesthetists. She moved to Los Angeles in 1917. [90]

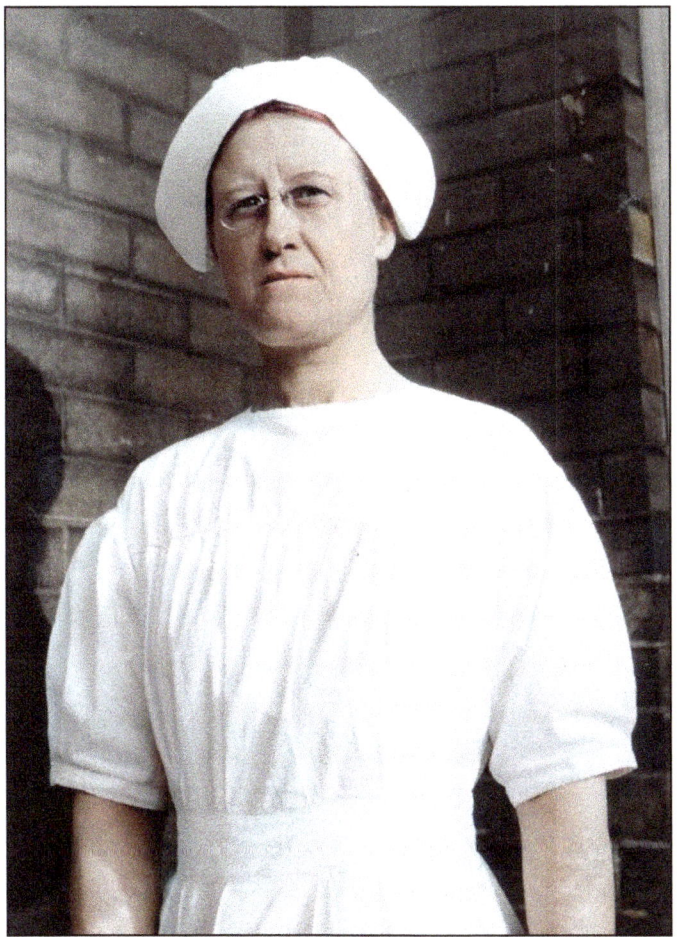

Figure 02.89. Florence Henderson in surgical attire, c. 1914. C. (Courtesy of the American Association of Nurse Anesthetists Archives)

Florence Henderson practiced at many hospitals in Los Angeles: St. Vincent's, the Angelus, Pacific, California, the French Hospital, and others. She started working with the Red Cross in 1918, acted as secretary for five years, and taught World War I nurses about anesthetics. She was treasurer of the Los Angeles Nurses' Club for three years. She became the first vice president of the California State Nurses Association, District 5 (Los Angeles), in 1921, and director from 1924 until 1926. She retired from anesthesia in 1923.[91]

In 1934 she was subpoenaed to testify in the trial against nurse anesthetist Dagmar Nelson. Henderson had retired in 1923, so she could not be held in violation of the 1933 Medical Practice Act.[92] Her last known address was 213 South Alexandria, Los Angeles.

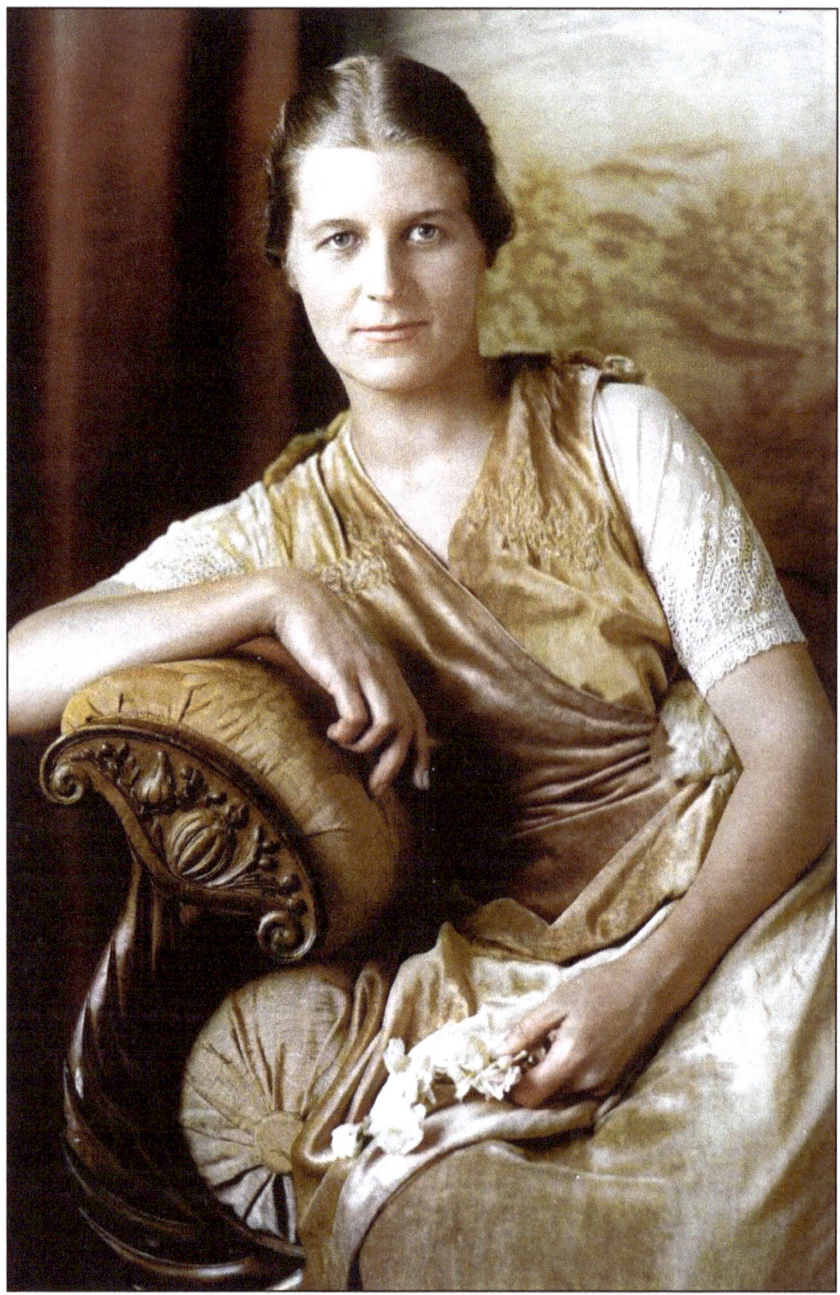

Figure 02.90. Dagmar Nelson, c. 1926. C. In July 1934, physician anesthetist Charles-Frances sued Dagmar Nelson for the "illegal practice of medicine in violation of the state's medical practice act." [93] (Courtesy of the History Center of Olmsted County)

Dagmar Nelson graduated from the two-year Mayo Clinic Training Program for Nurses in 1912—two months before the Titanic sailed off on its fateful cruise. She left Mayo after graduation and then returned in 1923 to study anesthesia under the supervision of Mary Hines—one of the three original nurse anesthetists. She learned the open-drop method and anesthesia by mask with oxygen and nitrous oxide. [94]

Nelson often worked with surgeon Vern Hunt at Mayo Clinic. Hunt later moved to Los Angeles and worked at St. Vincent's Hospital, but he did not like the quality of the physician anesthetists at St. Vincent's (doctors had not yet adopted the term anesthesiologists). St. Vincent's did not employ any nurse anesthetists.

Hunt remembered he liked the anesthesia care Dagmar Nelson administered at Mayo Clinic. He wrote to her and offered her a job at St. Vincent's. Nelson accepted. She moved to Los Angeles, rented an apartment two blocks from the hospital, and worked as Hunt's sole anesthetist.

In 1928, physician anesthetists convinced the California State Board of Examiners to produce a statement stating anesthesia was the practice of medicine despite that nurses had been the main providers of anesthesia since the Civil War. This was a veiled response to the diminishing income of physicians. Some nurse anesthetists continued to practice. Some quit.

The 1929 stock market crash increased competition. Physician anesthetist Charles-Frances filed an injunction, naming both St. Vincent's Hospital and Nelson, charging her employer-hospital for allowing her to illegally practice medicine without a license.

On 12 July 1934, the Charles-Frances v. Nelson trial began. Nelson's attorney argued that the most prestigious hospitals hired nurse anesthetists; hundreds worked in the United States, not just a few in Los Angeles. The evidence presented at the trial echoed the predominant view at the time: the dominance of the male physician over the female nurse, who was portrayed, even by the defense, as an extension of the surgeon who "has the power and therefore the responsibility to entirely control the surgery." [95]

After twelve days the judge said, "The administration of general anesthetics by Dagmar A. Nelson, pursuant to the directions and supervision of duly licensed physicians and surgeons, as shown by the evidence in this case, does not constitute the practice of medicine or surgery ... and ... constitutes the practice of nursing within the meaning of the laws of the State of California."

Nelson won her case on 31 July 1934. Had she lost, anesthesia as a nursing specialty might not exist today. [96]

Chapter Two

Sophie Winton joined the Red Cross in 1914 and left for the Army with Minnesota Hospital Unit #26. Her military training consisted of a two-week drill in New York City while staying at a local hotel. They assigned her to Mobile Army Surgical Hospital #1—the first MASH unit in the U.S. While in France, she worked with Dr. James Guathermey and the famous neurosurgeon Dr. Harvey Cushing. She offered her account of WWI:

> I gave anesthetics from the first day of June (1918) to November after the Armistice. How many anesthetics I gave during the World War I cannot determine, except that when the big drives were on, lasting from a week to ten days, I averaged twenty-five to thirty a day. The first three months I gave chloroform entirely, after which a ruling came that we were to use ether because there had been too many deaths from chloroform in inexperienced hands. Many a night I had to pour ether or chloroform on my finger to determine the amount I was giving, because we had no lights except the surgeon had a searchlight for his work. [97]
>
> When the shells fell close to the hospital, the surgeon and staff would duck under the OR table, but I would continue my anesthetic, holding one of the metal surgical trays over my and the patient's head.

Winton graduated from Swedish Hospital, in Minneapolis, in 1911. Her class was the first in Minnesota to ever take the state nursing board. She worked as an RN for two years and then began training as a nurse anesthetist at Swedish Hospital. She took frequent trips to the Mayo Clinic to share the techniques with anesthetists. Before joining the Army in WWI, she had already delivered anesthesia to 10,000 patients without a single death.

After WWI, Winton moved to Los Angeles. She never worked at a hospital. Instead, she bought a house on Wilshire Boulevard in Beverly Hills and opened her own dental and plastic surgery clinic. She converted the bedrooms to recovery rooms. Her clients included the celebrities of that era. [98] Her house in Laurel Canyon was filled with celebrities at her 100th birthday party—Governor Ronald Reagan called to congratulate her.

Winton was the epitome of the independent practitioner; she forged new ground for nurse anesthetists. She helped organize nurse anesthetists to prepare for the case against Dagmar Nelson; she lent both her psychological and financial support.

The French Government awarded a Croix de Guerre for her WWI service. She received the Agatha Hodgins Award for Outstanding Accomplishment from the American Association of Nurse Anesthetists. The Red Cross placed her pin, number 4442, in the Red Cross Archives in Washington, DC. [99]

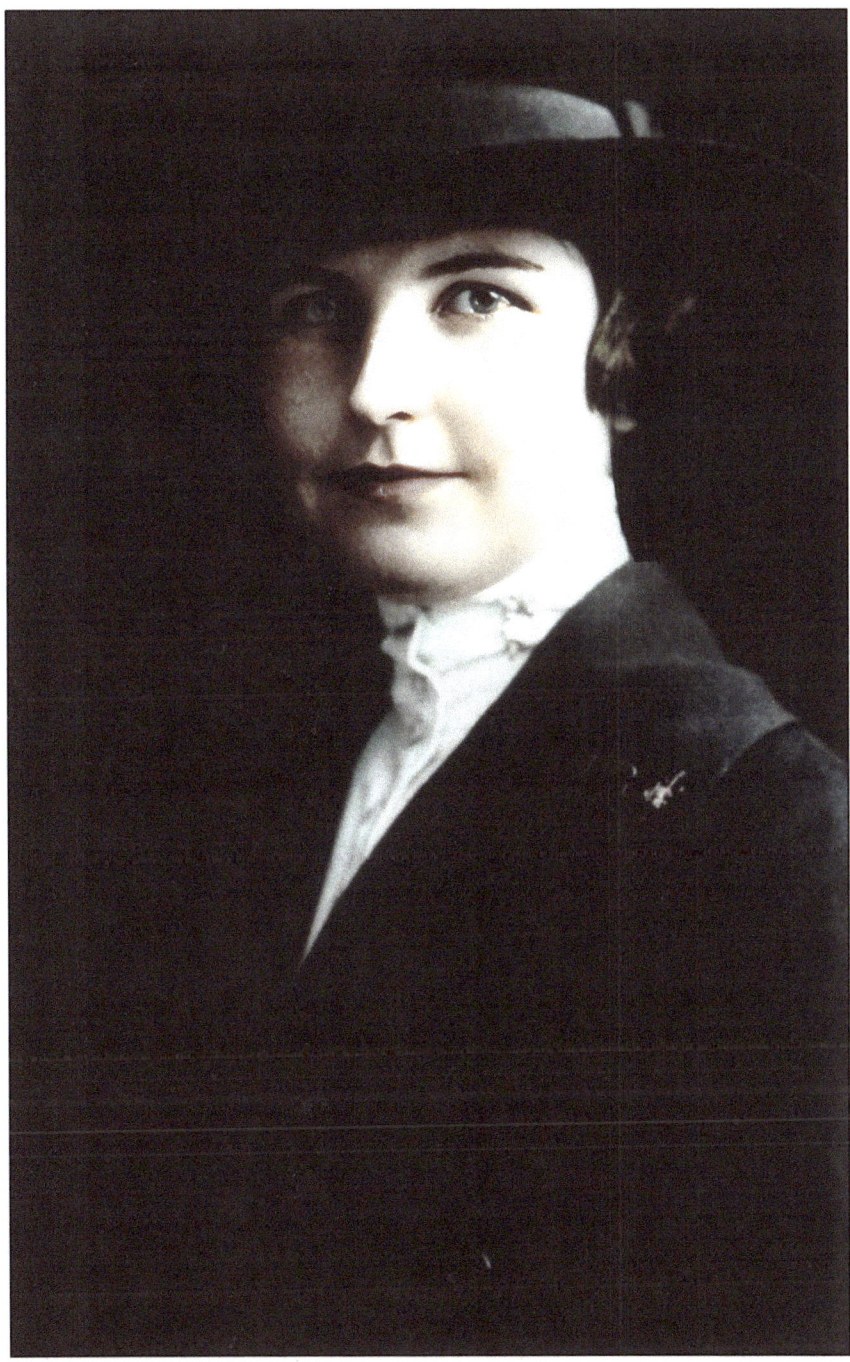

Figure 02.91. Sophie Winton in her WWI Red Cross Army uniform, c. 1914. C. (Courtesy of the American Association of Nurse Anesthetists Archives)

The History of Graduate Nurse Pins

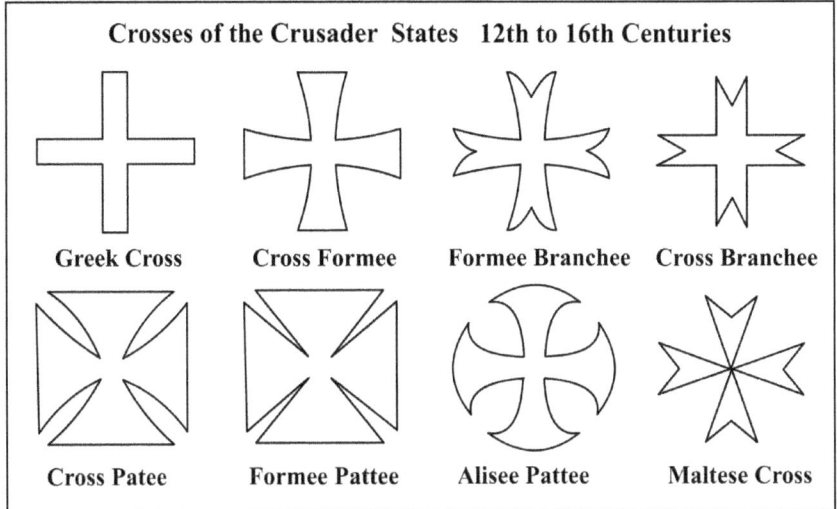

Figure 03.01. Knights Hospitaller cross shapes from the 12th to 16th century.

Beginning in the ninth century, the crusaders, nobility, wealthy, religious, and infirmed people made pilgrimages to Jerusalem. The pilgrims had no one to care for them if they became sick. Knights of the Order of the Hospital of Saint John the Baptist (the Knights Hospitallers) obtained permission from the Caliph of Egypt to build a hospital in Jerusalem to care for pilgrims. [1-2]

The Knights wore crosses on their habits. Many references state the Knights used a Maltese cross from the start of the hospital's inception. Edwin J. King, however, in "The Knights Hospitaller in the Holy Land," stated no evidence exists the Knights used a Maltese cross until they traveled to Malta in the fifteenth century. Early drawings depict Knights with a Greek Cross. [3-4]

Many schools of nursing, including Los Angeles schools, have used cross shapes on their graduate pins. Few used the actual Maltese cross shape, although many erroneously refer to their pin as a Maltese. They used the Vatican, Greek, and Lutheran crosses.

Pins often contained the double snake helix of the Caduceus (also called the magic wand of the Greek god Hermes) or a single snake with the staff of Asclepius. Modern schools often integrate the school seal. [5]

Schools incorporated the lamp of learning, an open book, laurel wreaths, or the pain-relieving poppy flower into their designs.

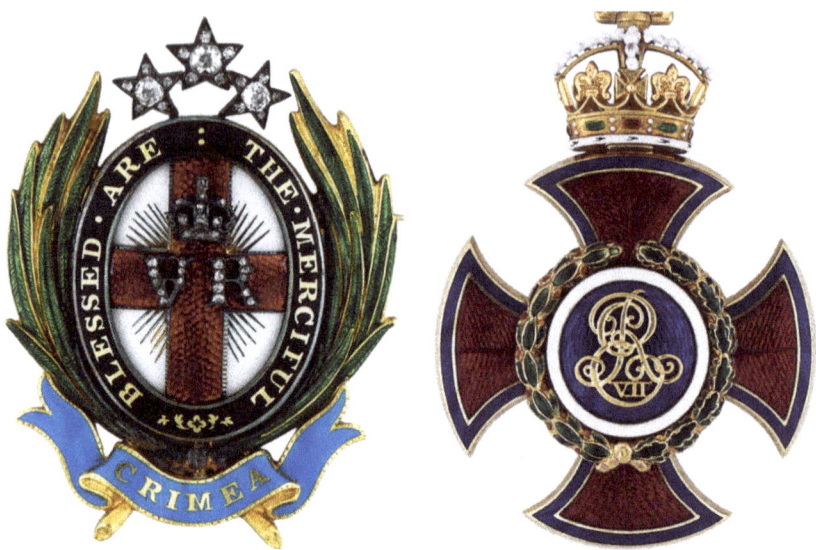

Figure 03.02. At left is the original Nightingale Jewel—a gold-enameled badge presented to Nightingale in 1855 for service in the Crimean War. Queen Victoria awarded Nightingale several royal badges; the shapes corresponded to the shapes of the crusader crosses.

The center piece is the Red Cross of Saint George (Greek Cross design). The crown, letters VR, and three stars were made of diamonds. Prince Albert, the Prince Consort, designed the brooch; R and S Garrard and Co. manufactured it in 1855. [6]

The back is engraved with a dedication from Queen Victoria: "To Miss Florence Nightingale, as a mark of esteem and gratitude for her devotion towards the Queen's brave soldiers, from Victoria R. 1855." This was the first known incident of a badge awarded to a nurse for excellent service. Nightingale adopted this tradition and gave gold and silver medals to her excellent students. Perhaps this created the custom of graduate nurse pins. [7-8]

Figure 03.03. At right is the Badge of Florence Nightingale, awarded to her in 1907 for the Order of Merit. Since its inception in 1902, the Order of Merit has admitted only eight women—Nightingale was the first. [9]

This prestigious Order was limited to British Sovereigns. A maximum of twenty-four members were admitted at any time. The Order comprised six admirals, six generals, and twelve civilians eminent in the fields of art, music, and literature. [10] The shape is an Alisee Pattée cross.

(Courtesy of the Council of the National Army Museum, London, England)

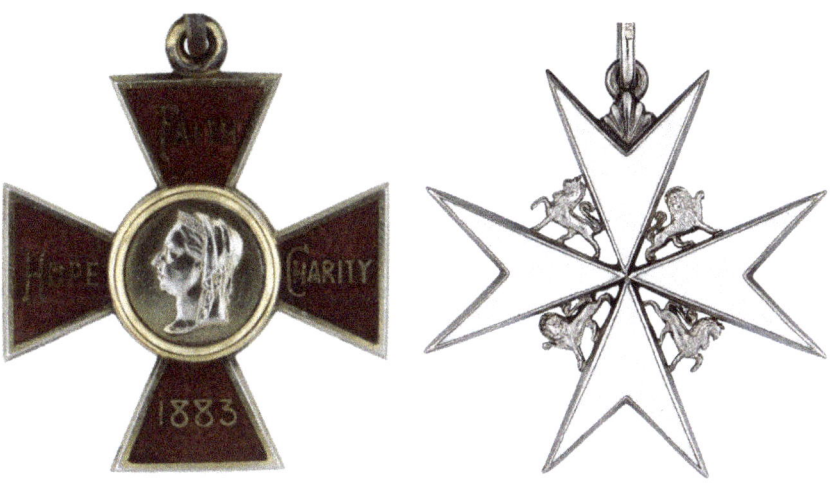

Figure 03.04. At left is the Royal Red Cross, 1st Class, Queen Victoria issue, presented to Florence Nightingale in 1883—a Formée Pattée shape. During the Crimean War (1854–1856), nurses were not eligible for campaign medals; the Zulu War of 1879 was the first campaign to recognize their service. [11]

Nightingale was one of the first thirty-one recipients of the Royal Red Cross, awarded specifically to women for special devotion in nursing sick and wounded servicemen. The decoration is now awarded to Army nurses for exceptional service, devotion to duty, and professional competence in British military nursing. [12]

Figure 03.05. On the right is the Order of the Hospital of St. John of Jerusalem, in England, Badge of a Lady of Grace, presented to Nightingale in 1904—a true Maltese Cross shape—given for the recognition of voluntary work in hospitals, ambulances, and relief work.

The Most Venerable Order of the Hospital of St. John of Jerusalem was incorporated by Royal Charter of Queen Victoria in 1888. The order traces its origins to the Knights Hospitaller in the Middle Ages, the oldest surviving chivalric order, considered founded in Jerusalem in 1099 and later known as the Order of Malta.

The Order of the Hospital of St. John of Jerusalem is now divided into six classes under the Sovereign and Grand Prior of the Order. [13]

(Courtesy of the Council of the National Army Museum, London, England)

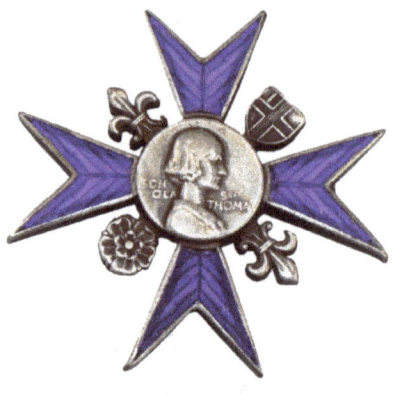

Figure 03.06. Nightingale Training School for Nurses badge, 1925.

The first association of a nurse to a badge was in London, 1724. Franks reported that "When the hospital first opened, the nurses came to the hospital for the day. Their only uniform was a round tin medal, inscribed with the name of the ward and the status of the nurse. The staff hung these around their necks over their own clothes." [14]

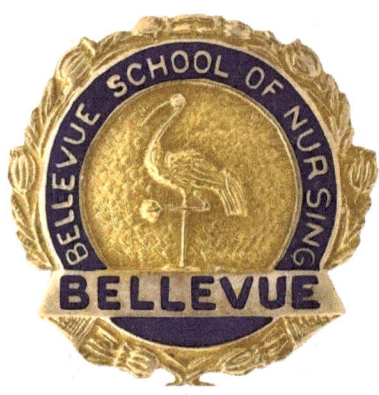

Figure 03.07. Bellevue School of Nursing Graduate Nursing pin, 1880.

The first pin awarded to nursing school graduates in the United States. Designed in 1880 by Tiffany and Company jewelers. The crane represented vigilance, and the wreath of poppies illustrated the role of nurses to allay pain and bring rest to the suffering. The blue circle signified consistency of care. [15]

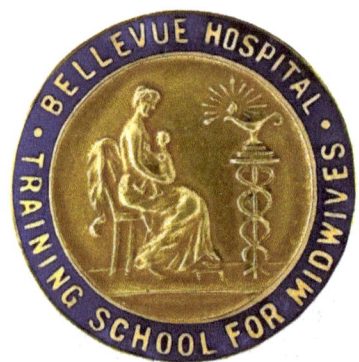

Figure 03.08. Bellevue School for Midwives pin, 1911.

Bellevue opened the first U.S. school for midwives in 1911.[16] It closed in 1936. Nightingale made this statement concerning the importance of the midwife: "Though everybody must be born, there is probably no knowledge more neglected than this, nor more important for the great mass of women." [17]

Graduate Pins

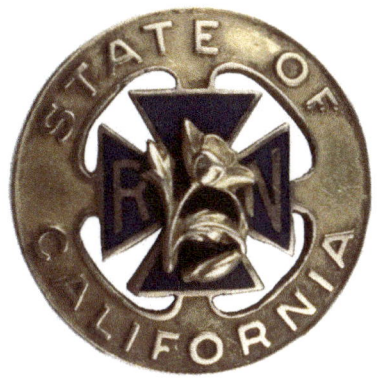

Figure 03.09. State of California Registered Nurse pin, c. 1910.

In the 1900s, the California State Board awarded nurses a state pin after they passed the licensing exam. Other states adopted the custom as well.

Eventually, states phased out the pins, and most of them were lost. The inset is a Formée Patée shape with a California Golden Poppy—the state flower.

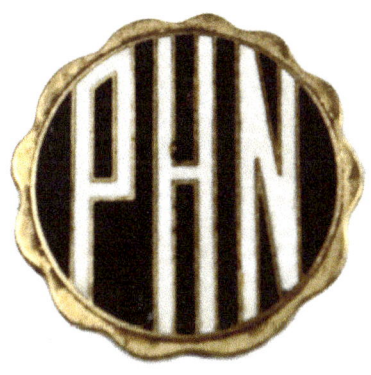

Figure 03.10. Public Health Nurse (PHN) pin, 1923.

Lillian Wald coined the term public health nurse in 1893 for nurses who worked outside of hospitals in the poor and middle-class communities.[18] PHNs received referrals from physicians and patients; they collected fees based on a patient's ability to pay. In 1898, Los Angeles became the first U.S. city to pay the salary of a district nurse (PHN).[19]

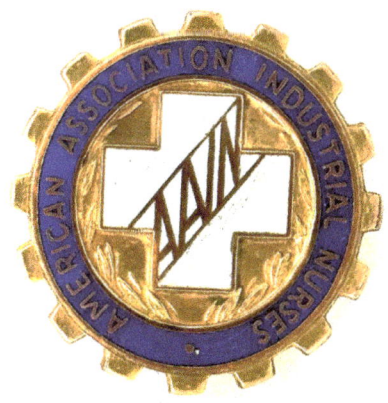

Figure 03.11. American Association of Industrial Nurses pin, 1946.

Industrial nurses, as PHNs, worked in factories, department stores, laundries, mining villages, and for insurance companies. In 1895, Vermont Marble hired the first industrial nurse.[20] The American Association of Industrial Nurses formed in 1942; in 1977 they renamed it the American Association of Occupational Health Nurses.[21]

Chapter Three

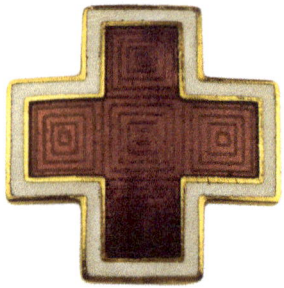

Figure 03.12. WW II American Red Cross Nurse cloisonné hat pin, c. 1944.

At the Geneva Convention, in 1882, the Red Cross created a legal document designed to protect the insignia of a red cross on a white background. Still, the American Red Cross (ARC) wasn't officially recognized until 1900.

Johnson & Johnson had used a red cross symbol on their products since 1887. R. W. Johnson and Clara Barton, the founder of the American Red Cross, discussed the trademark issue; in 1895 they signed an agreement recognizing Johnson & Johnson's right to use the logo.

In 1905, Congress granted the ARC exclusive rights to the symbol. Section 706, Title 18, U.S. Criminal Code, part 18 stated: Whoever… other than the American National Red Cross and its duly authorized employees and agents and the sanitary and hospital authorities of the armed forces of the United States, uses the emblem of the Greek Red Cross on a white ground…Shall be fined under this title or imprisoned not more than six months, or both.[22]

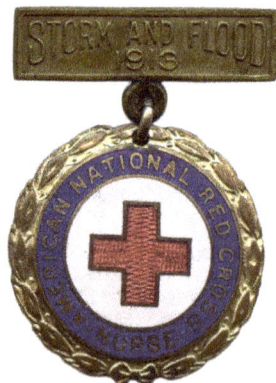

Figure 03.13. An American Red Cross Nurse uniform hanging badge, 1913.

A decade later, President Theodore Roosevelt signed legislation to protect the ARC's use of the mark, but he reserved Johnson & Johnson's rights to continue to use it on their products.[23]

Graduate Pins

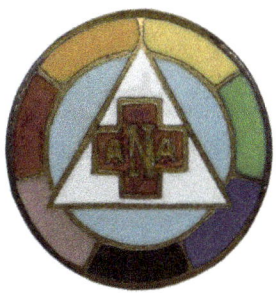

Figure 03.14. Nurses Associated Alumnae pin (predecessor of the ANA), n.d.

The Nurses Associated Alumnae of the United States and Canada began in 1896. In 1911, Canada disaffiliated, and the organization became the American Nurses Association (ANA).

Before the ANA formed, no accreditation, licensing, or unified organization existed. The organization's policymakers lobbied for the interests of nurses from the eight-hour working day in 1934, to the Fair Pay Act of 1995. In 1929, California led the U.S. in passing an eight-hour working day law.

The ANA has advocated for the interests of U.S. nurses and for the protection of public health issues from mental health to pandemics. They supported the recommendations of the National Academy of Medicine, enabling nurses to work within their full knowledge and scope of practice. They have promoted education and development. The ANA established the American Credentialing Center Certification Program (ANCC) in 1990. [24]

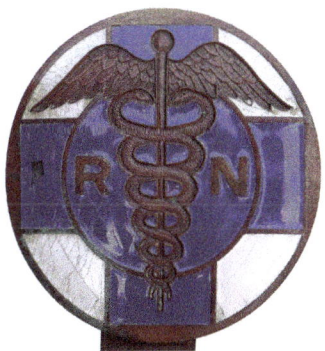

Figure 03.15. Decorative License Plate Topper for Registered Nurses, 1940.

From the 1920s to 1940s, companies used decorative license plate toppers for advertising. Police, fire chiefs, doctors, nurses, and pharmacists also used them to declare their status—and to avoid speeding or parking tickets. [25]

The Great War to the Great Depression: 1914-1929

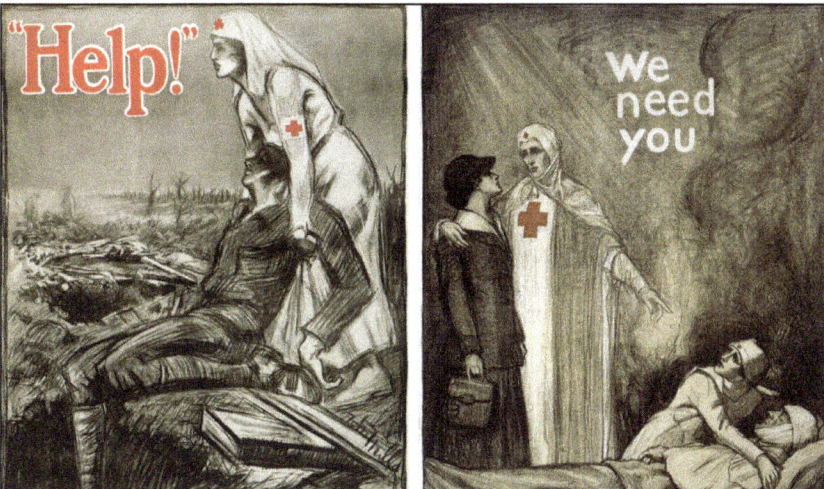

Figure 04.01. WWI Red Cross nurse recruitment posters, c. 1917.

The Army Nurse Corps began in 1901 and the Navy Nurse Corps in 1908. However, these two organizations did not contain sufficient reserve nurses to meet future war needs. Jane Delano witnessed the shortage of Red Cross nurses during the 1898 Spanish-American War.

In 1909 she organized the American Red Cross Nursing Service (within the Red Cross) into disaster response teams. Over 8,000 registered nurses were ready on 6 April 1917 when President Woodrow Wilson declared the United States would enter World War I. The Red Cross used posters to appeal to nurses' sympathy. [1]

By the end of the war, more than 30,000 female nurses had served in the Army, the Navy, and the Red Cross. Regardless of their sacrifice, women still were not allowed to vote. In September 1918, Wilson addressed the Senate, urging them to pass the 19th Amendment. He said this about women:

> Are we alone to ask and take the utmost that our women can give, service and sacrifice of every kind, and still say we do not see what title that gives them to stand by our sides in the guidance of the affairs of their nations and ours? We have made partners of the women in this war; shall we admit them only to a partnership of suffering and sacrifice and toil and not to a partnership of privilege and right? [2]

The vote failed. The amendment was not ratified until 18 August 1920.

Chapter Four

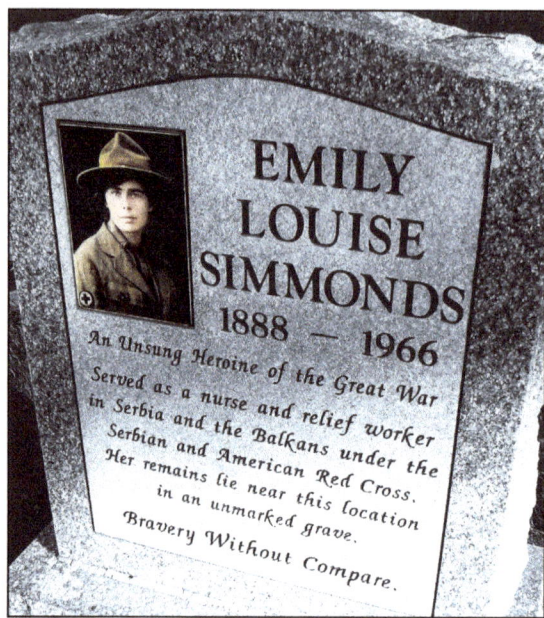

Figure 04.02. Emily Louise Simmonds' grave marker at the Pomona Valley Memorial Park, 2006. C. (Courtesy of Joe Blackstock)

World War I broke out in Europe in 1914, while Emily Louise Simmonds vacationed in Paris. Instead of returning home, she volunteered for the Red Cross. She treated battle victims in a military hospital in Kragujevac under horrific conditions.[3] In 1916, she single-handedly treated a cholera outbreak on a warship, saving hundreds of lives, and established a hospital in Corfu with war survivors. In 1917, she assisted starving women and children in Macedonia and distributed Red Cross supplies.

After a decade in Serbia, she went home to the U.S. She returned to Serbia later, carrying medical supplies, when a typhoid epidemic spread through the country. Doctors fell ill and died. Simmonds continued to work.

In 1951 she was working in Pasadena as a nurse. She died from pneumonia she developed after a fall in 1966. They cremated her but no one claimed her ashes; they placed her in an unmarked grave at Pomona Valley Memorial.

In 2005, Joe Blackstock wrote a column about Simmonds in the *Inland Valley Daily Bulletin*.[4] Patti French of Pasadena read it and contacted Louise Miller in Edinburgh, Scotland. The women decided she should not be forgotten. In 2006, they placed a marker at Pomona Valley Memorial Park, and the San Gabriel Pomona Chapter of the American Red Cross honored Simmonds with a special event.[5]

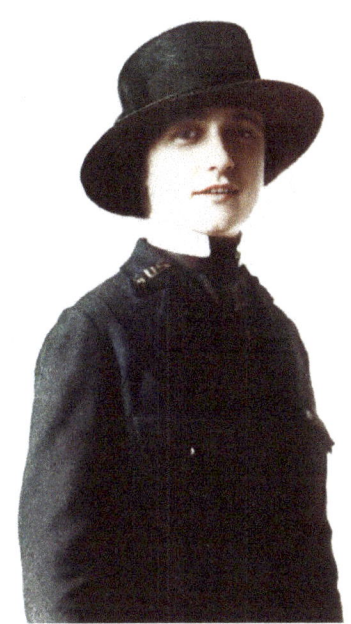

Figure 04.03. Grace Williams Major on duty with the Red Cross, 1918. C. (American Red Cross of Greater Los Angeles)

Grace Williams Major graduated in 1913, in the fifteenth class at the Hospital of the Good Samaritan School of Nursing; she worked there for many years. The history states that when the hospital moved to a new building in 1927, Majors was given the honor of locking the old building and unlocking the new one. [6]

During World War I, the Red Cross transferred Major to Mars-sur-Alliers, France. According to her journal, the soldiers arrived in poor condition:

> By September a considerable amount of flu and pneumonia had affected the corpsman. On November 1, trainloads of 1,500 to 2,000 patients arrived in boxcars, no dressings changed or faces washed.

Germany signed the armistice on 11 November 1918. General Pershing inspected 150–200 nurses and 2,000 corpsmen on 2 April 1919, and told them how proud he was of their work. Major was relieved from active duty on 23 July 1919. [7]

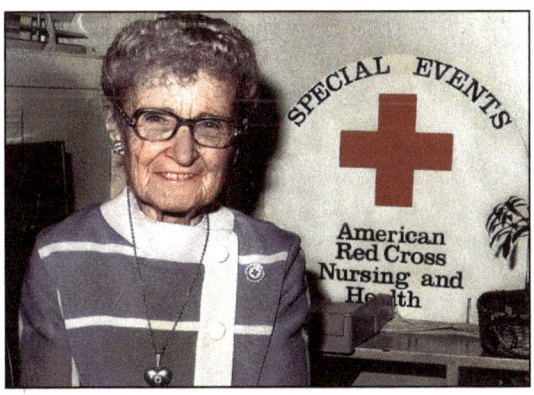

Figure 04.04. Grace Williams Major at a Los Angeles Red Cross event, 1981.

Chapter Four

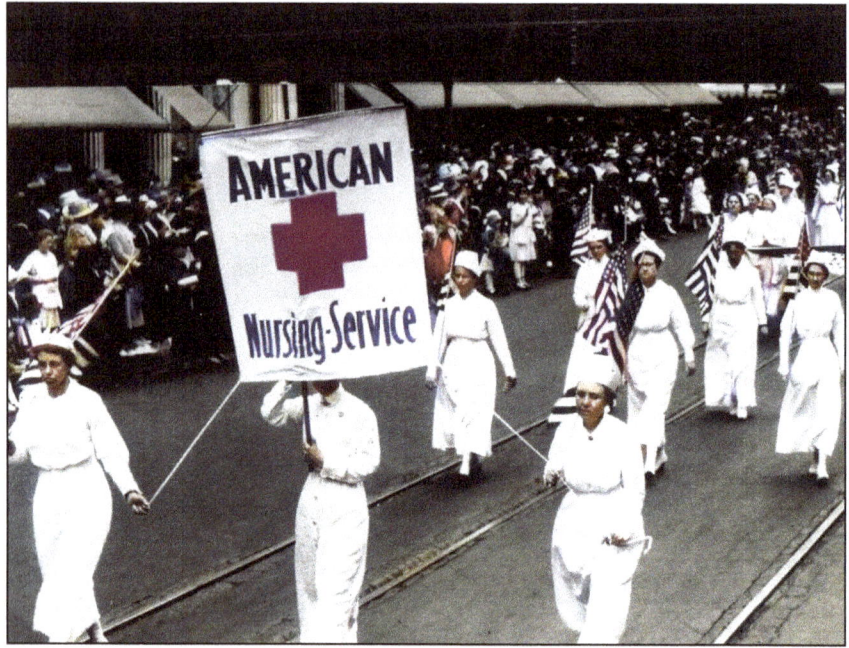

Figure 04.05. American Red Cross Nursing Service marching in the Los Angeles Parade, 1918. C (Shades of L.A. Archives/Los Angeles Public Library)

The 18 May 1918 Red Cross parade promised to be the greatest parade ever held in Los Angeles. The goal was to raise $750,000 for World War I. The parade started at 1:30 on Seventh and Hope Streets. The American Red Cross Nursing Service marched on the 600 block of Broadway, and other Red Cross divisions followed. Many major United States cities held Red Cross parades on the same day. [8]

County Hospital nurses and students carried a flag with stars for each of their nurses serving in the war. Superintendent Helen Muir led the procession. Nurses in the back held a sign, "City Nurses." Spectator nurses watched the parade from the upper windows. Ambulances followed.

Seven musical organizations marched, including the largest military band to ever parade in Los Angeles: the Consolidated Band of Camp Kearny, Elks Band, Whittier State School Band, Mrs. Danzinger's Band, Hamburger's Fife and Drum Corps, Scottish Band, and Women's Band. Fifty-one groups marched. A squadron of planes flew overhead. [9]

The Yellow Car rails were temporarily halted. A stuffed elk won the Most Beautiful Float prize. Other floats included trucks elaborately decorated with leaves, an ostrich pulling a woman in a cart, and a Liberty Bell reproduction.

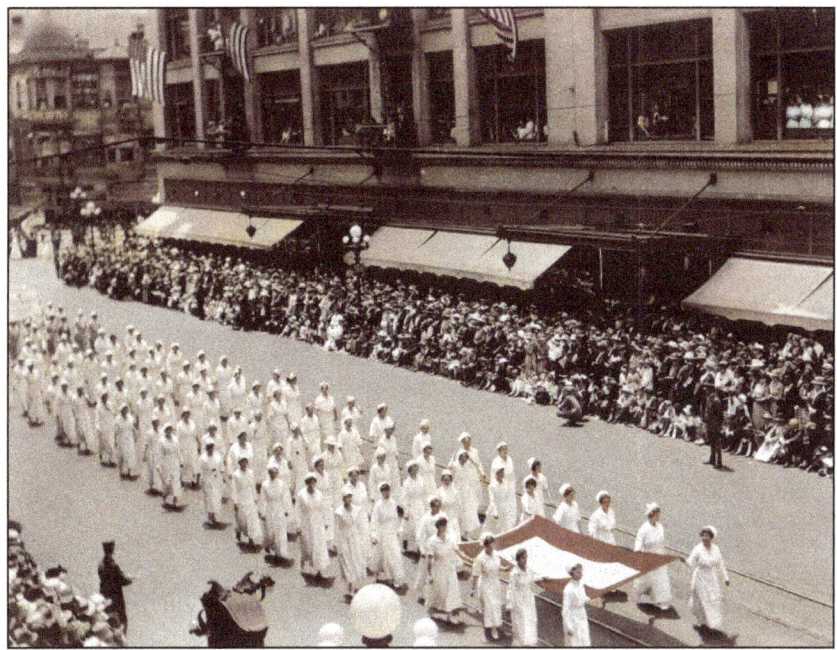

Figure 04.06. County Hospital nurses and students held a flag with a star for each of their nurses in the war. Superintendent Helen Muir led the group. C.

Figure 04.07. The largest military band to ever parade in Los Angeles. C.

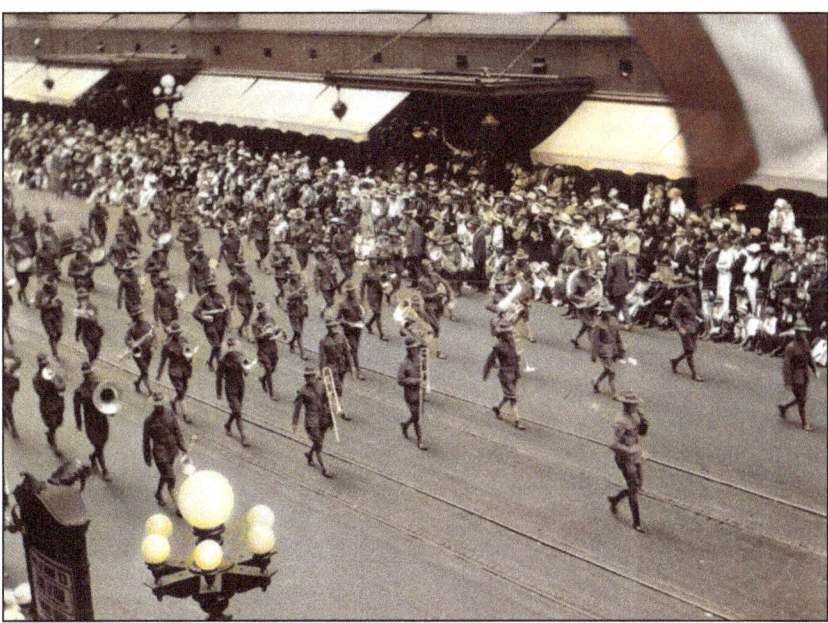

Chapter Four

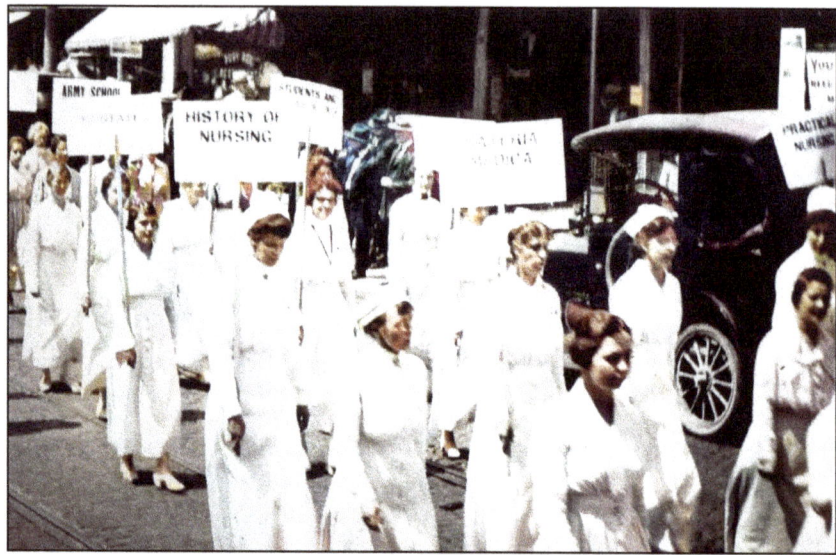

Figure 04.08. A Red Cross Parade down Main street in Poughkeepsie, New York, July 27, 1918. C. The Vassar Rainbow Division marched, carrying signs that designated the subjects they studied. (History and Special Collections, Louise M. Darling Biomedical Library, UCLA)

The Training Camp for Nurses at Vassar College in New York attempted to allay the shortage of nurses during World War I. The Council of National Defense and the Red Cross created a twelve-week camp called the Vassar Rainbow Division. The trainees had already obtained a college degree (in any discipline) and had been accepted into a school of nursing where they would continue training after the camp.

The camp recruited prestigious faculty from major eastern universities. Students attended classes eight hours daily; they were instructed in anatomy, physiology, bacteriology, chemistry, dietetics and cookery, hygiene, practical nursing, history of nursing, materia medica, psychology, and physical exercise. Trainees paid $95.00 for room, board, and instruction. At the end of the summer, 419 women had completed the camp. Fifty-eight percent completed their nurse's training and received a diploma.

Birdie May Adair attended the camp, moved to Los Angeles, and finished training at Good Samaritan Hospital. She had attended nurse's training at Boston University. She dropped out when she contracted diphtheria. She became a teaching nurse at San Pedro High School (1924–1930) and Franklin High School. She taught at Los Angeles City College and in Red Cross Teacher Training at UCLA. Adair said, "That training camp was probably the most interesting and worthwhile event of my whole life." [10]

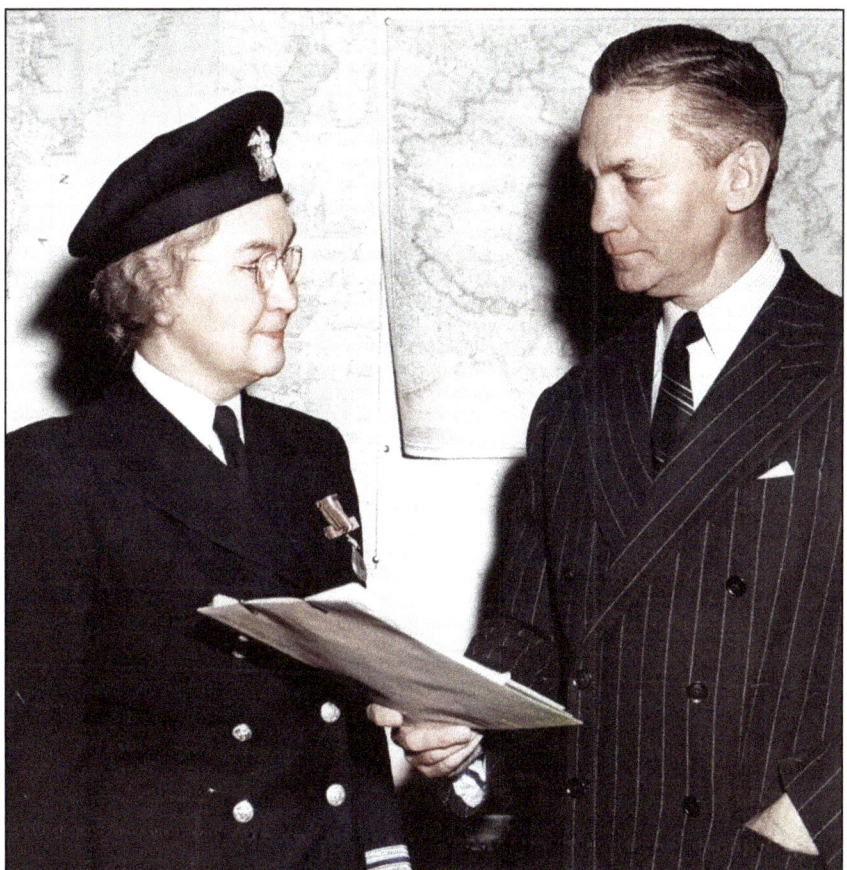

Figure 04.09. Secretary of the Navy, James Forrestal, presents Sue Sophia Dauser, left, the first Distinguished Service Medal awarded to a nurse, December 14, 1945. C.

Born in Anaheim, California, Dauser graduated from the California Hospital School of Nursing in 1914 and became superintendent of nurses. She joined the Navy Nurse Corps in 1917, served in Scotland during World War I as a chief nurse, and then worked aboard several ships during the 1920s. [11]

After World War I, Dauser headed the nursing department at San Diego Naval Hospital. She tended to President Harding during his fatal illness in 1923. One theory circulated that Harding's wife had poisoned him. Dauser said the story was "utterly ridiculous as no one could have poisoned the patient—someone was with him every minute." [12]

The Navy Nurse Corps appointed her to superintendent from 1939 to 1945. After the ranking laws changed in 1942, she received her captain's rank. [13]

Chapter Four

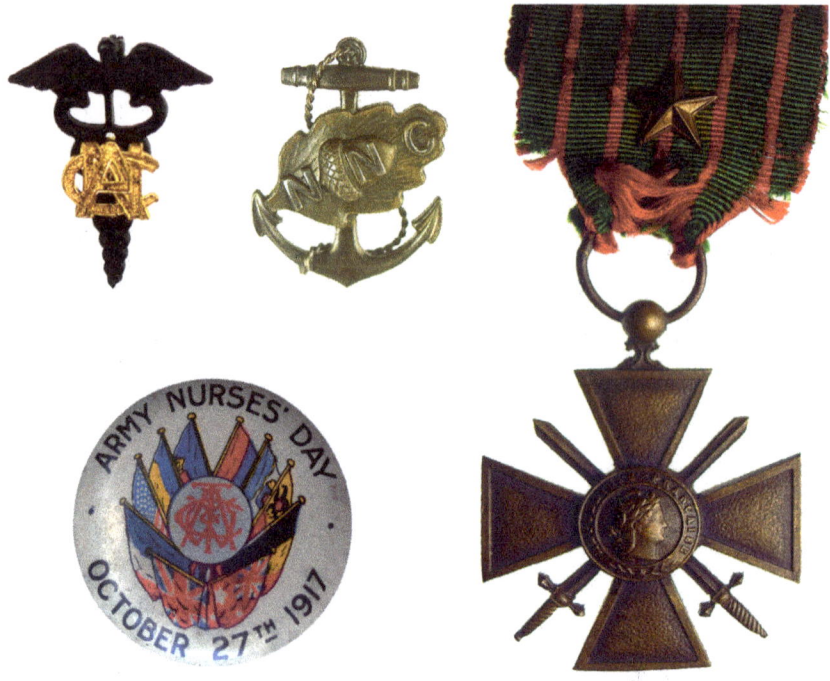

Figure 04.10. A 1917 Army Nurse Corps (ANC) pin, a 1917 Navy Nurse Corps (NNC) pin, an Army Nurses' Day pin, and a WWI Croix de Guerre medal. The center of the award depicts a woman wearing a Phrygian cap, which represents freedom and the pursuit of liberty. (Author photographed)

Louise M. Todd graduated from nursing school in 1896. She went to France in 1918 for World War I and served in Germany after the armistice. The French government awarded her the Croix de Guerre (Cross of War) for her gallantry. France awarded only twenty Croix de Guerre to nurses.

After she returned home, she married, became Louise LeBart, and moved to Los Angeles in 1925. On 4 January 1931, after being sought for weeks, the Los Angeles post office tracked her down at her job as superintendent of nurses in the Eye and Ear Hospital on 500 South Lucas Street. They presented her with another Croix de Guerre.

"I was given a Croix de Guerre before. Why do you suppose they would give it to me twice for?" she asked the *Los Angeles Herald*. The citation stated thus: Louise M. Todd, formerly a nurse, Army Nurse Corps, Field Hospital No. 7, American Expeditionary Forces. The medal carried a bronze star. Her organization served at Saint Mihlel and in Argonne. "I don't have the faintest idea on what incident the award was made," she said. "I don't know what it's for. Maybe for just being a nurse." [14]

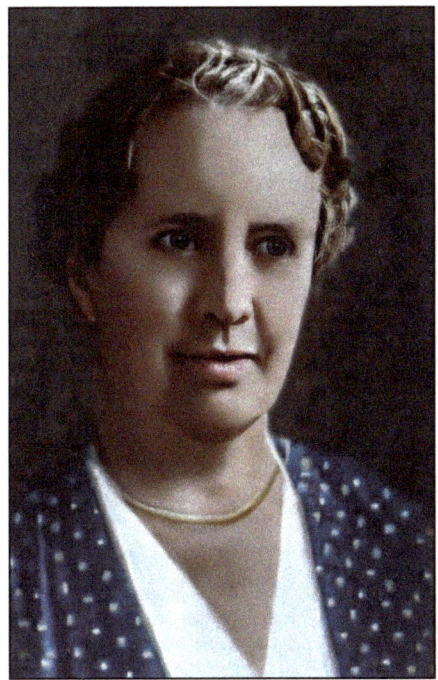

Figure 04.11. Edith Bryan, n.d. C.

In 1918, the Regents at the University of California, Berkeley, chose Pasadena Hospital nurse (class of 1910), Edith S. Bryan, to create a new Public Health Nursing Program. Bryan became the first nurse appointed to Berkeley as a member of the faculty.

For Bryan, however, her most prestigious historical event had yet to occur: in 1927 she became the first nurse in the United States to earn a PhD.

Bryan developed Berkeley's summer certificate program into an eight-month academic year offering. She took leave from 1925-1927 to attend Johns Hopkins University in Baltimore, Maryland, where she obtained a master's and a Doctor of Psychology and Counseling. [15]

She delivered a speech to spur the nursing profession to action at the National League of Nursing Convention in San Antonio, Texas, on 14 April 1932. She said that the professional service of nursing had three realms for research: pure science, applied science, and social science. She encouraged nurses to conduct research in these three areas. She explained further:

> The very term science denotes systemic observation and reasoning… If we develop the pure science of nursing as opposed to the applied science of nursing, we shall need to rearrange some of our old ideas and clarify our minds as to the field which can be turned over to the student who is interested in the pure science and not interested in the practice of nursing. [16]

Later that year, the *American Journal of Nursing* published her entire presentation in their July issue, "Methods of Research and Study." [17] Bryan became active in several professional nursing organizations: she simultaneously held offices in the California State Nurses Association (CSNA), the California League for Nursing Education, and the California League for Public Health Nursing. She served as president of the CSNA from 1935 to 1937 and remained involved until 1940. [18]

Chapter Four

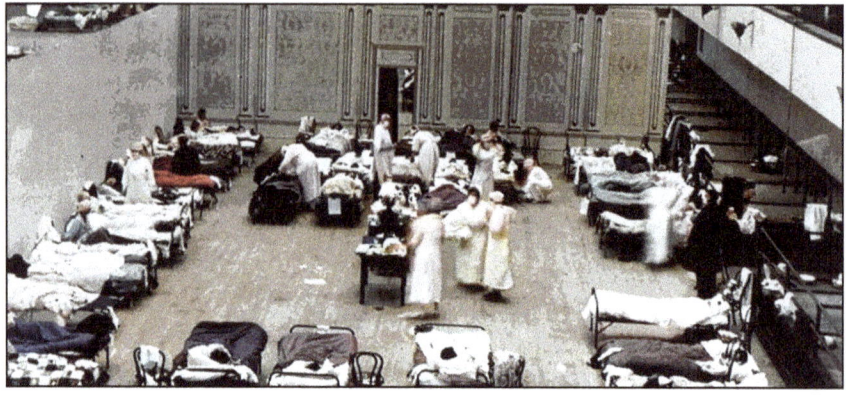

Figure 04.12. American Red Cross nurses caring for influenza patients in a California auditorium, staged as a temporary hospital, 1918. C.

The influenza pandemic of 1918 killed 700,000 people in the U.S.—more deaths than in World War I. Fifty million died worldwide. At first, Los Angeles seemed spared until September 1918, when a naval training ship arrived in San Pedro from San Francisco with 400 infected, healthy-appearing sailors. Los Angeles reported 680 cases within a few weeks. [19]

The first civilian cases appeared on 22 September: 55 students at Polytechnic High. [20] But influenza was not a reportable disease until 27 September. [21] Mayor Woodman declared a public emergency on 11 October. [22]

The City Council quickly appropriated $5,000 to outfit an emergency hospital at the Parent-Teacher Clinic on Yale Street. [23] In November, they spent $10,500 converting the Mount Washington Hotel into a convalescent home for recovering flu patients. [24] Additional makeshift hospitals appeared.

All large gatherings were discouraged. The government asked people to shop for Christmas by phone. [25] Theaters and churches shut down. Schools closed. Families were quarantined; doctors were required to post signs on the doors.

Many nurses died caring for infected patients, and nursing school enrollment dropped to historically low numbers. The *Los Angeles Times* ran frequent ads for nurses who were willing to risk working with patients with influenza. The Pasadena Red Cross conducted a house-to-house canvass for nurses. [26]

By November, cases fell to fewer than 800 per month. [27] Schools opened in February. [28] The epidemic in Los Angeles ended in March of 1919. The closures, bans, and quarantines resulted in 494 deaths per 100,000—lower than many other American cities, including San Francisco's 673 per 100,000 deaths, which relied on ineffective gauze face masks instead of closures. [29]

In 1918, the *Los Angeles Times* reported that student nurses had protested the admission of four Black students into the L.A. County Hospital Nurses Training Program.[30]

Despite protests by student nurses, the hospital admitted its first group of Black student nurses in 1919.

County records list the first Black nurse that graduated, in 1922, as Adele E. Kemp McGruder—no photograph of McGruder could be located. Black students and White students lived and ate meals in separate buildings until 1950, when the Director of Nursing, Nina Berthea Craft, integrated the student body.[31]

Figure 04.14. Nina Berthea Craft, the director of nursing, 1950.

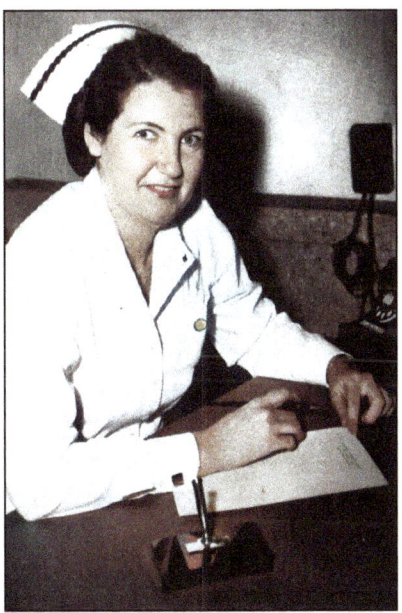

Nurses' Strike will Impair Efficiency, Says Martin.

Students Reinterate Threat to Resign in a Body.

With the resignation of 127 out of its 140 training school nurses about to become effective, because the girls object to the admission of four colored girls as student nurses, the Los Angeles County Hospital is facing a serious crisis.

Yesterday the nurses in the hospital were working double shifts to carry the heavy burden placed upon the institution by the prevalence of influenza here. Thirty nurses are listed as being sick with influenza, one ambulance driver is on the sick list and the other is working in spite of a severe cold. Fifteen new cases made application for admission to the hospital within two hours while both ambulances were at the harbor.

Mrs. Norman R. Martin, wife of the Superintendent, and the superintendent of nurses, were engaged in making beds all afternoon. One nurses, who volunteered her services for outside influenza work, died at the County Hospital Monday night, a victim of the disease she sought to stampt out.

The student nurses at the hospital have served notice on the Board of Supervisors that they will leave the hospital the first day of November if the board permits four colored girls to enter the institution as stu-

Figure 04.13. *Los Angeles Times* report of student nurses protest, concerning the admission of Black students, October 16, 1918.

Chapter Four

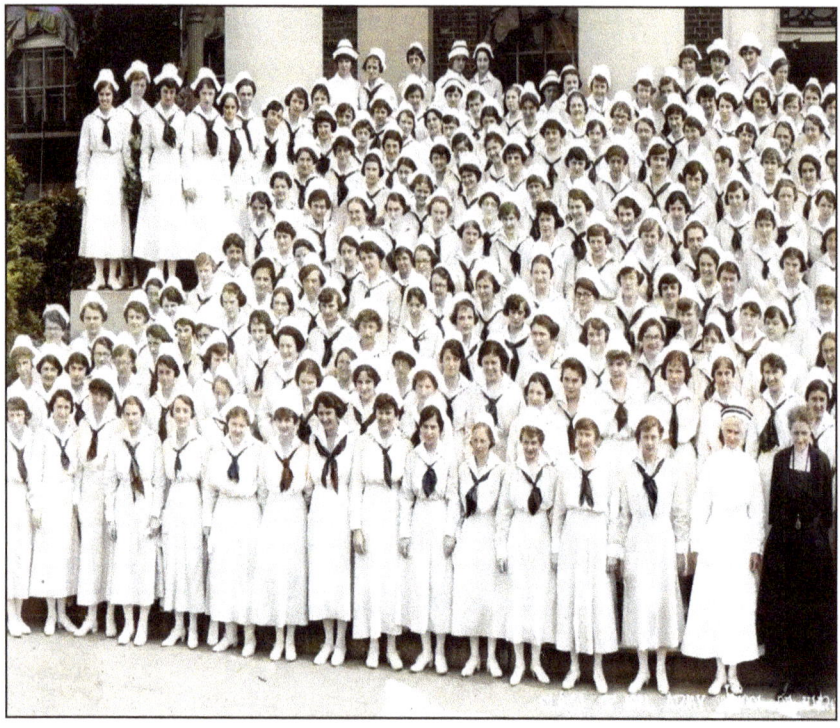

Figure 04.15. The first graduating class, Army School of Nursing, at Walter Reed General Hospital, Washington, D.C., June 16, 1921.

The distinct blue student uniforms earned them the nickname Blue Birds. First Lieutenant Anne Williamson, the chief nurse (in white), and Annie Goodrich, the first dean of the Army School of Nursing (in black), are front row and center. Goodrich founded Yale School of Nursing. On 25 May 1918, the Secretary of War authorized the Army School of Nursing as an alternative to utilizing nurse aides in Army hospitals.[32] Courses opened at several Army hospitals in July 1918. Students retained civilian status. In December 1918, there were 1,578 students enrolled in the schools.[33]

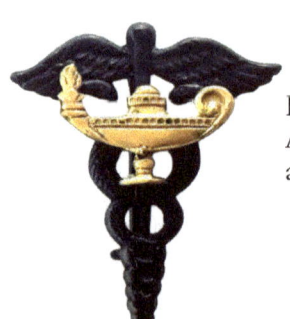

Figure 04.16. A 1921 nurse graduate pin from the Army School of Nursing—the wings of Mercury, a Caduceus, and a lamp of learning.

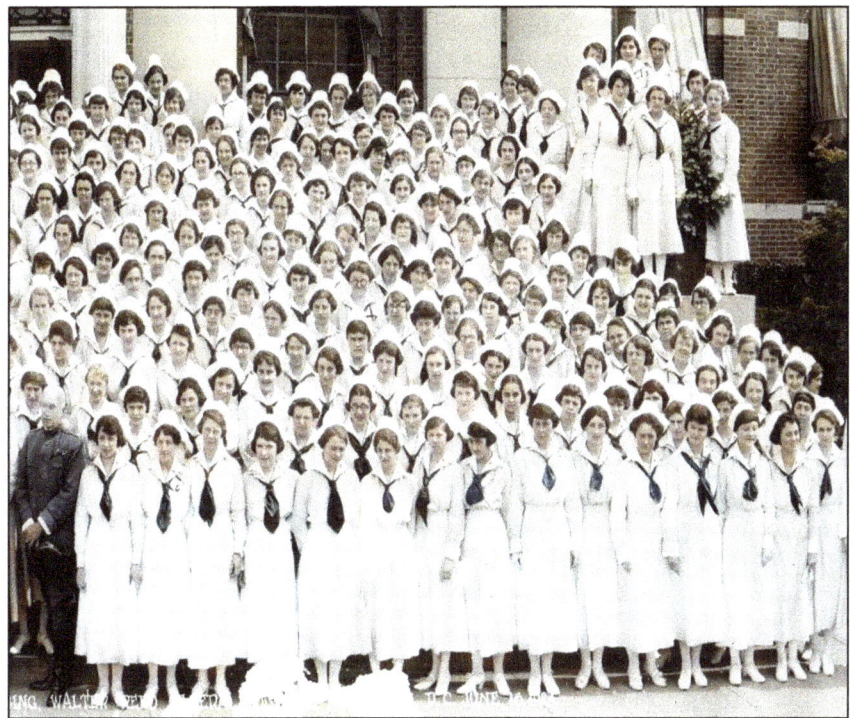

Within the group of 404 nurses, of the 1921 graduation class, were three Los Angeles nurses: Elise Alber, Helen Cross, and Eleanor Lowell.

By 1923, the Army had consolidated all Army schools to train at Walter Reed Army Hospital. Then the Secretary of War discontinued the school on 12 August 1931 as an economic measure because only a small percentage of graduates actually joined the Army. A total of 937 young women received the school's diploma. [34]

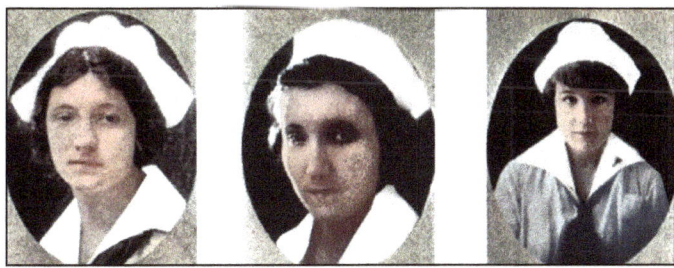

Figure 04.17. Los Angeles nurses Elise Alber, Helen Cross, and Eleanor Lowell. Editor notations were included in the *Annual*. Elise Alber: "A tremendous amount of energy." Helen Cross: "Her chief delight is the movies." Eleanor Lowell: "Just as beautiful in character as she is to look upon."

Chapter Four

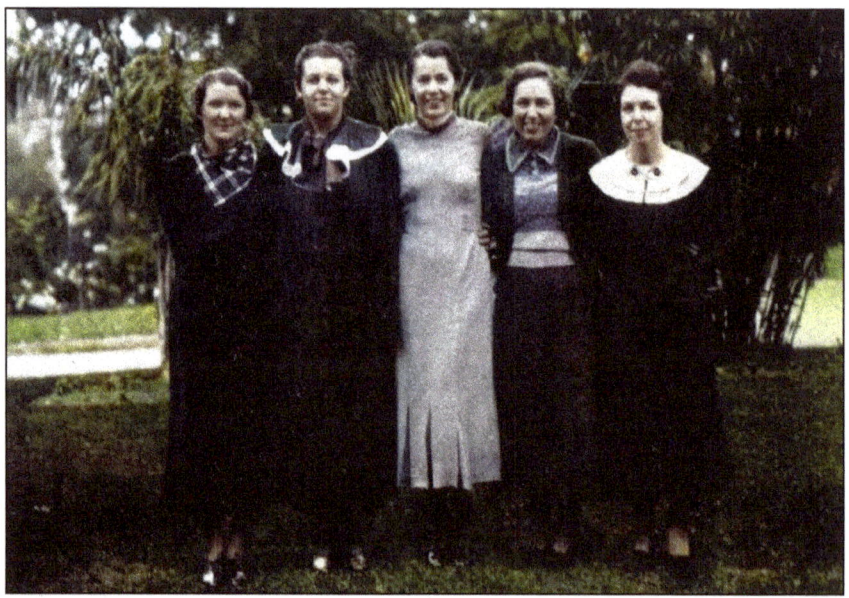

Figure 04.18. Five members of the 1935 Gamma Chapter, left to right, M. Van Buren, V. Watson, F. Honeyman, M. Connie, and P. Horner, 1935.

The professional nursing organization Alpha Tau Delta was founded on 15 February 1921 at the University of California, Berkeley. The third chapter, Gamma, was founded at the University of California, Los Angeles, in 1928.

They named the Gamma chapter in honor of Henrietta Muir, the 1917-1937 superintendent of nurses at Los Angeles County General Hospital. Gamma met frequently with the Zeta Chapter from the University of Southern California to foster unity among members in Los Angeles. They named the Zeta Chapter in honor of Harriet Cochran, chief nurse of the Los Angeles City Schools in the 1930s.

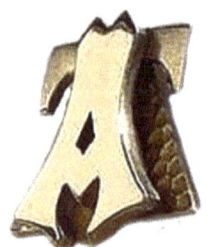

Figure 04.19. The Alpha Tau Delta induction pin. Memberships included college members, honorary members, alumni members, and members-at-large. Alpha Tau Delta (ATD) fostered an intra-fraternal spirit and promoted an environment of excellence for individual performance, advancement of education, character enrichment, and leadership.

Other chapters in the Los Angeles area included Alpha Theta at Mount St. Mary's College; Phi at California State University, Los Angeles; and Gamma Pi in Manhattan Beach. [35]

Great War to the Great Depression

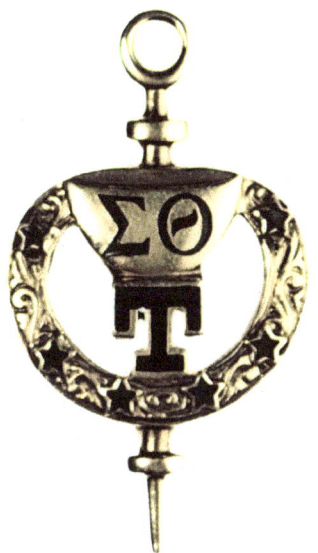 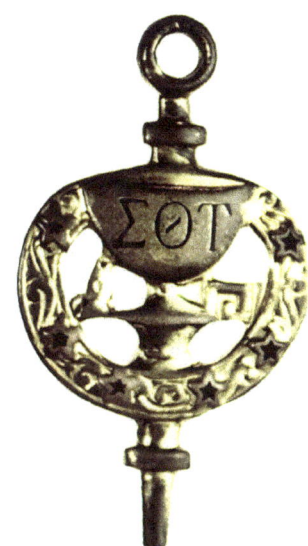

Figure 04.20. On the left is the original Sigma Theta Tau induction pin with six stars for the six founders and a large T. In 1967, leaders redesigned the pin: They removed the large T and replaced it with a lamp of learning—the pin on the right. [36]

In 1922, six nursing students at the Indiana University Training School for Nurses created Sigma Theta Tau, an honor society that recognized and encouraged scholarship and high achievement. They held the first induction ceremony for the Alpha Chapter on 16 October 1922. [37]

The society recognized nurses who excelled in their field. In 1936, the Society awarded the first national nursing research scholarship. The title, Sigma Theta Tau, was derived from the Greek words Storge, Tharsos, and Time (love, courage, and honor). In 1985, they became incorporated as Sigma Theta Tau, International Inc. Los Angeles County chapters included these schools:

- Gamma Tau-at-Large: UCLA/CSU, Northridge/CSU, Channel Islands
- Iota Eta: California State University, Long Beach
- Iota Sigma: Azusa Pacific University
- Nu Mu: California State University, Los Angeles
- Phi Lambda: Mount Saint Mary's University
- Xi Theta: California State University, Dominguez Hills
- Omicron Delta: University of Phoenix, Southern California Campus
- Alpha Alpha Psi: Charles R. Drew University of Medicine and Science
- Chi Beta: West Coast University, North Hollywood
- Xi Theta: California State University, Dominguez Hills

Chapter Four

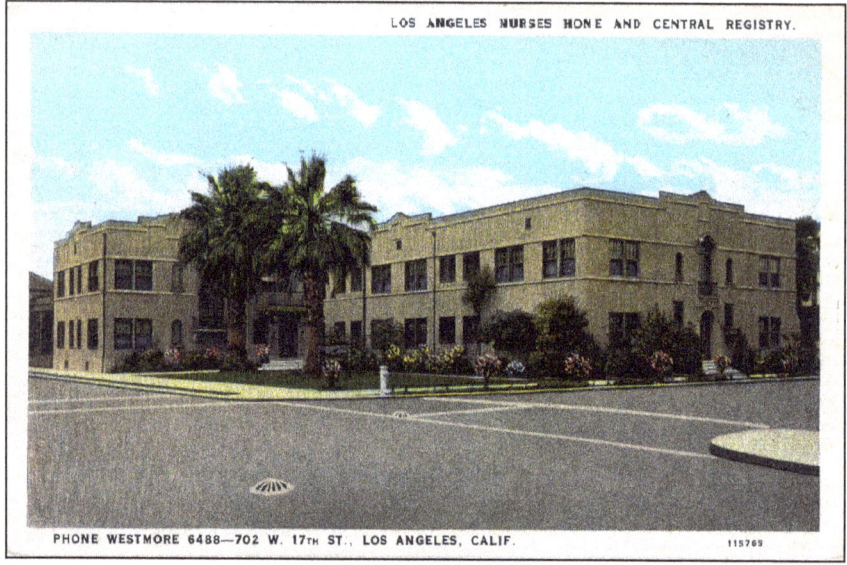

Figure 04.21. A 1920s postcard of the Nurses Home and Central Registry at 702 W. 17th Street, established in 1910. On the back of the card a handwritten note from a nurse said, "This is the Central Nurses Registry, which gives me all the work."

Before the Great Depression of the 1930s, most graduate nurses worked in private homes. Student nurses cared for hospitalized patients while learning to become nurses. Graduates worked for the hospital as instructors, superintendents, and in select specialties such as surgery and obstetrics. If the hospital could not attract enough student nurses, they hired graduates.

The hospitals gave students a room, meals, and some paid a small stipend. After students graduated, the hospital did not employ them—they had to find jobs in private homes or as special duty for a hospital patient. The "specials" slept on a cot next to the bed; post-op and critically ill patients could require the nurse to stay awake for twenty-four hours without sleep. Graduate nurses often lived in buildings called nurses' homes, with shared bathrooms and kitchens. These buildings were also central registries. When a family or doctor needed to hire a nurse, they called the registry.

Nurses were not happy with the custom of living in nurses' homes; they could not invite family or friends to stay overnight; they did not make enough money to rent a private apartment. Few nurses could find enough private cases to work full-time, which contributed to nurses' low incomes. Hospitals started several classes of students each year to meet the demand for cheap labor. This flooded cities with nurses and contributed to the inability of graduate nurses to find work. [38]

Great War to the Great Depression

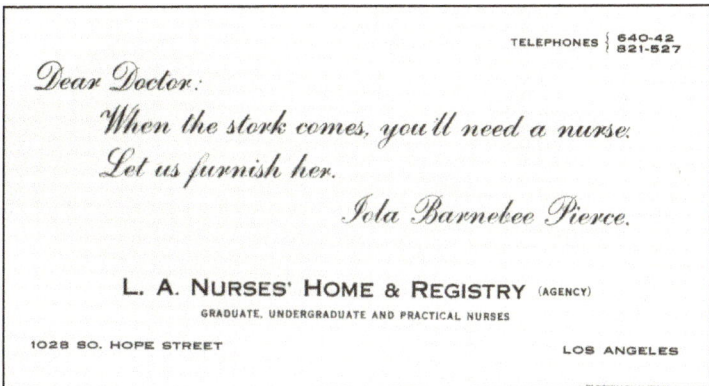

Figure 04.22. A tear-off business card with a memo pad and a button from the L.A. Nurses' Home & Registry on 1028 South Hope Street, c. 1930. They advertised graduate, undergraduate, and practical nurses for hire.

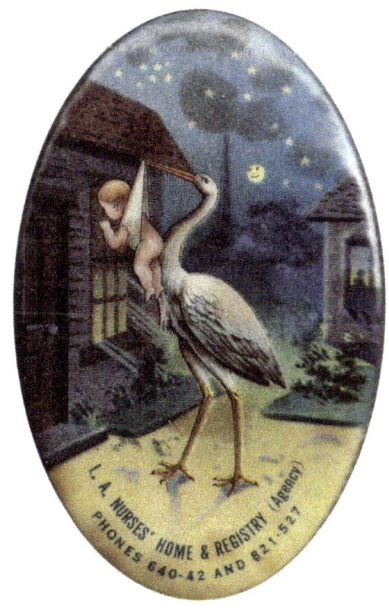

Chapter Four

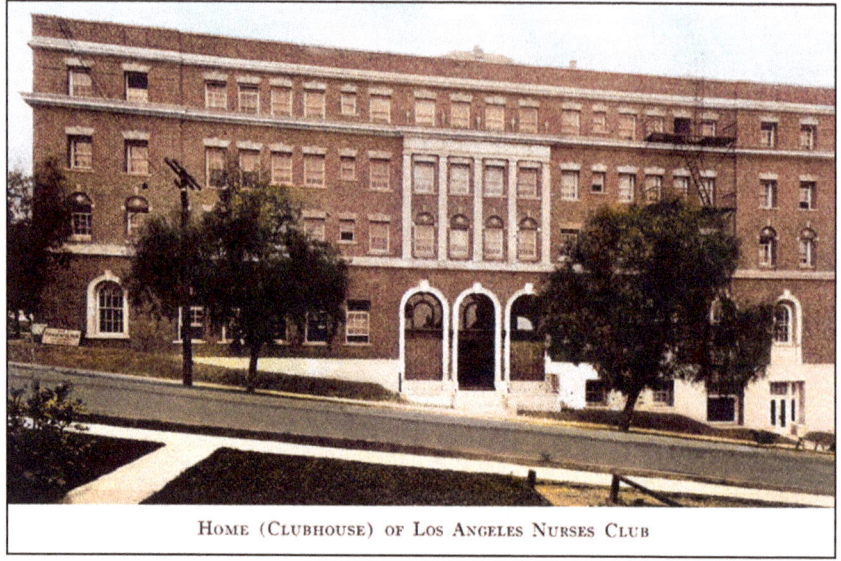

Figure 04.23. Los Angeles Nurses Club & Apartments, 1924. C.

In 1921, a group of Los Angeles nurses financed their own clubhouse and apartment building—the only one in the United States financed entirely by nurses. They held fundraisers. They met with architects and lawyers. In July 1923, the building at 245 South Lucas Avenue was completed for $160,000.[39]

The Los Angeles Nurses Club had a living room with a fireplace, library, auditorium, and apartments for one hundred nurses. The building functioned as a central registry with twenty-four-hour telephone service.[40]

In the cornerstone of the building, the nurses placed a copper box (a time capsule) filled with items from hospitals and schools of nursing: graduation pins, hospital histories, photographs of first graduation classes, bylaws, and yearbooks from nine Los Angeles hospitals. The "Angelus Sextette," comprised of nurses from Angelus Hospital, sang at the dedication ceremony in 1923. The celebration dance lasted well into the evening.[41]

The nurses eventually sold the building for a profit. It still stands at 245 South Lucas Avenue, as the Los Angeles Nurses Club & Apartments—now a building of low-cost rental rooms with shared baths and kitchens. The entrance to the basement auditorium was covered with concrete, and the living room is a dusty storeroom, but the building is mostly unchanged. Current residents use the original bathtubs and small gas heaters.[42] The Los Angeles Cultural Heritage Board designated the building as a Historic-Cultural Monument in April 1985, and the National Register of Historic Places added it to its protected list in 1995.[43]

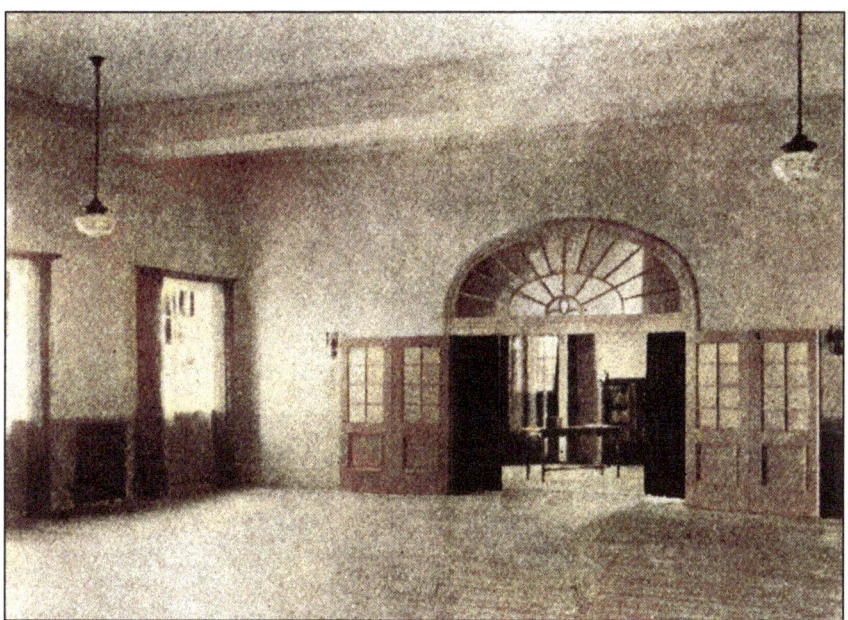

Figure 04.24. The auditorium. Nurses used the room for meetings, as a ballroom for dances, or for taffy pulls. C. Figure 04.25. The living room, 1924. C. (Courtesy of the *American Journal of Nursing*)

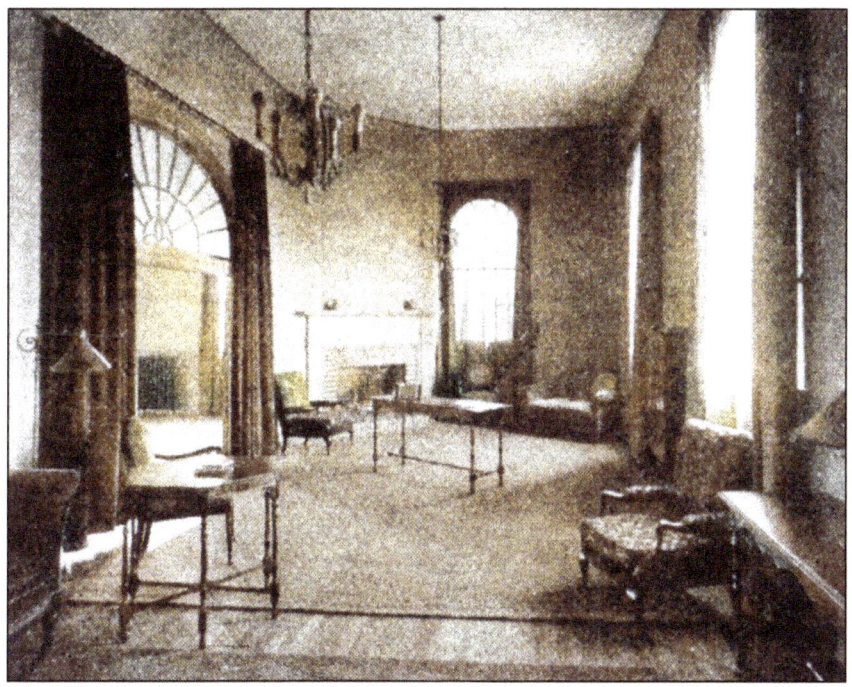

Chapter Four

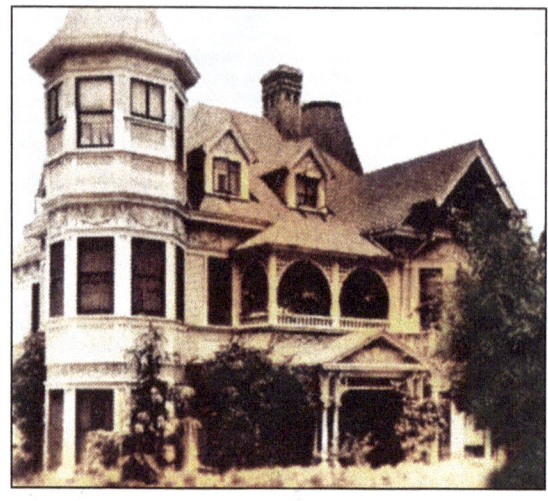

Figure 04.26. The Cope House, 1925—the year the Franciscan Sisters of the Sacred Heart bought it for their first hospital. The following year, the student nurses moved in.

The deed was issued as St. Joseph's Home and Hospital, but they called it Queen of Angels.

The first few patients were elderly and chronically ill. Some had upper respiratory infections, and some had cancer. If they had funds, patients paid $3.00 per day for nursing care, meals, linens, and medicine. The Sisters were the nurses and cooks. They engaged in the Franciscan exercise of begging for alms on the street to raise money to care for patients.

Figure 04.27. The Franciscan Sisters on the Cope House porch, 1925. C. Sister Superior M. Luitguardis headed the contingent of nuns. One year later, in 1926, they excavated down to the foundation and moved the house to the center of the property in preparation for a new hospital wing.

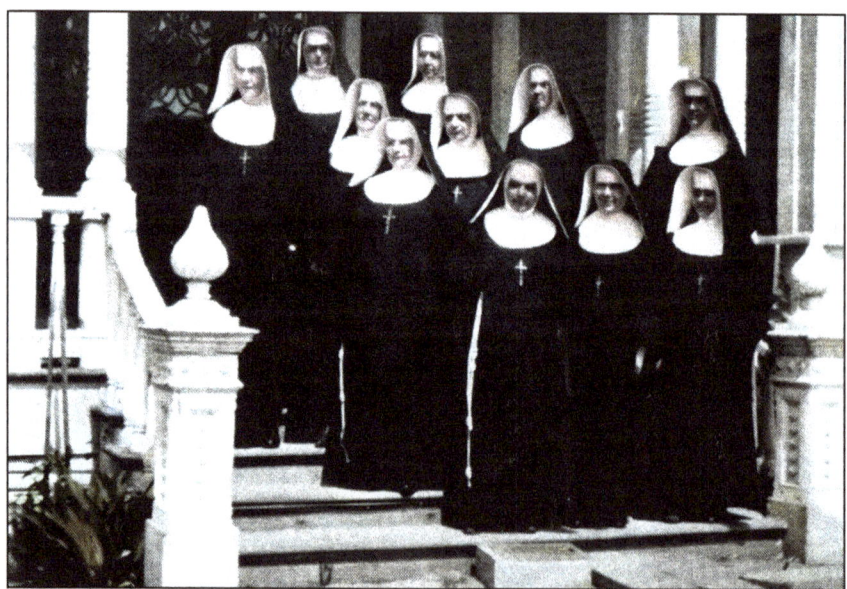

Figure 04.28. The completed first unit of the new Queen of Angels Hospital. C. The original Cope House building is visible in the lower-left corner.

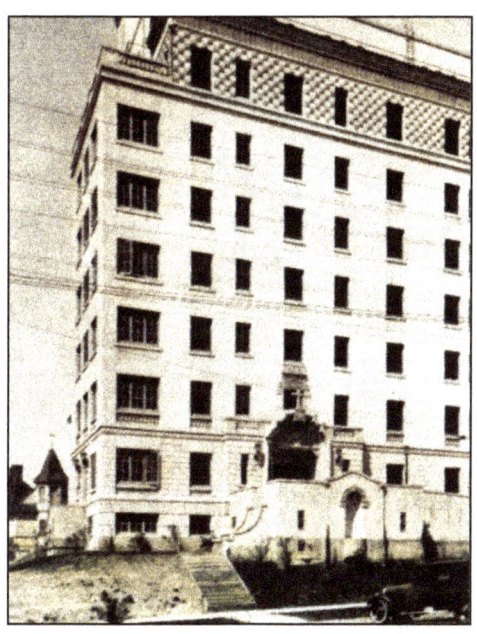

The Sisters chose this location, on Bellevue Avenue and Kent Street, for many reasons: it was adjacent to Sunset and Temple streets, close to the streetcar routes, and "it was located on a plateau elevation that allowed a Model T automobile to turn onto Rosemount from Temple, in high gear, and accelerate up the eight-percent grade."

The Sisters borrowed $600,000 from the Bank of Italy (now Bank of America). The bank did not require references or security collateral. They laid the cornerstone on 16 April 1926, and the deed was changed to Queen of Angels. They opened Queen of Angels Training School for Nurses in September 1926. Students worked eight hours in the hospital, followed by four hours of classroom study in nutrition, chemistry, and English at Belmont High School. They scrubbed the new building to make it hospitable and then transferred patients. The Sisters moved to the hospital, and the students moved to Cope House. 44

Figure 04.29. First students at Queen of Angels Training School, 1926. C. Nellie Gordon Sepulveda, of Los Angeles, was the first student, and Mary Roncell Barnes received the first diploma. Their instructor, Mary Keating, stands between the two Sisters. (Hollywood Presbyterian Medical Center)

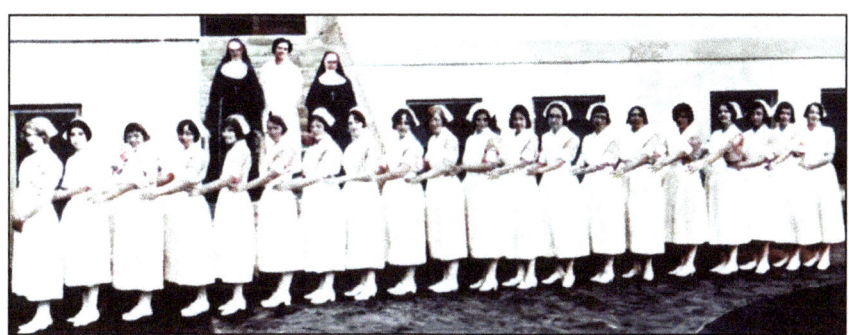

Chapter Four

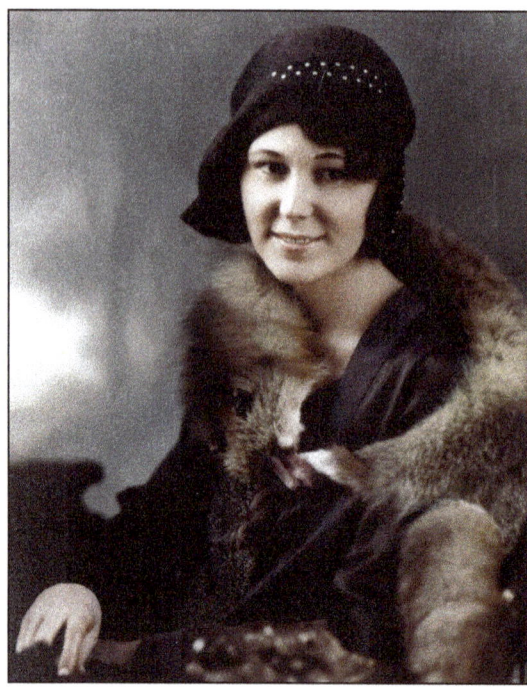

04.30. Anna Lois Lackey, dressed in flapper fashion, during her training years at the Hospital of the Good Samaritan School of Nursing, c. 1926. C.

Lackey's mother lost three children during the flu epidemic. Anna survived. Her parents did not want her to become a nurse, but when the Hospital of the Good Samaritan School of Nursing accepted her into their training program, she went anyway.

She lived in the nurses' dorm during the week and rode the electric Red Car from Los Angeles back to her parents' home in Ontario on the weekends. She told her daughter Susan that her parents would have made her quit school if they had known the seedy neighborhoods she had to walk through from the Red Car station to the hospital.

Figure 04.31. A Good Samaritan Hospital student nurse, a graduate nurse, and Anna Lackey during their training weeks at Childrens Hospital, 1926. C

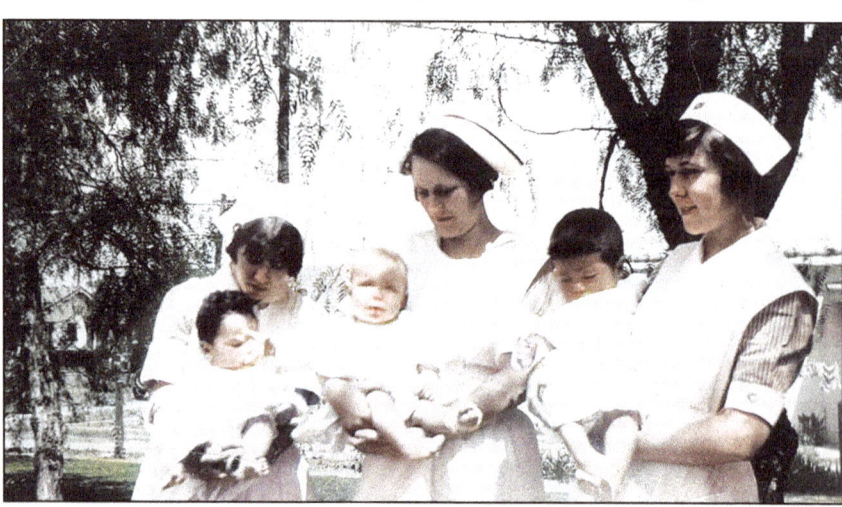

Great War to the Great Depression

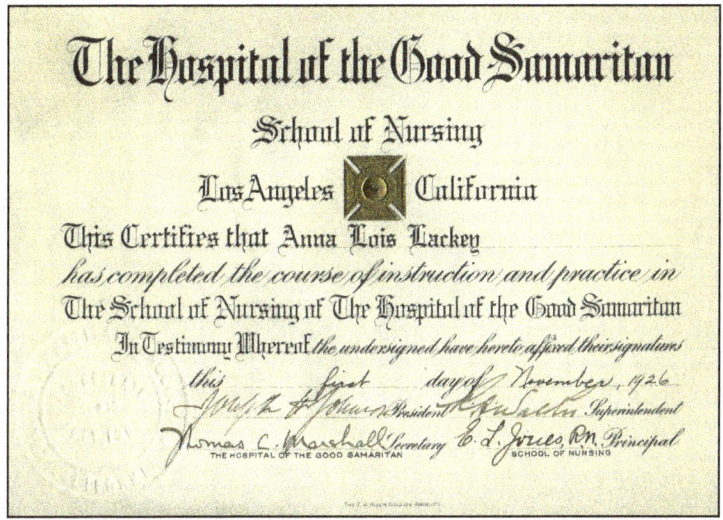

Figure 04.32. Lackey's 1926 diploma for the Hospital of the Good Samaritan.

Good Samaritan would have expelled Anna Lackey if they had known her secret—in Lackey's senior year she became Anna Lackey Wickham. In the early years, nursing schools forbade marriage, so Wickham hid her marital status. Her license was issued in the last year the Board of Health certified the licensure (1913–1927). In 1975 Anna Lackey's daughter, Susan Purdy, received her nursing degree from Chaffey Community College in Alta Loma.

Figure 04.33. Anna Lackey graduated in 1926. She still used her maiden name on her 1927 license. (Courtesy of Susan Purdy)

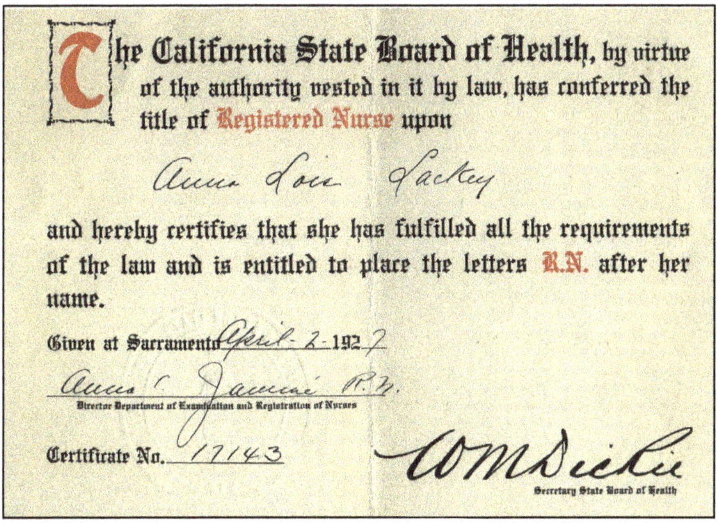

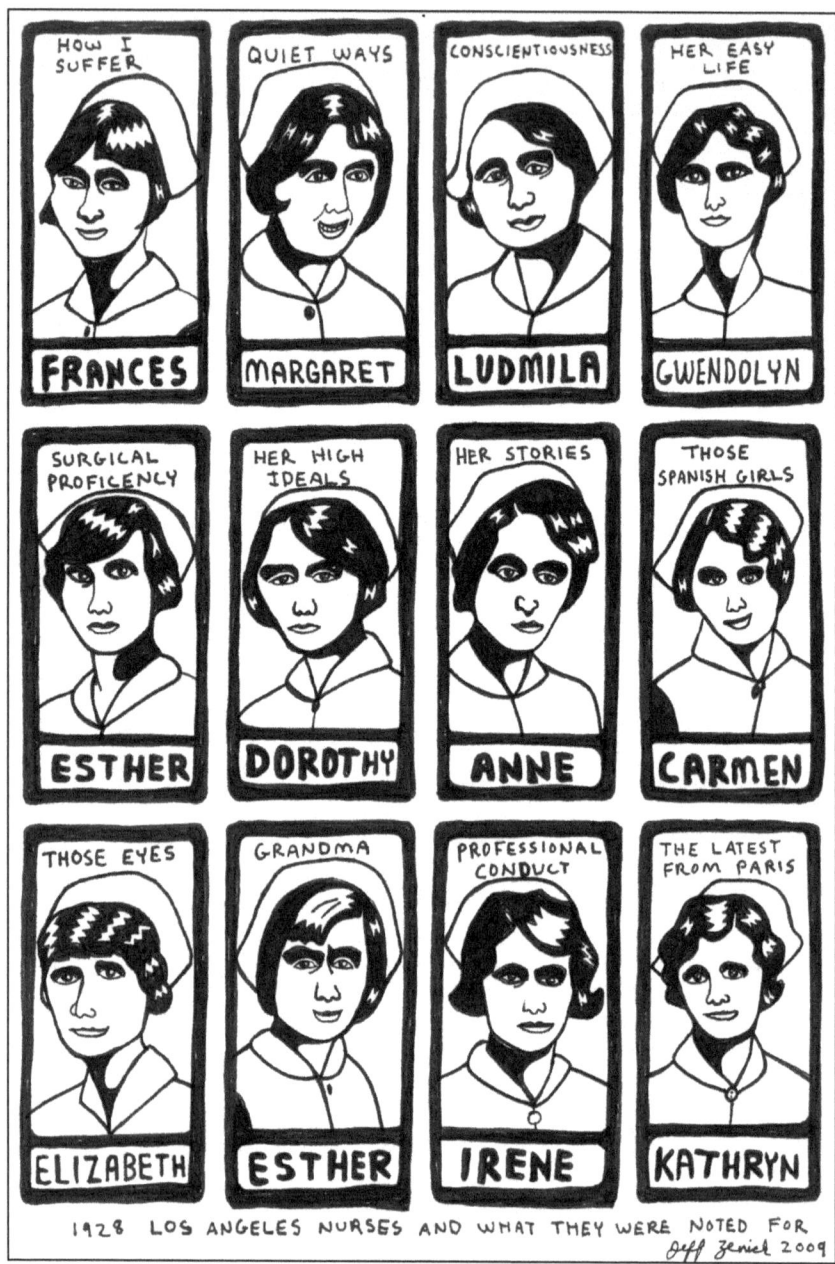

Figure 04.34. A pen and ink drawing by Jeff Zenick, based on a page from the 1928 Good Samaritan Nursing School yearbook, *The Stethoscope*, 2009. Most training schools for nurses printed annual yearbooks. In the early books, a phrase was written about each graduating nurse, often a humorous quote. Zenick's art parodied vintage yearbook pages. (Courtesy of Jeff Zenick)

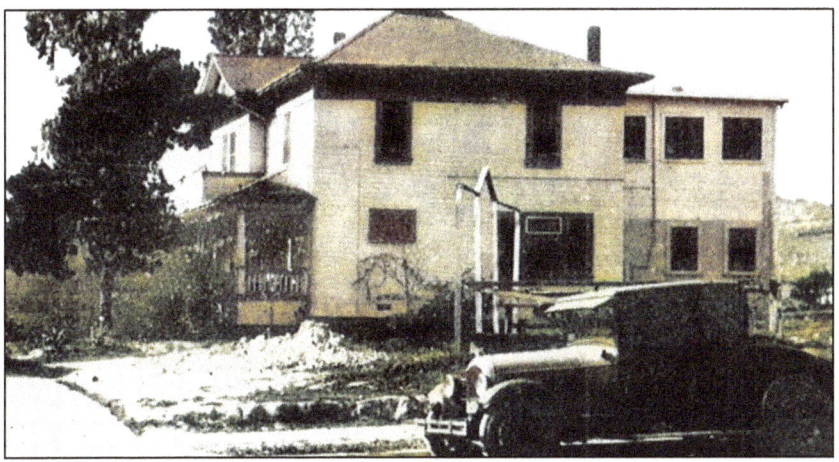

Figure 04.35. Mount Sinai Home for Incurables in Boyle Heights, 1928. C.

The Bikor Cholim Society founded the Bikor Cholim Hospital in 1920 after the influenza epidemic ended. In 1925, they secured a larger home and called it the Home for Incurables. In 1929 they changed the name to Mount Sinai Home for Chronic Invalids—a forerunner of Mount Sinai Hospital and Clinic, which later became Cedars-Sinai Medical Center. [45]

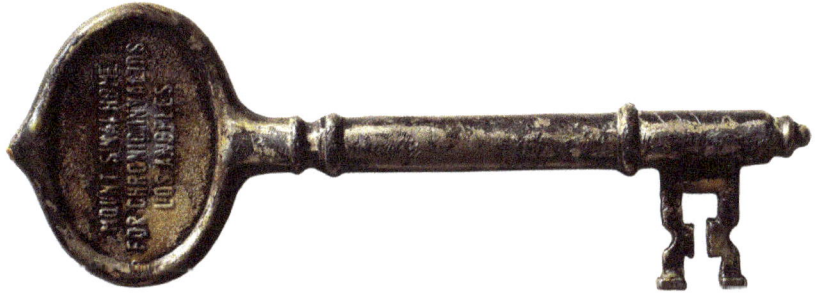

Figure 04.36. A one pound, twelve-inch key used in the dedication ceremony for the Nurses' Home at Mount Sinai Home for Chronic Invalids, 1937.

Philanthropic-minded individuals donated funds to construct a building for sixteen nurses on the grounds of the Mount Sinai Home for Chronic Invalids in the Boyle Heights section of Los Angeles.

On 14 March 1937, the hospital dedicated the new nurses' home. Civic leaders attended, and Hollywood stage and film stars performed at the location of the institution—831 North Bonnie Beach Place—on a platform built specifically for the ceremony. [46]

Chapter Four

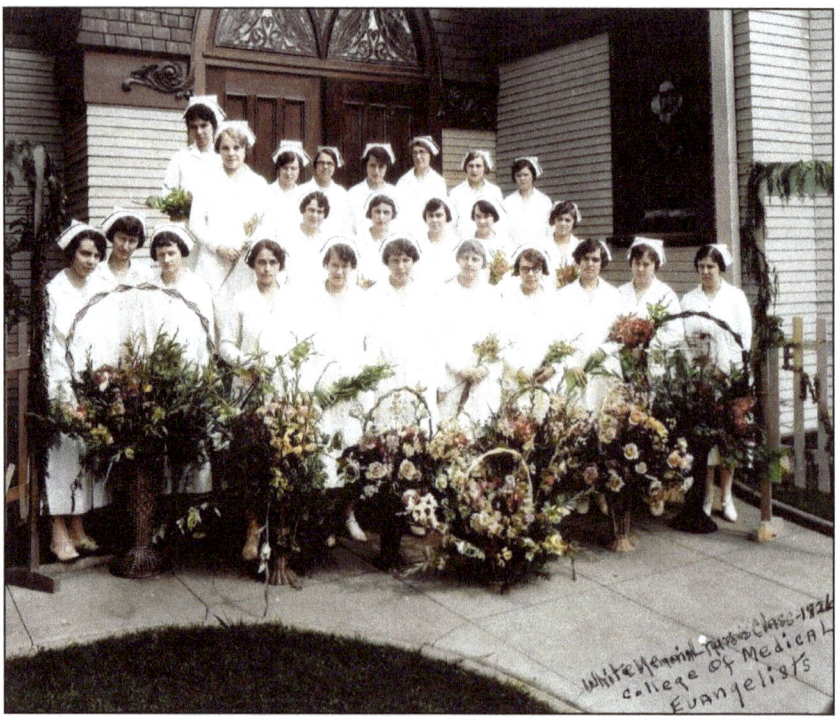

Figure 04.27. The first graduating class, White Memorial School of Nursing, at the College of Medical Evangelists, 1926. C. It began in Los Angeles in 1923. In 1948, the school moved to Loma Linda School of Nursing in Loma Linda, California. [47] (University Archives, Loma Linda University)

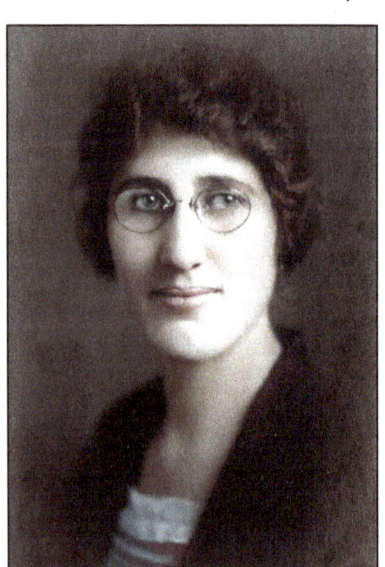

Figure 04.28. Martha Borg, the White Memorial Hospital Superintendent of Nurses from 1918 to 1942. C.

Borg was so integral to the development of the hospital that Martha Borg Hall, dedicated to her memory, was located within the building. [48]

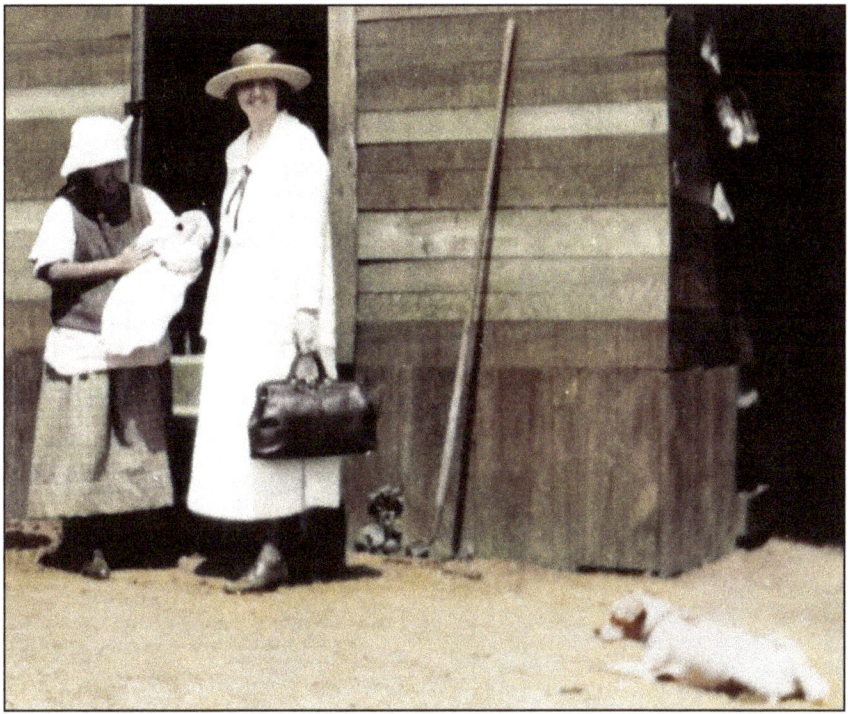

Figure 04.29. Ellen White Nurse on an obstetrical home visit during the Great Depression, c. 1930. C. (University Archives, Loma Linda University)

Doctors accepted eggs, chickens, and groceries in return for their services during the 1929 depression era. The city and county were drained of relief funds. As a public service, the College of Medical Evangelists organized a nurse corps (Ellen White Nurses) to offer home services to the poor who could not afford a hospital. Many nurses were also unemployed, but they donated their time—the hospital fed them, and the county paid their carfare. [49-50]

Figure 04.30. The depressed neighborhood and homes they visited, c. 1930.

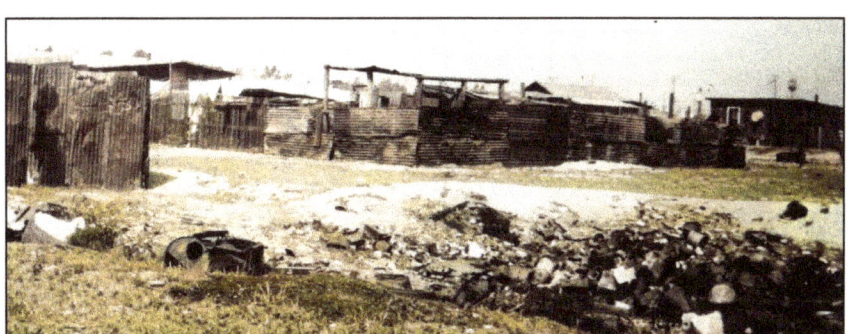

Nurses Take Off: 1930-1941

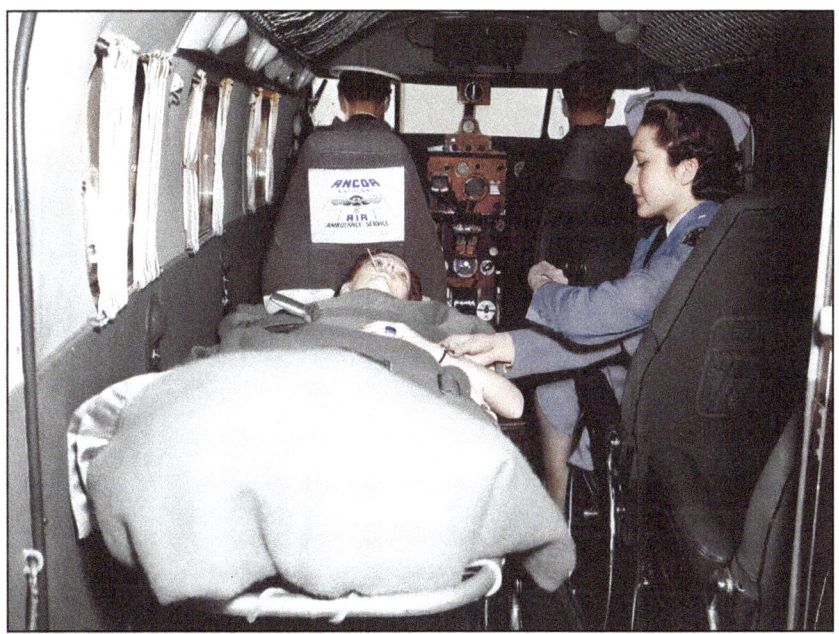

Figure 05.01. Aerial Nurse Corps of America member, Jeanne Lipis, RN, transporting a patient aboard a Lockheed Electra, c. 1938. C. (MMM)

In 1929, while flying over a tornado-damaged site in Ohio, a young pilot, Lauretta Schimmoler had an idea: isolated towns could receive medical attention quickly if nurses, trained in aspects of aviation, could fly in and render immediate care. She started planning. She chose the name as the Emergency Flight Corps; however, she never organized that group in Ohio.

Schimmoler moved to Los Angeles in 1933. In Los Angeles she found ten interested and dedicated nurses, and she changed the group's name to the Aerial Nurse Corps of America. They became the first nurse-staffed and speciality trained civilian group of air ambulances in the United States. [1]

Nurses volunteered. The requirements were restrictive: age 21–35, no young children, immune to airsickness, and qualified as Red Cross First Reserve.

Nurses trained for three years studying medicine and aeronautics. Schimmoler's auxiliary group of lay business and professional women, the Aviation Emergency Corps, assisted as a ground crew. By 1941, the Corps had more than 600 members with companies in fourteen states. [2-3]

Chapter Five

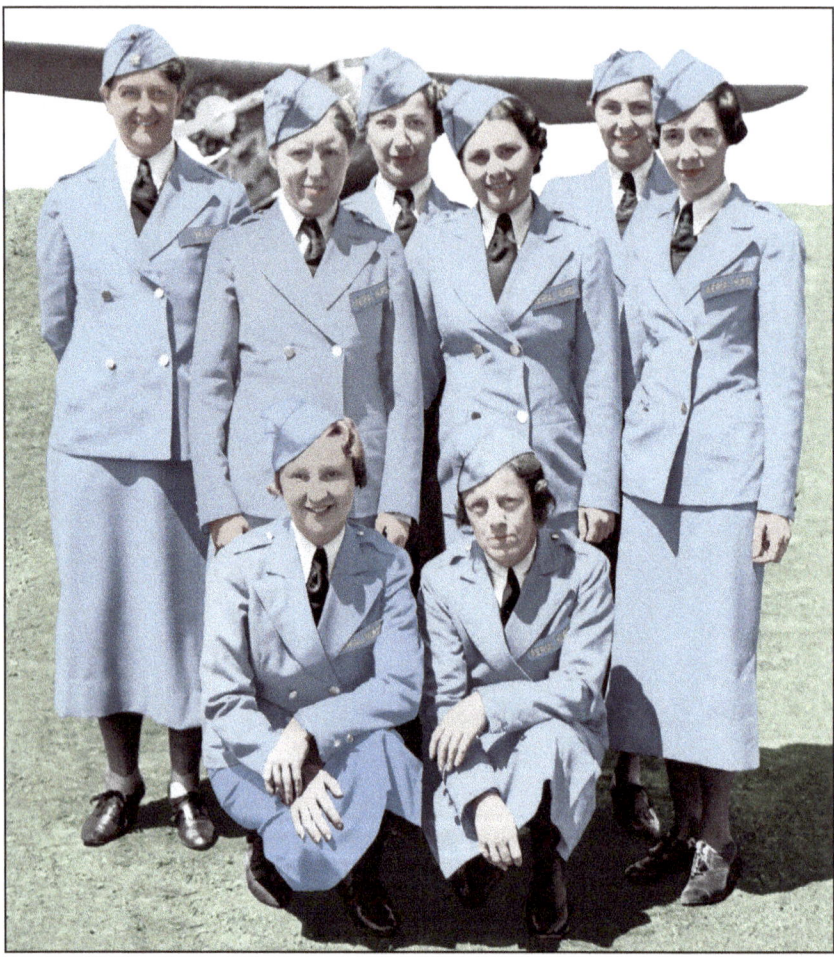

Figure 05.02. Seven of the first ten nurses of the Aerial Nurse Corps of America (ANCOA) on duty at the National Air Races in Los Angeles—their first official post, 1936. C. Kneeling in the first row: Cecelia Getsfred and Edna Yarnell. Second row: Velma Cook, Rose Marie Cummings, and Edwardine Malone. Third row: Lauretta Schimmoler, Amy Koening, and Ava Brook. C. (Courtesy of Bucyrus Historical Society)

Lauretta Schimmoler attempted to coordinate the Corps with the Red Cross and the military. Neither group was interested. The national director of the Red Cross told her, "There would seem no point in making an attempt to organize a special group of nurses for these purposes." The military said any nurse could fly when needed; they didn't need special training. However, when WWII began, they realized the importance of trained nurses. Many ANCOA nurses signed up for the military, including several who helped form the first Military Flight Nurse groups.[4]

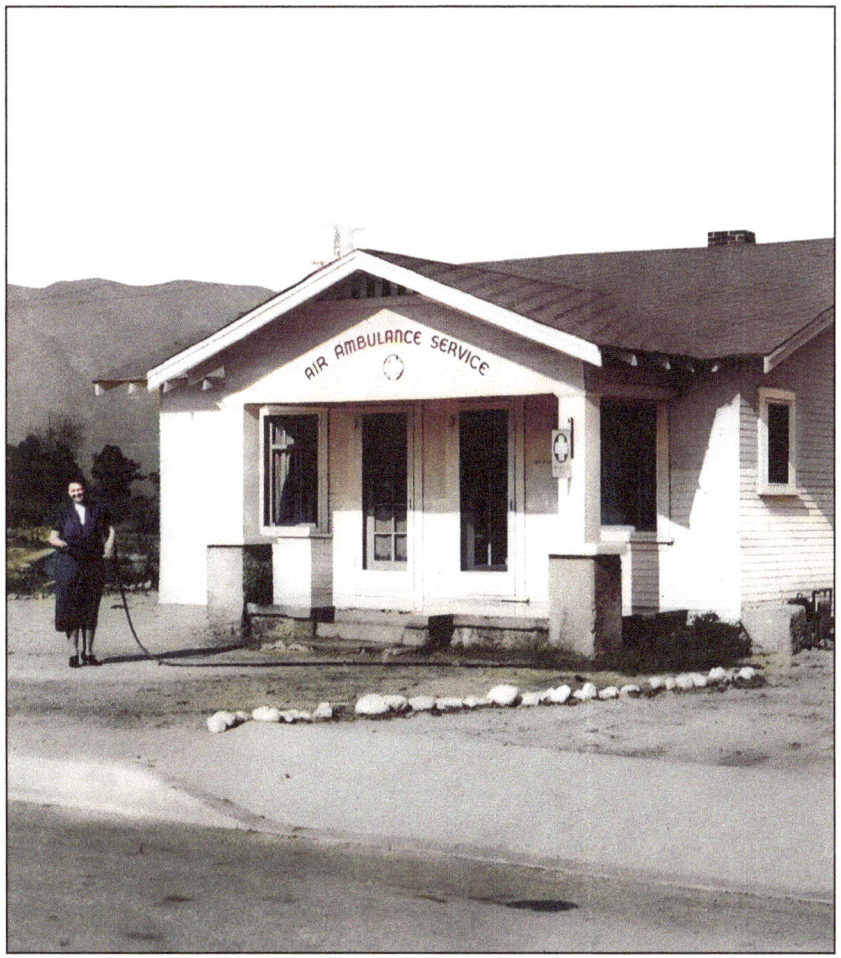

Figure 05.03. Lauretta Schimmoler at the ANCOA National Headquarters at 2711 Empire Street in Burbank, CA, 1937. C . She rented the house from her good friend Amelia Earhart and famous Hollywood stuntman, Paul Mantz.

Both Schimmoler and Earhart were early members of the Ninety-Nines—a group of female pilots who began the club in 1929. Schimmoler served as secretary-treasurer, and Earhart as its first president. Earhart became the most famous female pilot in history. She disappeared en route to Howland Island on 2 July 1937, while attempting to circumnavigate the globe.[5]

Earhart had been an ANCOA supporter. Both Earhart and Mantz agreed on the importance of establishing a formal air ambulance, with specially trained nurses, to benefit society. Mantz's fame allowed him to organize a meeting at Union Air Terminal with Los Angeles medical and aviation dignitaries to discuss forming the Southern California Aviation Medical Advisory Board.[6]

Chapter Five

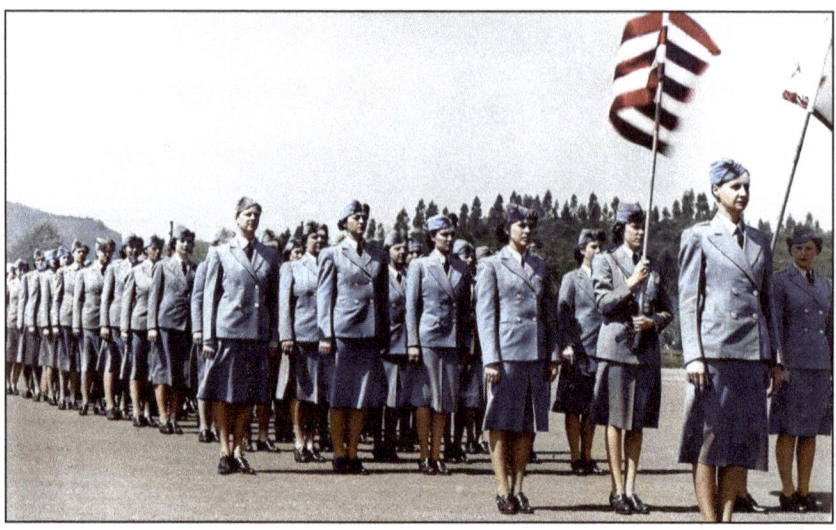

Figure 05.04. Los Angeles, West Los Angeles, and Glendale Platoon Color Guards marching, as extras, in the movie *Parachute Nurse*, 1942. C. (BHS)

In 1942 Columbia Pictures released *Parachute Nurse*—a movie about a fictional group of nurses who parachuted into remote areas to administer medical attention to soldiers. Schimmoler secured the position of technical director and the role of Captain Jane Morgan, poised to whip into shape any nurse who might stray from the military's impeccable requirements. [7]

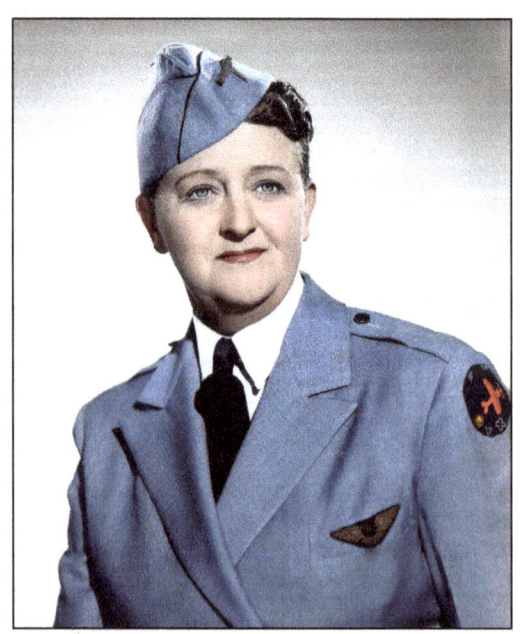

Figure 05.05. Lauretta Schimmoler performing as Captain Jane Morgan in the movie *Parachute Nurse*, 1942. C. (BHS)

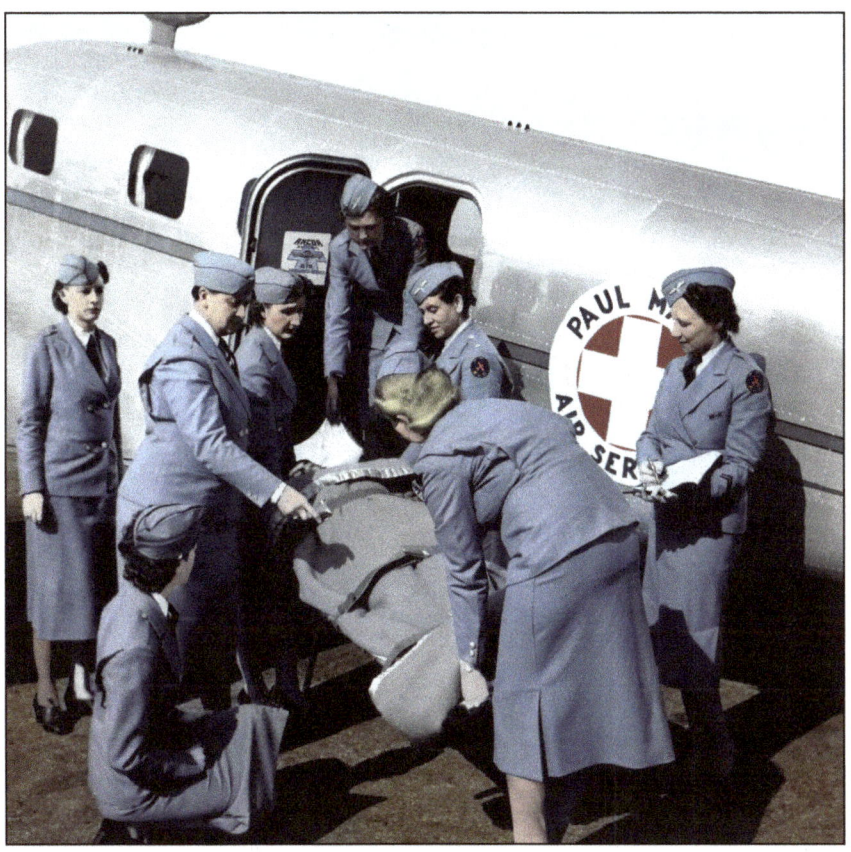

Figure 05.06. Los Angeles ANCOA loading a patient into a Mantz plane, 1938. C. (BHS). Schimmoler is pointing to a stretcher she designed that could fit through the narrow doorways and crowded interiors of the planes.

The Aerial Nurse Corps functioned for eight years—they disbanded primarily because of WWII. Many nurses joined the military, and civilian planes were grounded. [8] The remaining few members performed assignments at airports for the Civil Air Patrol and the Los Angeles County Sheriff's Department. [9]

Schimmoler, not a nurse, could not join her fellow nurses in the military. Instead, she joined the Woman's Army Corps as an aircraft dispatcher. The military adopted her idea of nurse-staffed medical air transport. One night while on duty, she witnessed the first C-54 military transport plane as it landed at Fairfiel-Suisan Air Force Base. "And they said it wouldn't be done," she said out loud. [10] Her nurse-staffed air ambulance dream became a reality.

In 1966 the Air Force nurses honored her at a ceremony as the pioneer of the Flight Nurse concept and awarded her Honorary Flight Nurse wings #1. [11]

Chapter Five

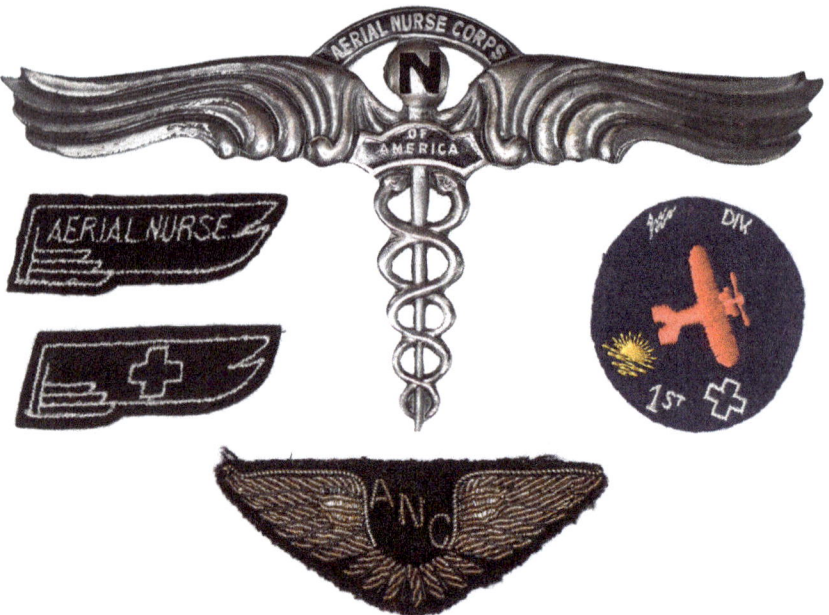

Figures 05.07-11. ANCOA cap pin for nurses. Aerial Nurse pocket patch and Aviation Emergency Corps pocket patch. Shoulder insignia with a 1st for the division and a white first aid cross. The Commander's pocket patch with wing insignia and ANC letters. (Author photographed)

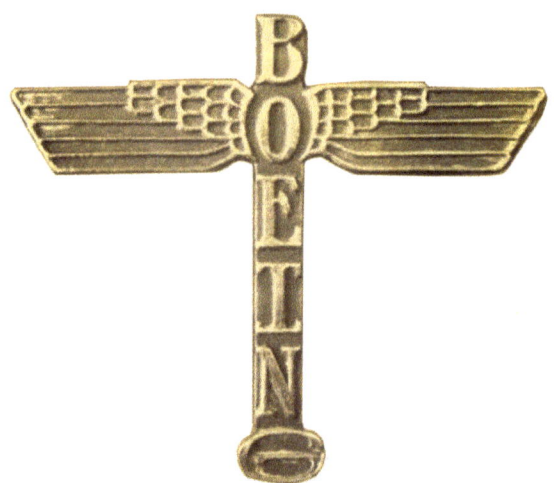

Figure 05.12. A Boeing Bug nurse-stewardess pin. (Author photographed).

The original eight nurse-stewardesses at Boeing (on the facing page) wore pins on each lapel in the shape of a Boeing 80 airplane. They called the pins Boeing Bugs.

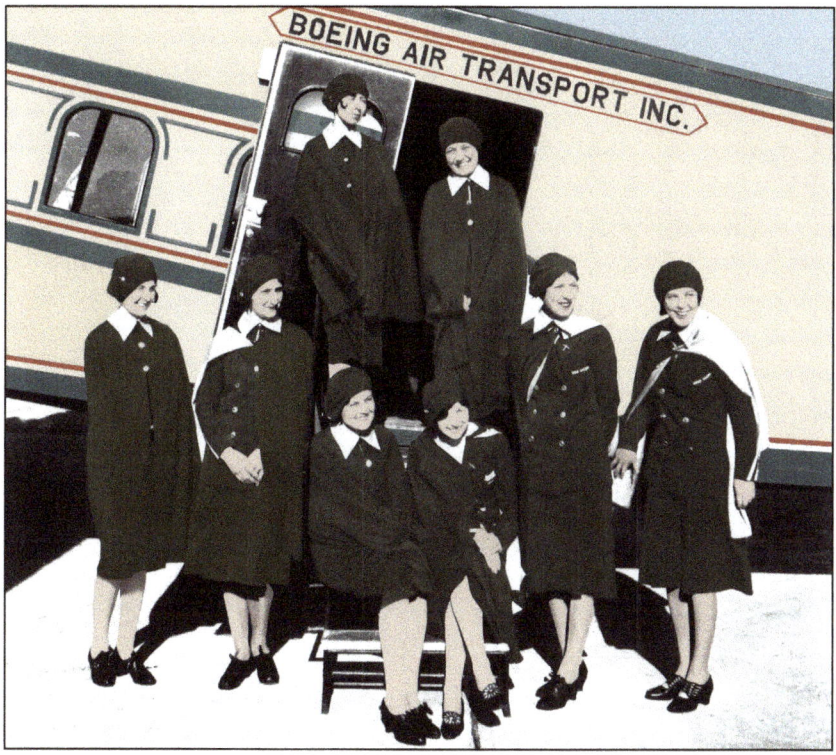

Figure 05.13. The original eight nurse-stewardesses for Boeing Airlines: Ellen Church (top left), Margaret Arnott, Jessie Carter, Ellis Crawford, Harriet Fry (a Los Angeles nurse), Alva Johnson, Inez Keller, and Cornelia Peterman, May 15, 1930, C. (Courtesy of Ethel Pattison, United Airlines)

The original eight took their first working flights aboard a Boeing 80, one nurse per airplane, in May 1930. The year before, a registered nurse, Ellen Church, met Boeing Traffic Manager Steve Stimpson while taking flying lessons in San Francisco. Stimpson told her he'd considered hiring young Filipino men as onboard stewards; Church told him nurses skills would be valuable in the air. Stimpson convinced Boeing to hire nurses. [12]

The planes were small; Boeing required a height limit of 5'4" and a weight of less than 115 pounds. The salary was $125.00 per month. If passengers became nauseous, nurses offered the barbiturate Secanol to sleep off nausea. Boeing merged with three other airlines in 1931 to become United Airlines.

Church learned to fly and completed 13 solo hours; however, she never obtained her pilot's license because she moved to Wyoming to work with Boeing. In 1940, she joined the ANCOA in Wisconsin. She joined the Army when WWII began and became one of the first military flight nurses. [13]

Chapter Five

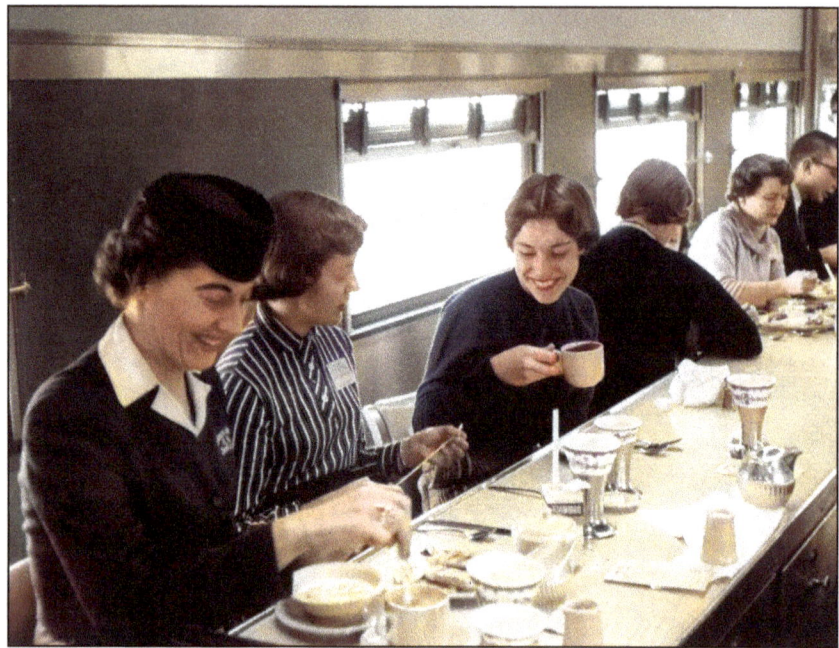

Figure 05.14. Marguerite Branyen, RN, of Los Angeles, the first Union Pacific railway nurse, [14] dines with State University of Iowa students prior to their arrival in Pasadena, CA, c. 1936. C. (Kansas State Historical Society)

In August 1935, the Union Pacific Railroad selected graduate nurses from Los Angeles, Salt Lake City, and Omaha hospitals to serve on the Luxe Coach train. The railway stewardesses launched a new branch of public health and industrial nursing. The applicant's main requirements were adaptability and experience because the nurse was the only medical service on the trip. Most employers expected railway nurses to have a college degree and a membership in the American Nurses Association.

Similar to air-based nurses, the requirements included age, height, a weight category, and physical stamina examinations. The shifts lasted 18 to 24 hours—day and night call. Snowstorms often stranded trains for days, and the nurse was the only source to handle medical emergencies. Nurses were asked to administer insulin, deliver babies, manage asthma, observe chronic cardiac conditions, teach good health habits, monitor accidents, manage heart attacks, and treat train derailment injuries. [15]

Railway nurses made independent decisions; they functioned with standing orders from the chief surgeon and a well-stocked medical kit. [16] Other railroads added nurses later, including Santa Fe Railroad, which owned a large hospital in Los Angeles. Santa Fe named their nurses Courier Nurses.

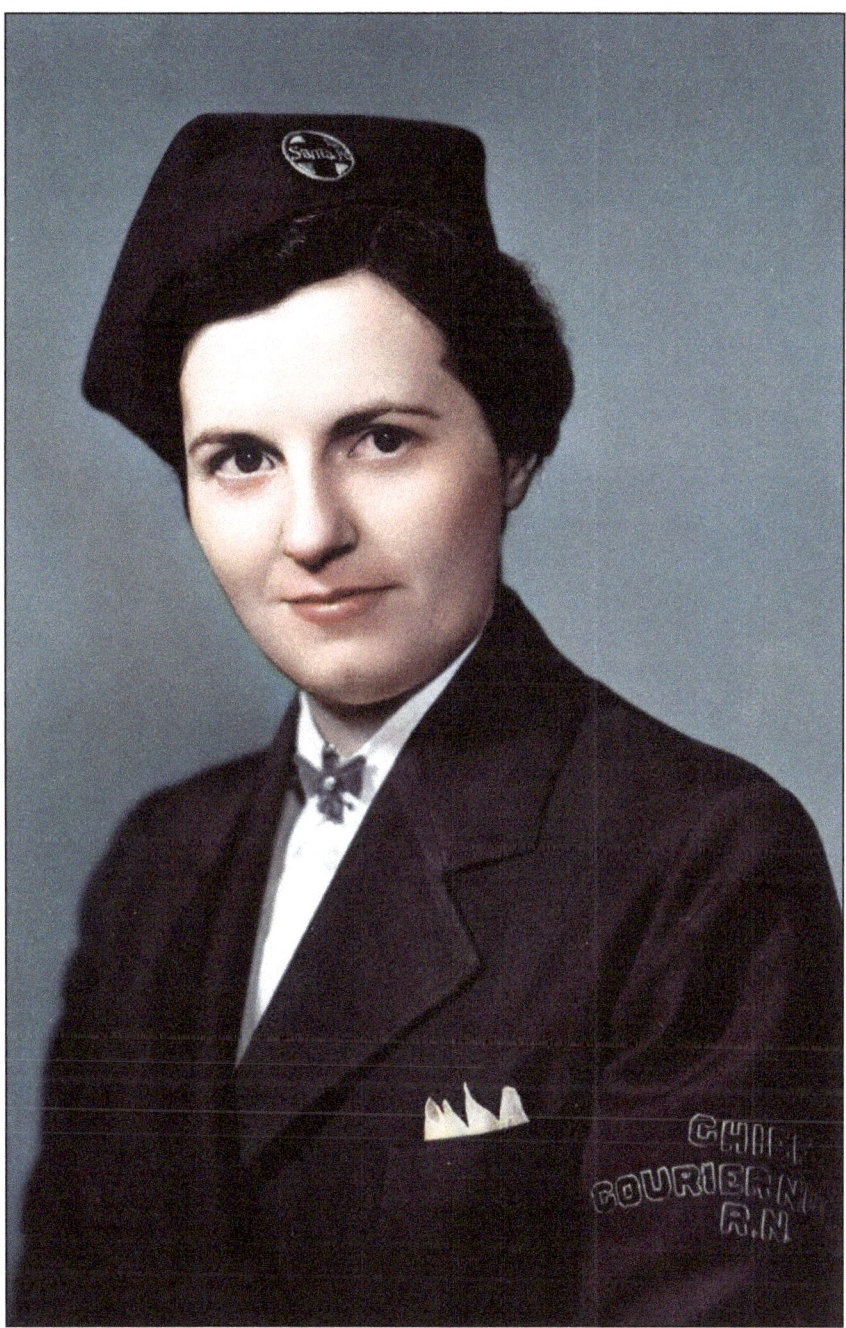

Figure 05.15. Chief Courier Nurse, Delma Frazer, RN, Santa Fe Railroad, c. 1940. C. (Kansas State Historical) The railway nursing service halted during WWII but returned in 1947. [17] Nurses served on railways for 38 years. [18]

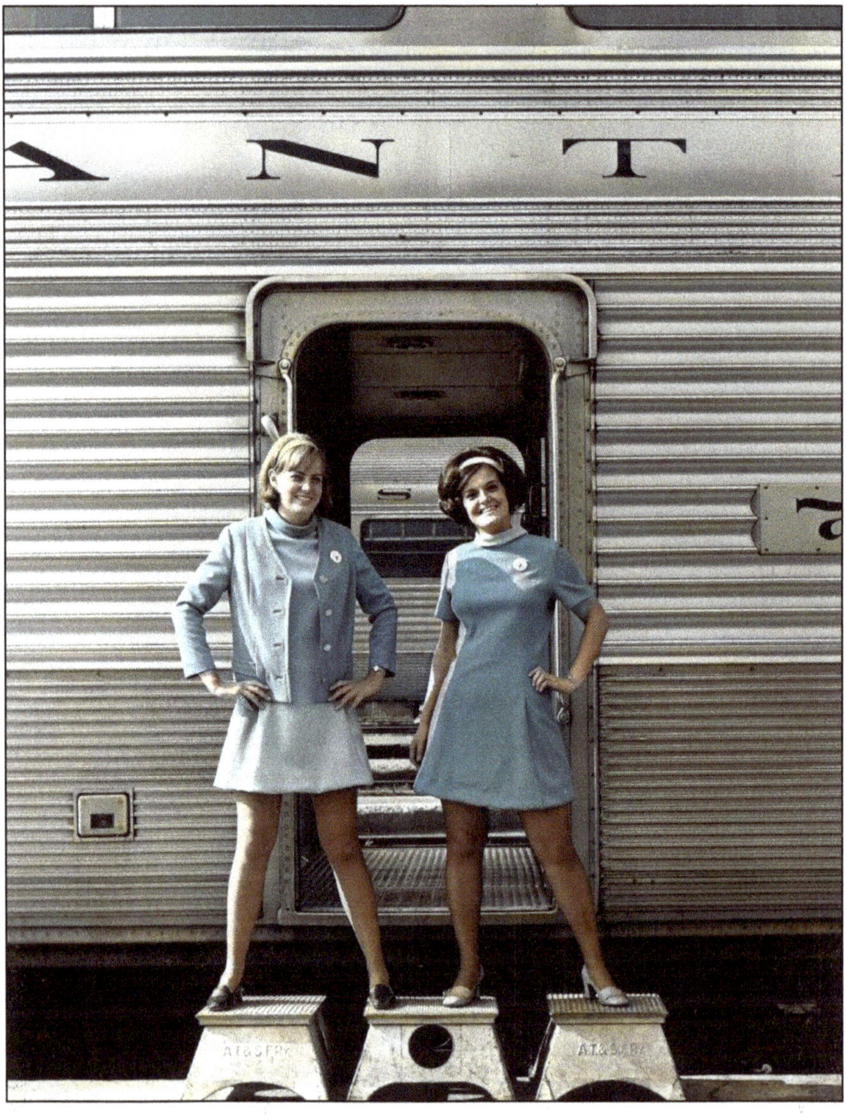

Chapter Five

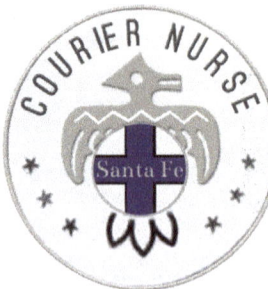

Figure 05.16. Courier nurses, Santa Fe Railcar, 1969, C. Figure 05.17. The 1960s Courier Nurse Pin. (Kansas State Historical Society)

In the '60s, Courier nurse uniforms changed to reflect the style of the decade. Nurses wore turquoise and mesa blue dresses to add a Southwestern touch aboard the El Capitan Santa Fe Railcar—a first-class railcar that traveled between Chicago and Los Angeles. [19]

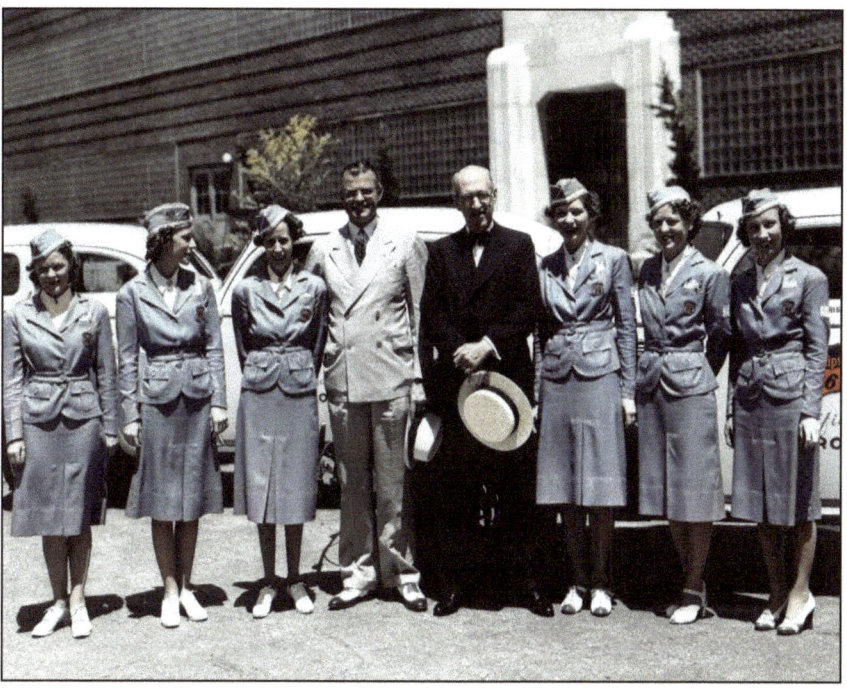

Figure 05.18. Six Highway Hostesses with their vehicles. Boots Adams, the president of Phillips, is center right, and one of the founding brothers, Frank Phillips, is center left, n.d. C. (ConocoPhillips Corporate Archives)

The Phillips Petroleum Company launched a campaign to clean up service station restrooms in 1939. The company employed local registered nurses and called them Highway Hostesses.

The nurses made surprise visits to Phillips 66 stations to inspect the restroom facilities and certify them for cleanliness throughout Phillips's territory. Restrooms were known to be filthy, and Phillips marketing plans assured customers their restrooms were hospital clean.

The nurses could administer first aid and acted as company ambassadors; they cheerfully aided motorists in distress and directed tourists to restaurants and hotels.

The Highway Hostesses wore light-blue uniforms with a Phillips 66 patch, military-style hats, white shoes, stockings, and a vest pocket handkerchief. They drove cream and green patrol-style vehicles with the Phillips 66 logo and the phrase "Certified Restrooms" on the doors. [20] The Phillips 66 logo looked similar to the famous Route 66 sign; probably not a coincidence. Route 66 started in Chicago and ended 2,448 miles later in Santa Monica. [21]

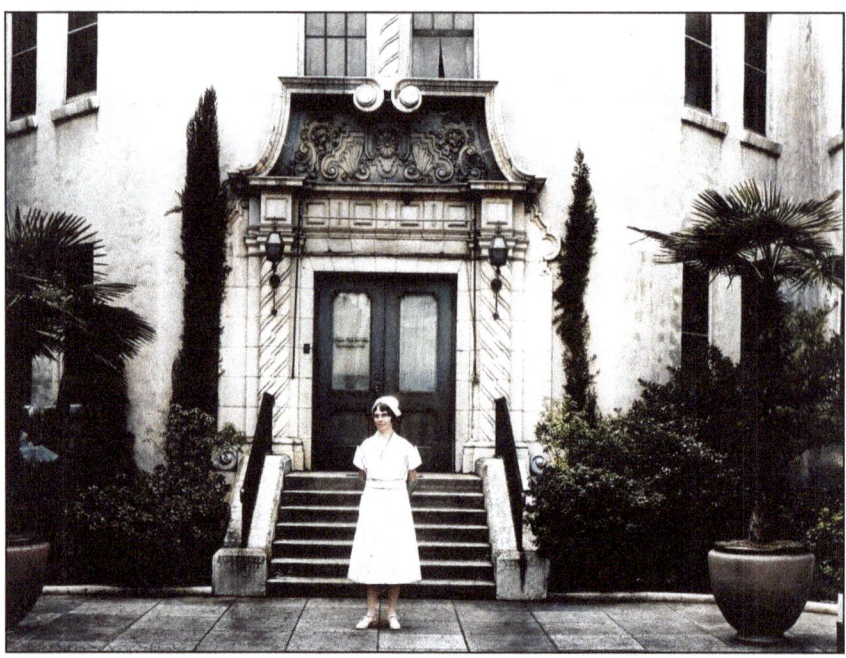

Figure 05.19. Clara Kramer, RN, at Golden State Hospital, 417 Towne Ave, July 31, 1934. C. (Shades of L.A. Archives/Los Angeles Public Library)

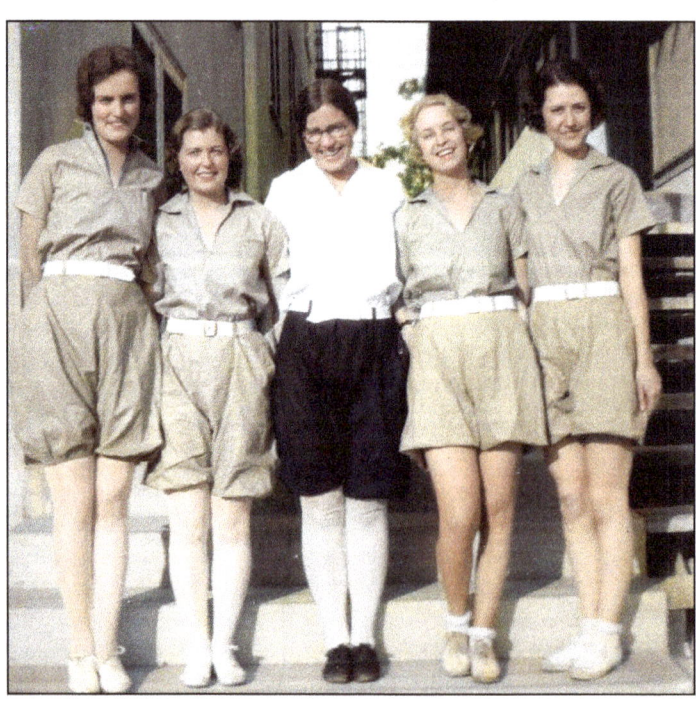

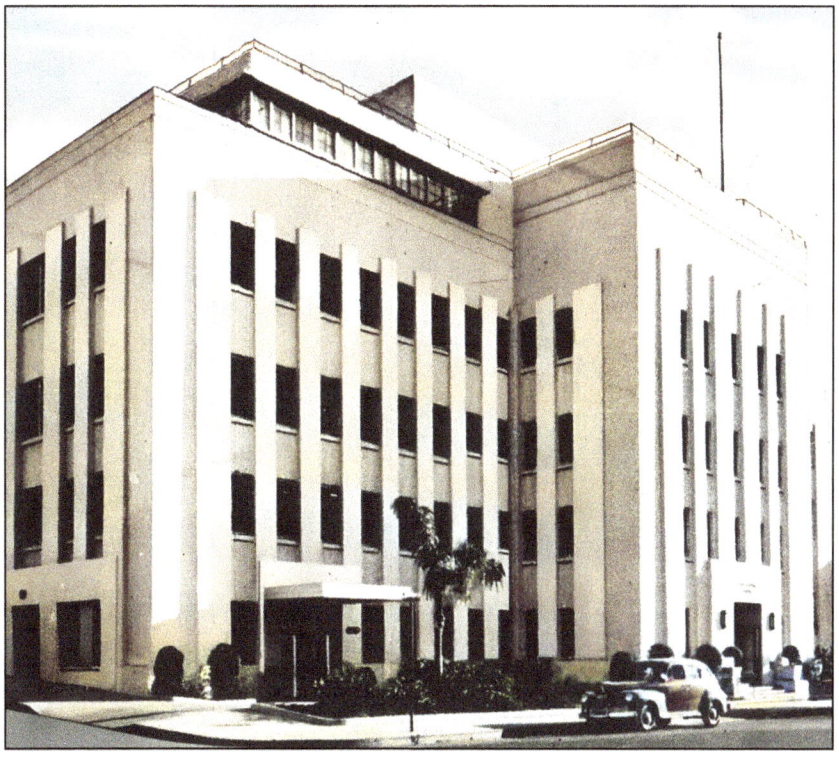

Figure 05.20. Photo postcard of White Memorial Hospital on the corner of Boyle and Michigan Avenues, Los Angeles, 1937. C. The building opened in 1918; they named it in honor of Ellen White. Loma Linda University/ White Memorial School of Nursing began in 1923. The school moved to the Loma Linda campus in 1948. In 1962, they transferred the hospital's ownership to Southern California Conference of Seventh-day Adventists.[22]

Francis Allen graduated from White Memorial Hospital in 1935. During her final year in school, she eloped to Ensenada, Mexico, with surgical resident Edison French. Nursing students were not allowed to marry, so she kept it secret—her sister Gladys had been expelled the year before when she married.

After graduation, the French family moved to San Luis Obispo, California, and Edison French began a surgical practice. When World War II started, he joined the Navy. Camp San Luis Obispo lacked on-base housing for married couples; Francis opened her home to officers and their wives while Edison was stationed overseas.[23]

Figure 05.21. (Facing page) Francis Allen French, right, with her classmates in their student exercise uniforms, c. 1933. C. (Courtesy of Jim French). Early nursing schools included daily exercise classes.

Chapter Five

In June 1936, eleven thousand nurses met in Los Angeles, from every state, to attend a week-long convention of three nursing organizations: the American Nurses Association (ANA), the National League of Nursing Education (NLNE), and the National Organization for Public Health Nursing (NOPHN).

Army nurses, Navy nurses, public health nurses, hospital and private nurses arrived by car, train, bus, airplane, and ship. Forty Sisters added interest: Sisters of Mercy, Sisters of the Holy Cross, Sisters of Charity, Sisters of the Charity of Providence, and Sisters of the Incarnate Word. The conference theme was "Nurses as Part of Tomorrow's Community Health Service." [24-25]

The first vanguard of executives arrived on 18 June wearing evening gowns. Aurelia Reinhart, dean of Mills College; Alma Scott, director of the ANA; Amelia Grant; and ANA President Susan Francis were among the many dignitaries to attend the welcoming dinner in the Arcady Hotel at 2619 Wilshire Boulevard.

A tribute to Florence Nightingale at the Hollywood Bowl kicked off the first event on 20 June. A chorus of 250 uniformed nurses sang compositions dedicated to Nightingale. Kay Francis, who played Nightingale in the *White Angel* movie, wore the costume of Nightingale as she addressed the group. She said she loved the role but felt unworthy standing in front of thousands of real nurses. [26] Annie Goodrich, founder of the Yale School of Nursing and first dean of the Army School of Nursing, presented the tribute. [27]

The Navy Hospital Ship, *Relief*, entertained nurses in Los Angeles Harbor. Nurse groups held ninety-six sessions at the Shrine Auditorium, the Biltmore, and the Ambassador Hotels. Boy Scouts helped keep the convention running smoothly at the Shrine. [28-29]

One of the subjects of discussion was the creation of the eight-hour shift—which began in Los Angeles in 1929—fifty percent of groups in all fifty states had already adopted the idea. They discussed a standard for wages: four to seven dollars for an eight-hour shift, five to eight dollars for ten hours, and six to nine dollars for twenty-four hours. [30]

Speakers called for the abolition of child marriage and child labor, the development of nursing bureaus, vocational and placement services, and the importance of scientific education for students. All three organizations voted in new officers: Susan Francis was re-elected as president of the ANA.

One thousand attended a high-mass service at St. Vincent's Cathedral. Virginia Dunbar, from UCLA, was named the first American graduate to win the prestigious Bedford College of London University Scholarship.

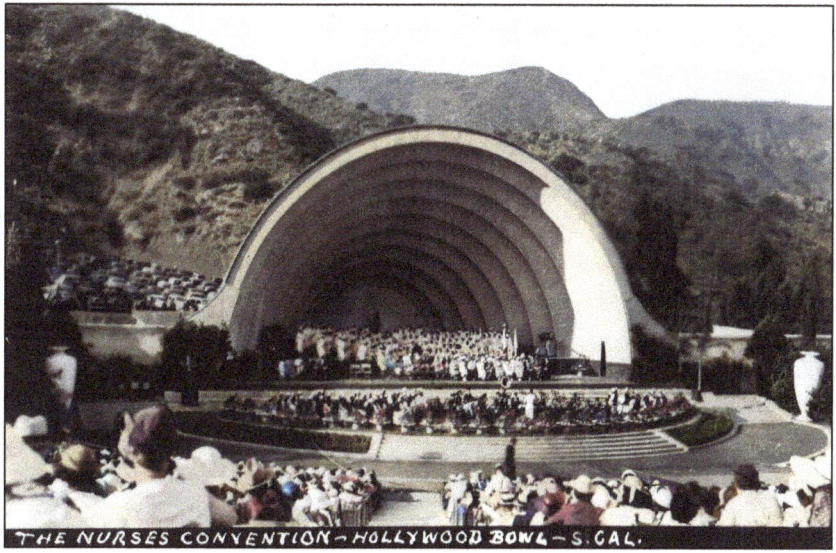

05.22. Photo postcard of the nurses gathered at the Hollywood Bowl for the tribute service to Florence Nightingale, June 20, 1936. C.

As a special tribute to the nursing profession, Warner Brothers arranged a pre-release screening of *The White Angel* for conference attendees at Warner's Hollywood Theater.

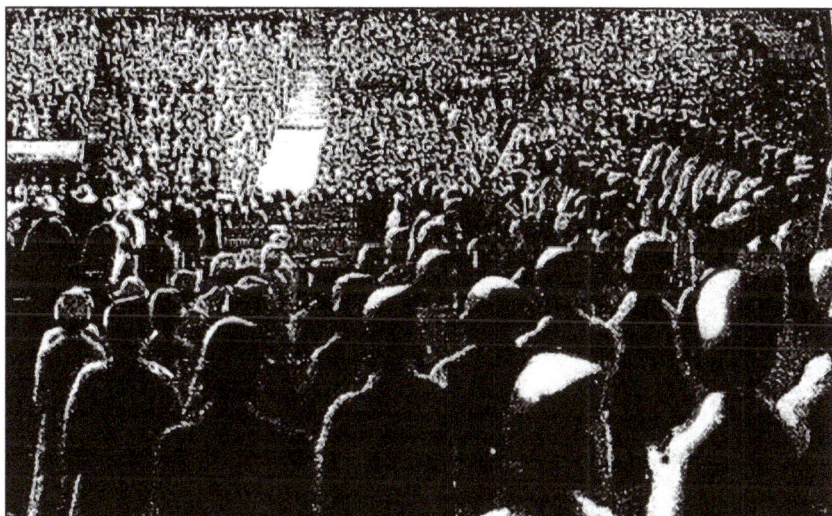

Figure 05.23. A section of a lost photograph of nurses singing, taken from inside of the Hollywood Bowl and looking toward the audience of nurses and guests.

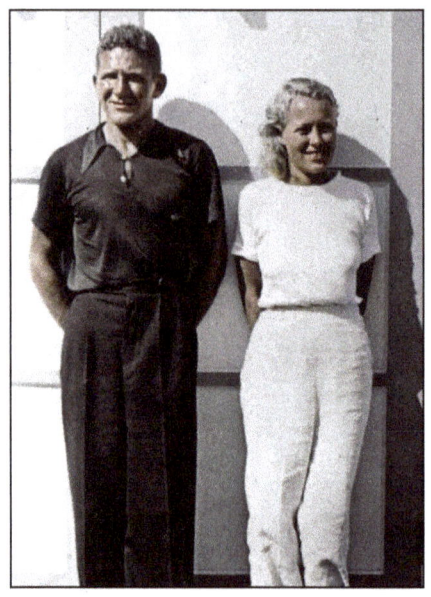

Figure 05.24. Betty Runyen, RN, Kaiser Permanente Hospital's first nurse, and Sidney Garfield, MD, at Contractors General Hospital, 1934.

While working in the delivery room at Methodist Hospital in 1933, Betty Runyen received an offer to become the first nurse at Contractors General Hospital—a twelve-bed hospital at a remote construction site in the California desert. Doctors Gene Morris and Sidney Garfield started the hospital for the 5,000 Colorado River Aqueduct construction workers. Runyen wanted an adventure.

She thought working with men might be an interesting change from the women and babies on the maternity floor she'd worked on since graduation. And the job paid more.

The hospital had ten beds in one ward and two beds in a semi-private room. Garfield's office doubled as the staff lounge and became his bedroom at night. Runyen had a small room. A married couple, who had their own room, functioned as housekeeper and orderly. After Garfield began to receive pre-payments, he hired a second nurse named Nadine Cherry. [31]

Figure 05.25. Contractors General Hospital surrounded by cactus and Cholla bushes. Nadine Cherry standing, an unidentified woman sitting, c. 1934. C.

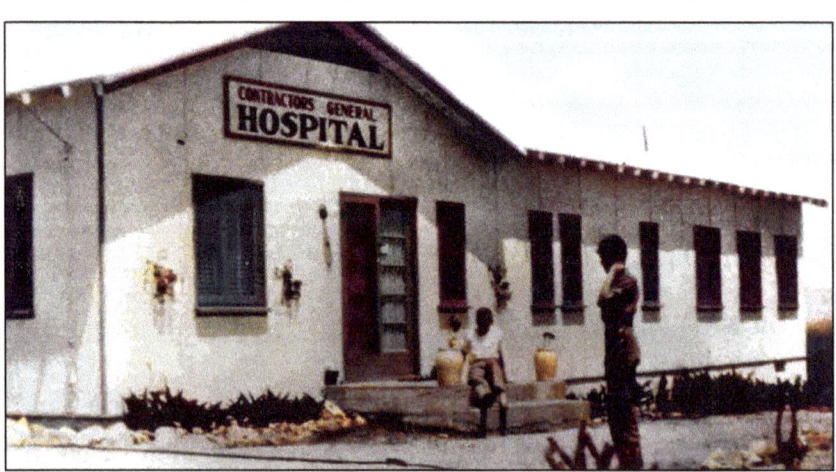

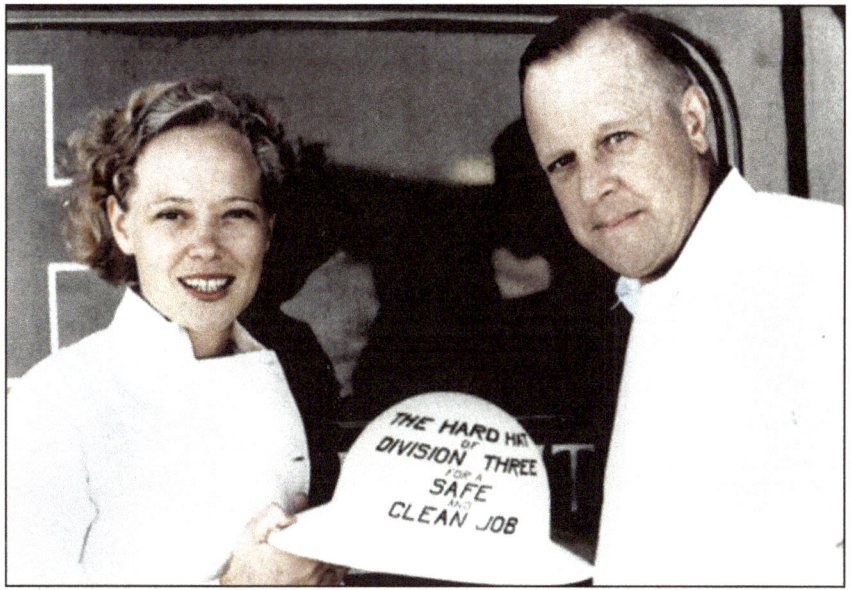

Figure 05.26. Betty Runyen awarding the safety prize of a hard hat to the foreman. (Photos courtesy of Steve Gilford)

Fractures were a common diagnosis at Contractors General. Powder headaches, a frequent complaint, were caused by the workers close proximity to dynamite explosions while blasting through hard rock in the mountains. Many complained of back pain, although sometimes they faked illness to garner rest and collect Workmen's Compensation.

Contractors General Hospital held safety contests to decrease injuries and lower costs. Runyen often drove the ambulance. Nurses did not insert intravenous lines in the 1930s, but Garfield had trained Runyen so she could start one during emergency calls.

After one year, the hospital began to run out of money because insurance underwriters often discounted charges. Garfield struck an agreement to cover the medical expenses of all 5,000 workers for a guaranteed fee of five cents per worker, per day.

This guaranteed a payment system at Contractors General and became the model for Kaiser Permanente's health maintenance organization (HMO). Garfield and other doctors later started Kaiser Permanente Hospital and continued this prepayment model.

Runyen graduated from the Los Angeles Methodist Hospital School of Nursing in the early 1930s.[32]

Chapter Five

Poliomyelitis began in the late 1920s and persisted until the late 1950s. The U.S. polio epidemic reached every segment of the population. Initially, the disease appeared in poor and overcrowded areas; however, it soon became a threat to everyone.

President Franklin Delano Roosevelt contracted polio. In 1938, he used his power to create the National Foundation for Infantile Paralysis. [33]

From 1934 to 1936, approximately 150 nurses contracted polio while working at Los Angeles County General Hospital. In 1937, the California State Nurses Association studied all the cases—many nurses had recovered by then, but 106 remained partially or completely disabled. [34]

In the beginning the nurses were cared for at County General. After 1935 the hospital transferred them to rest homes in each nurse's district. Many facilities were not equipped to care for paralyzed patients; the nurses were on bed rest for three years.

Other nurses were not paralyzed, but they did not have the physical capacity to return to hospital work. Some of the affected were student nurses who had years of education remaining, and the special college classes they had taken, for diploma nurses only, did not transfer to other college degrees.

The nurses complained about substandard care in the rest homes. During a 1937 court hearing, several paralyzed nurses testified that the food was bad and they were given incorrect medications. The rooms were never cleaned. Some buildings were converted garages, and since they were level to the ground, bugs crawled in.

One nurse reported they were supposed to take curative baths; however, frogs inhabited the pool. They thought they would recover if they could return to County General for rehabilitation. Many families could have cared for some of the nurses at home, but if transferred to home, they would lose medical care payments.

A group of nurses received salary compensation of sixty-five to ninety-five percent of weekly wages for 240 weeks. Others received much less. Many had worked long hours during the polio epidemic; fatigue had lowered their resistance. The hospital had not given training in communicable diseases.

In 1937 the grand jury made its recommendations: nursing personnel should be protected during future epidemics; they should be allowed to live in private homes; satisfactory compensatory pay should be given to low-paid graduate nurses and student nurses; and they should be given rehabilitation with job retraining. [35]

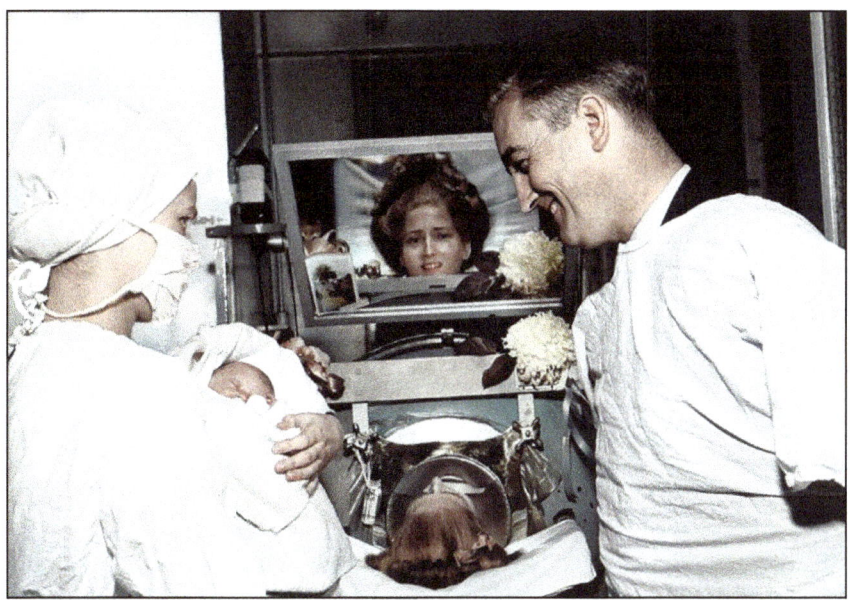

Figure 05.27. County General student nurse, Martha Talbert, holding a baby just born to his mother, who lived in an iron lung, November 1951. C.

Figure 05.28. Geraldine Stanyar attending to General Hospital's youngest polio patient, a two-year-old, in an iron lung (artificial respiration device). Multiple iron lungs were present in the background, 1948. C. (Shades of L.A. Archives/Los Angeles Public Library)

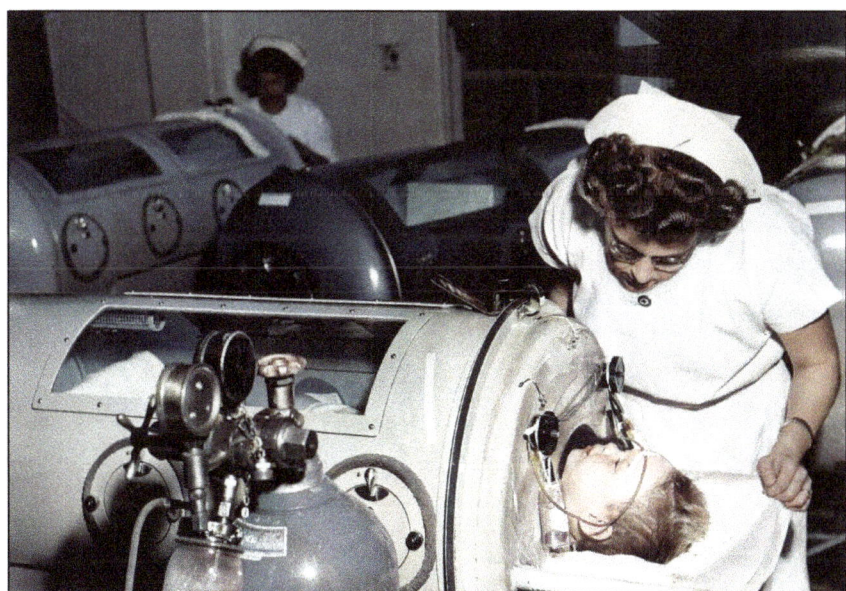

Chapter Five

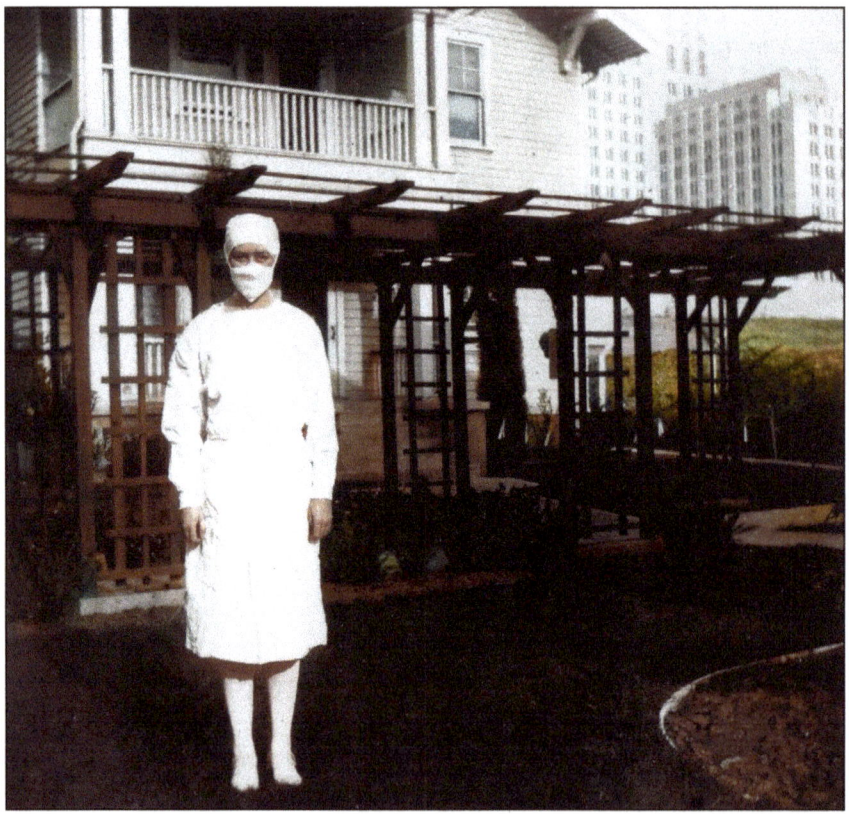

Figure 05.29. Student Nurse Helen Ackley, dressed for surgery, standing in front of Cottage 31 which she shared with her roommates at Los Angeles County General Hospital School of Nursing, November 1929. C. The student nurses lived in these nearby cottages. The new County General building (under construction) is visible in the upper corner. (Author's collection)

Surgery was one of the first specialties for nurses. This was one area where hospitals did not depend on student nurses—they hired experienced graduate nurses, and operating nurses were often chosen before head nurses. Correct nursing knowledge was so important to the success of operations that student nurses often spent three months or more in surgical studies.

Helen Ackley kept a journal throughout her training. Her 1931 grade card shows nurses still studied massage as a full course, and Materia Medica was the term used for the study of pharmaceutical drugs. One of the handbills in her collection is for a recital and service to honor the 110th anniversary of the birth of Florence Nightingale at the Cathedral Church of St. Paul on Figueroa Street, 1930. A notation in her journal stated that students from all Los Angeles nursing schools attended the service. [36]

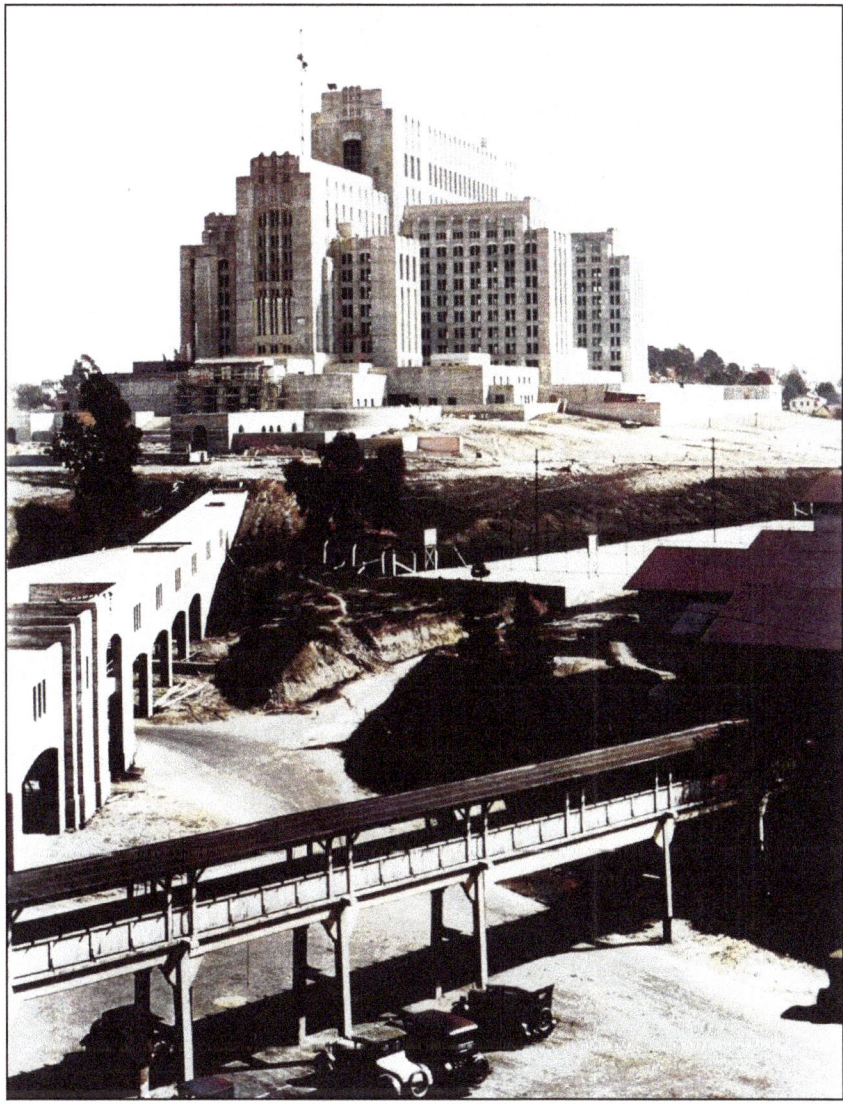

Figure 05.30. County General Hospital, still under construction, as student nurses saw it from their cottages, 1927. C. (Author's collection, Helen Ackley's student nurse journal)

Actress Mary Pickford laid the cornerstone for the new County Hospital building on December 7, 1927, which opened in December of 1933. Students walked many times a day on this long, covered bridge, nicknamed the Bridge of Sighs, from the old County Hospital building where they trained to the cottages where they lived (the cottages are in the shade on the right side). Cottage #185 was reserved for sick doctors and nurses. [37]

Chapter Five

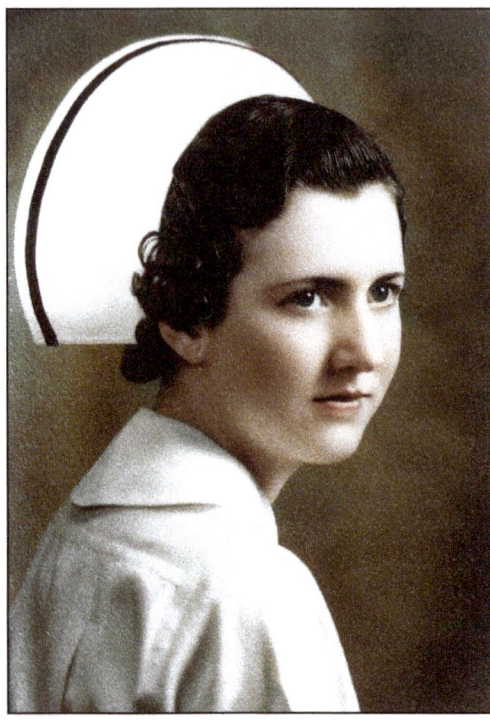

Figure 05.31. Nurse Margaret Anderson's graduation photo, 1936. (Courtesy of Margaret Anderson Freed)

Margaret Anderson started nursing school the first year Los Angeles County General Hospital opened the new building in 1933. A new hospital should have made students flock to the nursing program, but the polio epidemic frightened many from applying.

The student nurses often accompanied police when they were called to attend an emergency—Anderson once delivered a baby while on a police call.

She met Arnold Freed, a young medical student, during her training. He became infected with tuberculosis during the first year of his residency and was sent to Barlow Sanitarium for three years to recover. He had to postpone medical training. Anderson visited him while he recovered in Barlow, and a romance began. They married three days after his release from Barlow. She developed a mild case of polio during her training; she still graduated on her scheduled date. [38]

She was a literary editor of her senior yearbook; her writing was sprinkled throughout the book. This is an excerpt from one of her poems: [39]

Friendship's Picture

Some friends are like stalwart trees;
'Neath their shade we find rest.
And like the trees are heaven sent
That our lives may be blest.

Other friends resemble the rocks
Smoothed with life's rippling stream.
Some in our lives cast a shadow,
And are not just what they seem.

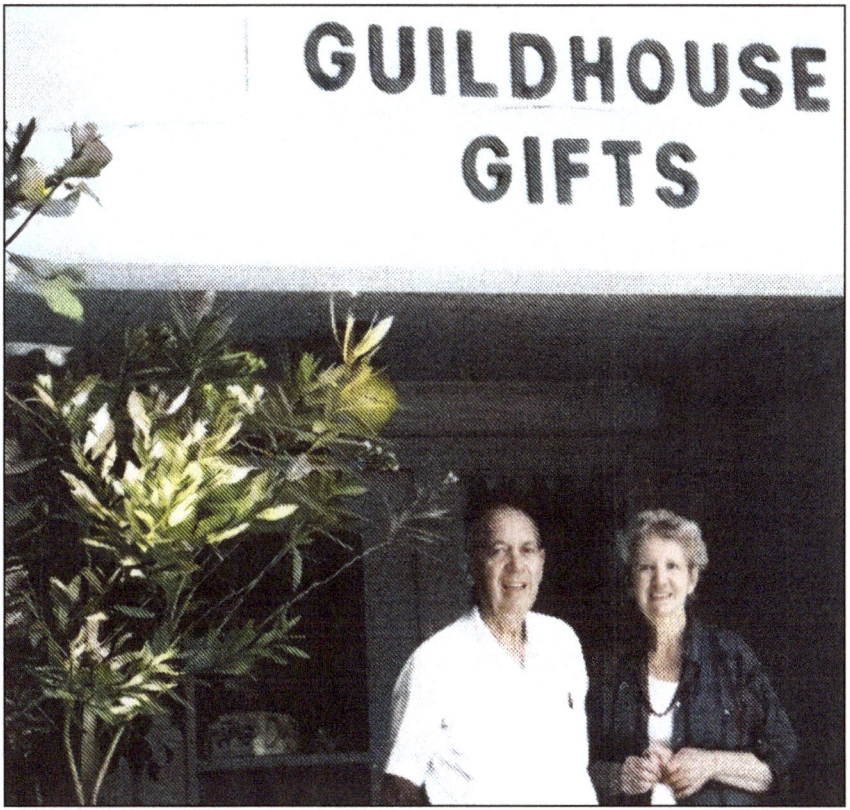

Figure 05.32 Arnold and Margaret Freed in front of Guildhouse Gifts. (Courtesy of Barlow Respiratory Hospital)

Arnold Freed finished his medical training. Margaret worked with him in his office on Wilshire Boulevard for thirteen years, but patients never knew they were married.

The Freeds returned to Barlow Sanitarium as volunteers, and in 1975 they started Guildhouse Gifts. They found an abandoned dormitory called the Men's Help Home. "It was full of junk," Margaret said, "with an old autopsy table in front of the fireplace." Guildhouse Gifts raised money to purchase equipment and other patient items that insurance did not cover.

Margaret attended conferences to purchase unique items to sell in the shop. "Arnold was particularly good at choosing items that would sell," she said. After he died, her granddaughter Amy Poulos helped her choose items. In 2006, Barlow, later named Barlow Respiratory Hospital, honored Margaret for sixty-plus years of volunteer service. Representatives from the city council, Barlow staff, and 100 community residents attended the ceremony. [40]

Girls Who Dreamt to Become a Nurse

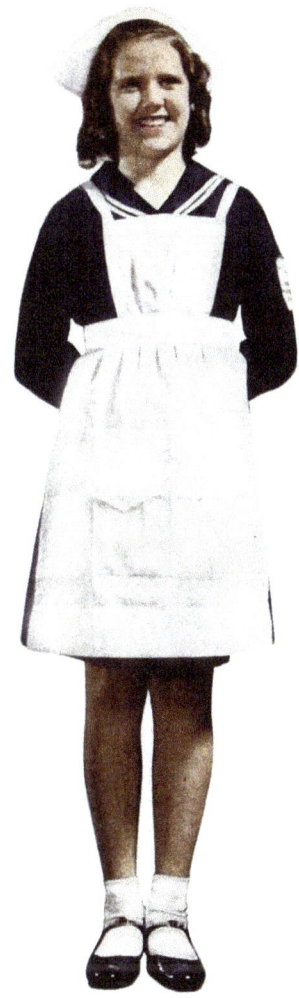

Figure 06.01. National President Dorothy Hart, in her Sunbrite Junior Nurse Corps uniform, c. 1937. C.

In 1936, CBS radio introduced teen nursing student Dorothy Hart and the Sunbrite Junior Nurse Corps, sponsored by Sunbrite Cleanser. Young Dorothy Hart and her Aunt Jane solved problems, dramatized adventures in nursing, and presented facts on prominent figures in medicine and nursing history.[1]

Many of Dorothy's sanitation dilemmas were remedied using Sunbrite Cleanser. Dorothy encouraged listeners to save their Sunbrite Cleanser labels and mail them to join the Sunbrite Junior Nurse Corps.

Girls could save labels to buy the official ring, toothbrush, bracelet, first aid kit, and more. Dorothy motivated girls to practice cleanliness, to learn first aid, to form Junior Nurse Corps groups, and to tell their moms to buy Sunbrite Cleanser.[2]

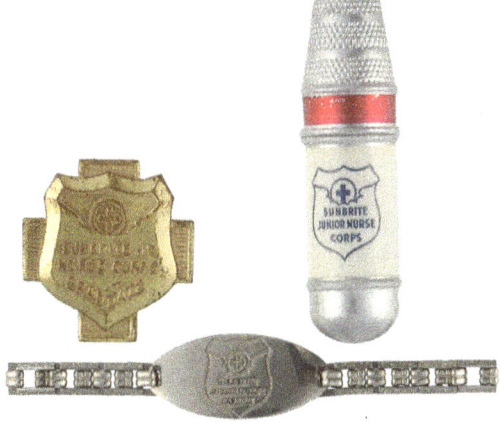

Figure 06.02. The radio show premiums: the pin, a bracelet, and a first aid kit. (Author's collection)

Chapter Six

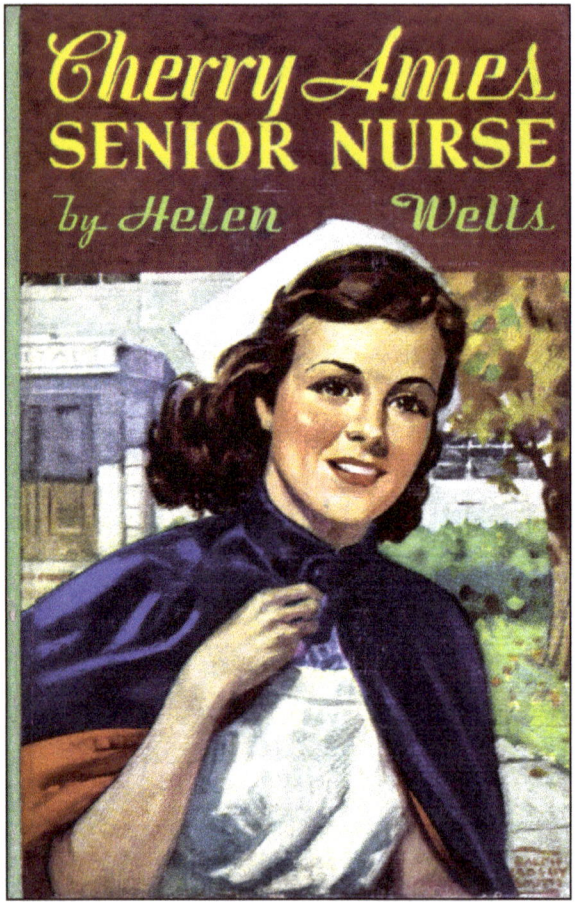

Figure 06.03. *Cherry Ames, Senior Nurse* Cover, 1944. (Springer Publishing)

Many young women wanted to become nurses after reading the stories of Cherry Ames. She solved mysteries while job-hopping from 1943 to 1968. Author Helen Wells created her; the books were sold in the United States as well as in Great Britain, Norway, Sweden, Denmark, Finland, Iceland, Japan, France, Italy, Holland, and Bolivia.[3]

Ames learned many specialties: flight nurse, army nurse, veteran nurse, private duty nurse, cruise nurse, clinic nurse, dude ranch nurse, rest home nurse, island nurse, rural nurse, jungle nurse, ski nurse, and others.

Springer Publishing reprinted several Cherry Ames titles in 2005. Her story, "The Big Wind" (*Cherry Ames, Girls Annual*, 1960), stated she was on her way home from a case in Los Angeles. Thus, the globetrotting Cherry Ames was a nurse of Los Angeles.

Girls Who Dreamt to Become a Nurse

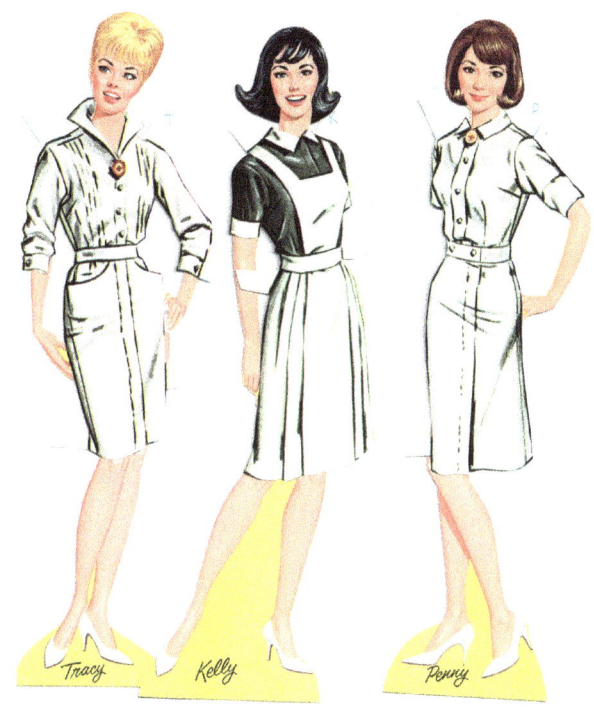

Figure 06.04. Paper doll cut-outs of the three Scott sisters, Tracy, Kelly, and Penny, 1965.

The three Scott sisters were characters in a fictional book series, *The Nurses Three*. Each sister had her own set of books.

Tracy, the oldest, was the self-assured, artistic one interested in pediatrics. The middle sister, Penny, was a tomboy who plunged herself into danger. The baby of the family, Kelly, was the sensitive one who tried to cope with the pressures of being a student nurse and her family's expectations. [4]

Figure 06.05. Paper cut-out outfits, 1965. The Whitman Publishing Company created two unique sets of paper dolls with many outfit changes. [5]

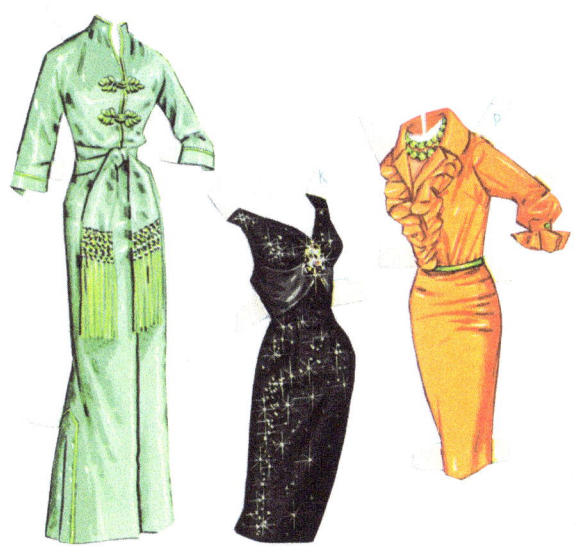

World War II: 1942-1945

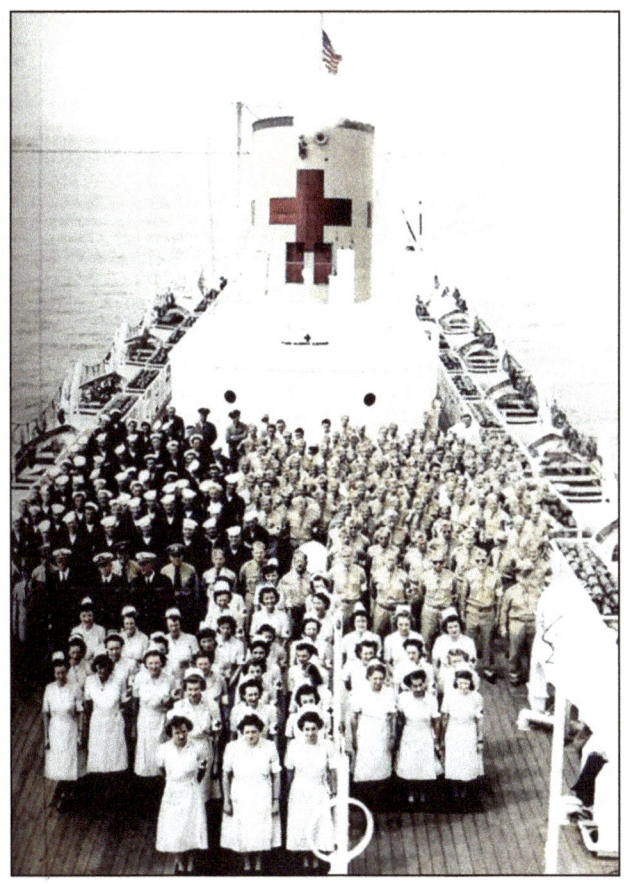

Figure 07.01. USS Comfort, AH-6, in Los Angeles Harbor, June 1944. C. Army Medical Personnel and Navy Crew on deck of the *Comfort* hospital ship prior to their trip to the Pacific Theatres. U.S. Army-controlled and U.S. Navy-built, the *Comfort* had a patient capacity of 400. On 28 April 1945, a kamikaze pilot stuck the *Comfort* with his plane, loaded to capacity with wounded from Okinawa. One hundred died, including six Army nurses.[1]

More than 60,000 nurses served stateside and overseas during WWII. In 1942, Japanese soldiers in the Philippines captured sixty-seven Army nurses and detained them as prisoners of war (POWs) for more than two and a half years. A second group of eleven Navy nurses were interred in Philippines for thirty-seven months. Five Navy nurses were captured on Guam and imprisoned for five months until they were exchanged. Nurses from Los Angeles were included in all three groups of POW nurses.[2]

Chapter Seven

Figure 07.02. Dorothy Still in her senior yearbook, 1935. C.

Dorothy Still graduated from the County General Hospital School of Nursing in 1935. After graduation, she joined the Navy and worked in Los Angeles, dating young doctors and aviation cadets, until she received orders to report to the Naval Hospital at Canacao, in the Philippines. She enjoyed the Philippines and started a journal of her journey.

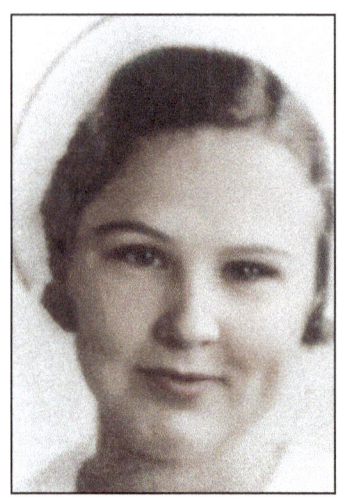

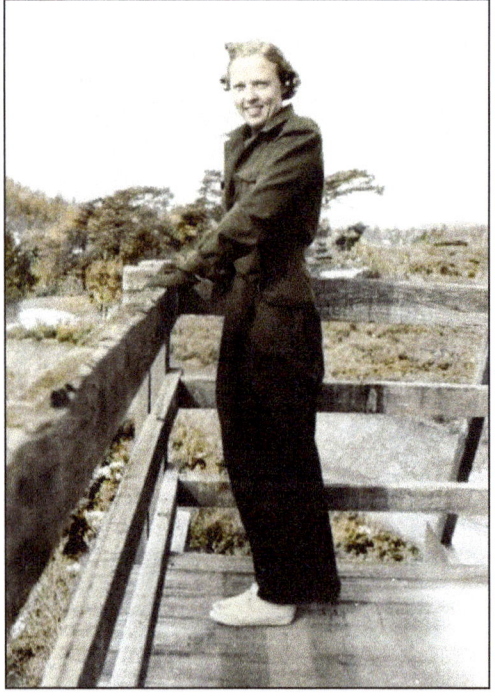

Ten hours after the Japanese attacked Pearl Harbor in 1941 they bombed the U.S. Naval Yard in the Philippines, and Still's life changed. Fatalities overwhelmed the hospital.

The Japanese captured and interred Still and eleven other Navy nurses for more than three years at Los Banos.

The Japanese fed them only 500 calories per day. However, under the command of their meticulous chief nurse, they continued to care for the sick with whatever medical supplies they could find.

Figure 07.03. Lieutenant Dorothy Still after her rescue, 1945. C. (National Naval Medical Center). The nurses were liberated in a harrowing rescue when American paratroopers dropped behind enemy lines.

In 1995 she married, became Dorothy Still Danner, and published her journal, *What a Way to Spend a War: Navy Nurse POWs in the Philippines.* [3]

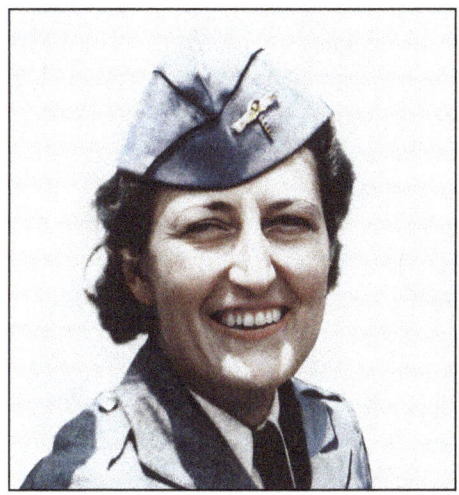

Figure 07.04. Edith Corns in her Aerial Nurse Corps of America uniform, 1936. C.

Edith Mary Corns graduated from Los Angeles County General Hospital School of Nursing in 1935. Corns and Still trained in the same nursing class. After graduation, in 1936, she joined the Aerial Nurse Corps of America, member #12. She became their first chief of staff and the first commander of Wing #1 and Division #1. [4]

When WWII began, Corns joined the Army, was stationed in the Philippines, and was captured and interned in 1942. The Army nurses set up two hospitals in the jungle. They cared for more than 7,000 sick and injured soldiers in 12 to 18-hour shifts, despite their own illnesses and severe weight loss. Corns lost thirty pounds. The Army nurses were also liberated in February 1945.

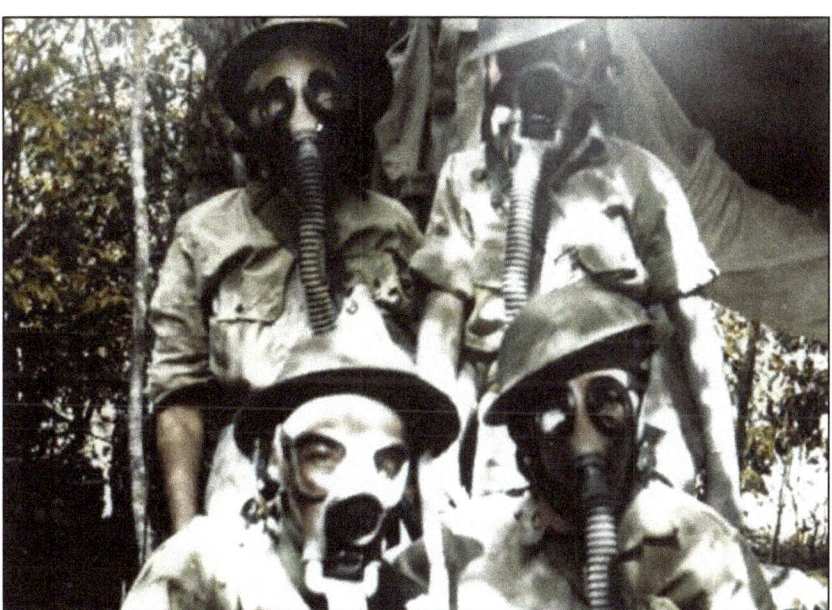

Figure 07.05. Army nurses Rose Rieper and Mary Moultrie (standing) with Edith Corns and Beth Veley pose in their helmets and gas masks in the Nurses' Quarters, General Hospital #2, Bataan, Philippines, 1942. C. (Army Nurse Corps Collection, Office of Medical History)

Chapter Seven

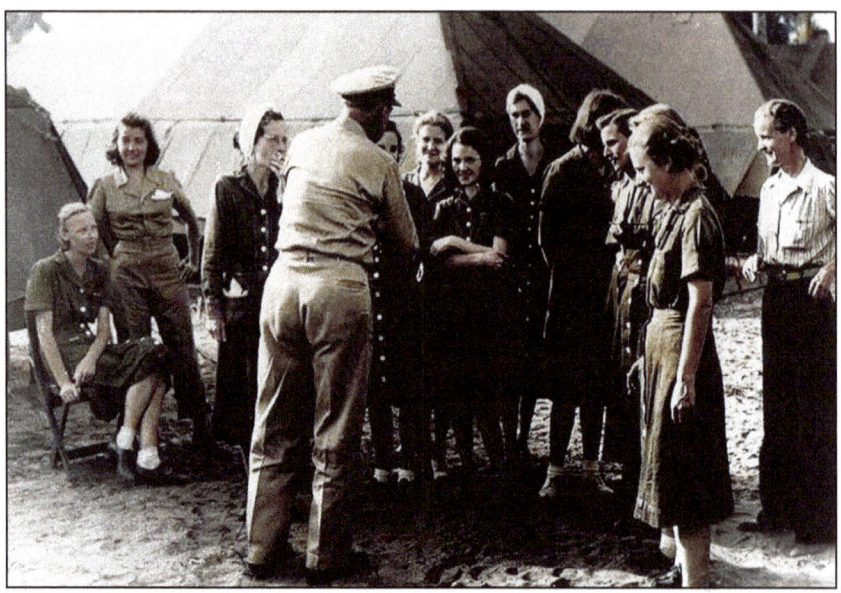

Figure 07.06. Admiral Kinkaid briefs the nurses after liberation, 1945. C. Dorothy Still (sitting in the chair) had developed the vitamin B1 deficiency beriberi and couldn't stand. "Now it was one blinding flashbulb after another as we neatly posed with Admiral Kinkaid," Still said, "until I messed up the arrangement for further pictures by fainting." [5]

In the early 1940s, young nurses joined the military to seek adventure. Most thought they had found paradise in the Philippines: beautiful beaches, a balmy climate, ball gowns from Josie's dress shop in Manila, and formal dances under thousands of stars.

Ten hours after the Japanese bombed Pearl Harbor, they flattened the Navy Yard in Manila Bay. The United States had never sent nurses to the front lines of a war; in the Philippines, the front lines came to them.

Eleven Navy nurses were taken prisoners of war and sent to Santo Tomas Internment Camp in Manila. They cared for 3,500 civilians until they voluntarily moved to Los Banos to establish a primitive hospital. The Japanese captured Army nurses on Corregidor and sent them to Los Banos to join the Navy nurses. The nurses tended to the injured despite constant fatigue from lack of food. They ate anything they found, including rats and swamp weeds. Eighty-two Army and Navy nurses were captured in the Pacific Theatre.

On 23 February 1945, the military received information that the Japanese planned to massacre everyone in the camp. In a daring attempt behind enemy lines, paratroopers rescued them after thirty-seven months of internment.

WWII

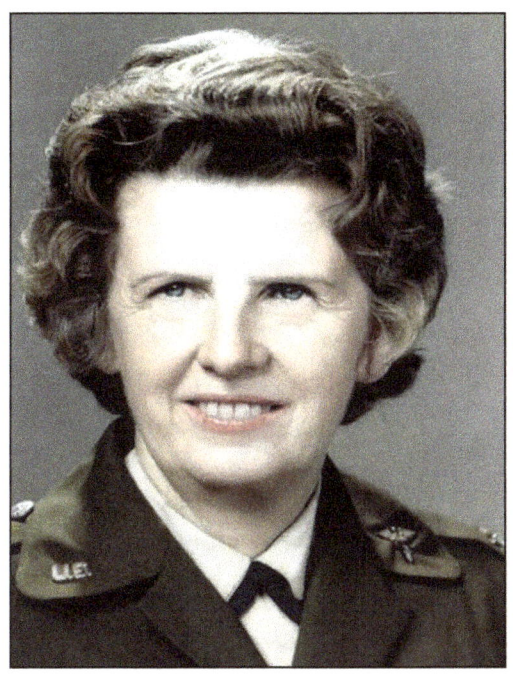

Figure 07.07. Colonel Ruby Grace Bradley, the director of nursing activities, Brooke Army Medical Center, Fort Sam Houston, Texas, n.d. C.

Bradley graduated from nursing school in 1933 and entered the Army Nurse Corps as a surgical nurse in 1934. She was serving at Camp John Hay in Baguio in the Philippines when the Japanese Army captured her three weeks after the 7 December 1941 attack on Pearl Harbor. She was the first nurse under fire.

Bradley assisted with 230 operations and delivered thirteen babies of prisoners; for one delivery she used tea strainers, gauze, and ether to anesthetize a woman in labor. They called her the Angel in Fatigues.

The POWs subsisted on one half-cup of rice twice a day; however, Bradley shared her rations with the children. She weighed 86 pounds when the U.S. liberated Manila in February 1945.

When she returned to the U.S., she completed her Bachelor of Science in Nursing Education at the University of California, Los Angeles, in 1949.

In 1950 the Army sent her to Taegu, South Korea. The North Korean Army overtook Taegu, but she refused to leave until she confirmed all the wounded had been loaded onto the last plane. She jumped aboard just as her ambulance exploded from enemy shells. The Army placed her in charge of all five hundred nurses in the Korean theater of war.

With thirty-four awards, she was the Army's most decorated female soldier. They promoted her to the rank of colonel in 1958—one of the first two women to hold the permanent rank of colonel. She retired in 1963. [6]

Bradley bought a ranch in Riane County, West Virginia, and worked 17 years as a nursing supervisor. In 1954 she was featured on the television show "This is Your Life." She told the reporter, "I want to be remembered as just an Army nurse." [7-8] She was buried in Arlington National Cemetery. [9]

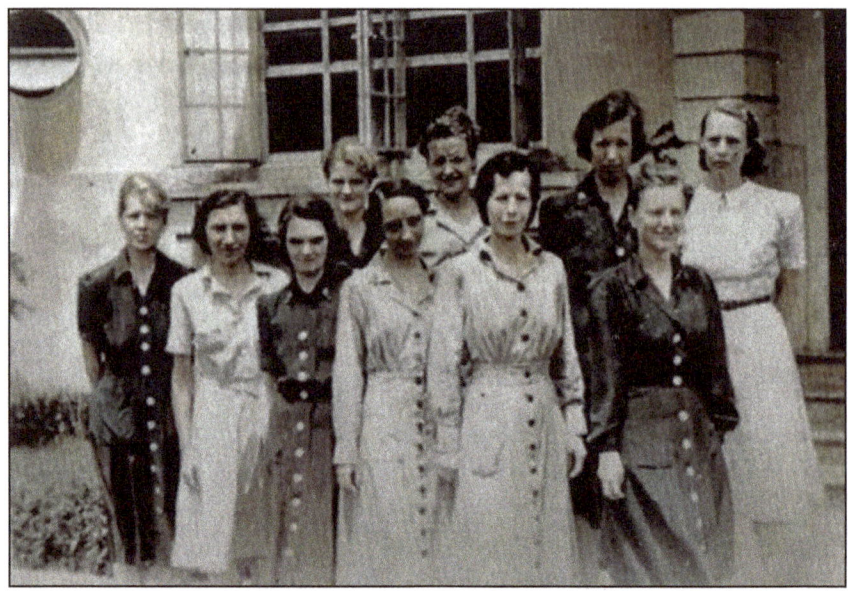

Figure 07.08. In front of the main building at Santo Tomas, a civilian POW internment camp. Photo by a Japanese guard, April/May 1942. C. L to R, Susie Pitchard, Helen Gorzelanski, Margaret Nash, Eldene Paige, Edwina Todd, Mary Rose, Harrington Nelson, Goldia O'Haver, Bertha Evans St. Pierre, Dorothy Still Danner.

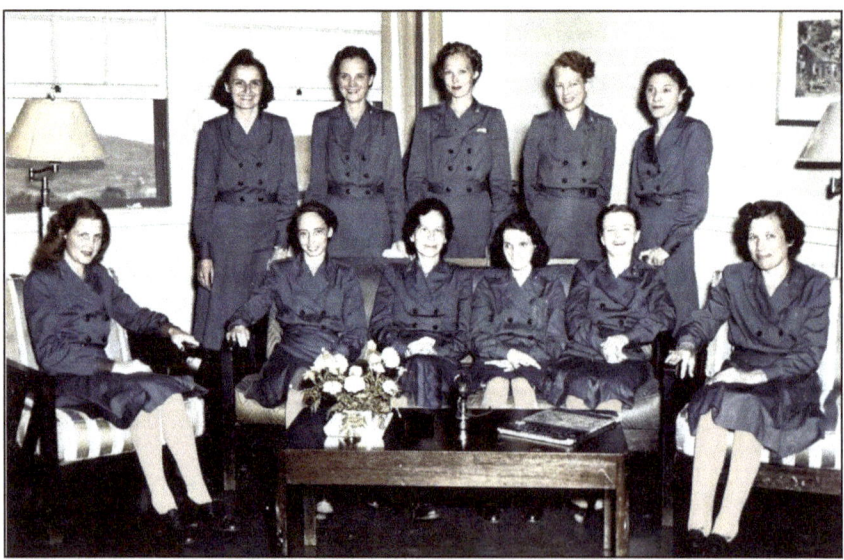

Figure 07.09. Navy nurses at Aiea Naval Hospital, Honolulu, March 1945. Edwina Todd seated fifth from left, Dorothy Danner standing third from left.

WWII

U.S. Army troops of the 11th Airborne Division and Filipino guerrillas stormed Los Baños by land and parachute on 23 February 1945. [10]

"Protect the babies with all your life," a supervisory U.S. Navy nurse told Lieutenant Edwina Todd as they crawled aboard a tractor. [11] Todd and colleague Elizabeth Nash moved two days-old infants and their mothers. Stray bullets flew in every direction. A small tractor brought them to the beach to larger amphibious tractors (Amtracs). One nurse covered a baby with a big hat and lay down on the sand over her. [12]

A soldier crawled over and told them, "When they stop shooting, with all the strength God gave you, grab the baby and get to the waiting Amtracs." On the bumpy ride to the beach, Todd and Nash held the babies while the other Navy nurses continued to care for the sick and injured. [13]

Japanese fired as the nurses scrambled to protect the patients. They finally made it to an Amtrac, but it sped off before the doors were properly closed. Water rushed in. "We held the babies over our heads," Nash said, "and wondered if we were going to drown. Someone closed the doors just in time. The Amtracs outran the gunfire, and we made it to a safer shore." [14]

Lieutenant Todd (1911-1996) grew up in California, graduated from Huntington Memorial Hospital School of Nursing in 1936, and joined the Navy Nurse Corps.

They assigned Todd to Canacao Naval Hospital at Cavite Navy Yard in the Philippines, eight miles southwest of Manila. Japanese bombers destroyed Cavite shipyard on 10 December 1941, three days after Pearl Harbor. Casualties filled the hospital; they had to operate on the floor and on steps. [15]

U.S. forces retreated to Corregidor when the Japanese landed in Luzon. The Navy nurses were forgotten, left behind. The Japanese invaded the hospital, and the nurses became POWs. One Navy nurse escaped aboard a submarine.

In March of 1942, the Japanese transferred the nurses to a 45-acre civilian internment camp at the University of Santo Tomas in Manila. They next transferred them to a camp called Los Banos; ten Navy nurses cared for 200 patients every day, including the Japanese guards, until U.S. and Filipino forces employed that daring land and parachute rescue in February.

During the Korean War, the Navy commissioned Todd as chief nurse and the first female commander of a Navy hospital ship, USS *Consolation* (later called US *Hope*). She remained in the Navy for 30 years, ending her highly decorated service in 1966 with the rank of captain—the highest rank a nurse could hold at the time. [16] Todd is buried in Arlington National Cemetery.

Chapter Seven

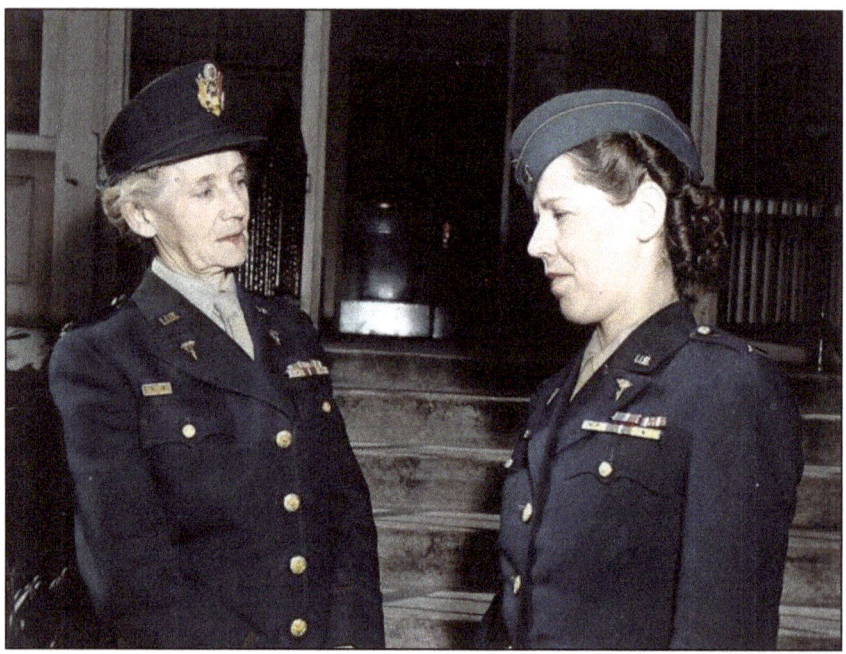

Figure 07.10. Major Maude C. Davison, left, and Lieutenant Eunice F. Young, ANC, at Letterman General Hospital in San Francisco, 1945. C. Davison was the commanding officer and the principal chief nurse in charge of POW Army nurses imprisoned in Santo Thomas, Philippines, during WWII. Young was also a WWII nurse POW. (AMEDD)

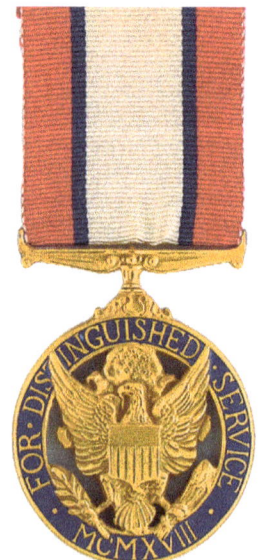

Figure 07.11. Army Distinguished Service Medal awarded to Davison, posthumously, on August 20, 2001. POW nurses credited Davison for their survival.

After the war, ANC officials nominated her for an Army Distinguished Service Medal; the War Decorations Board denied the honor—they incorrectly determined she did not work independently.[17] In 2001, Brigadier General Connie Slewitzke, Senator Daniel Inouye, Beth Norman, and the surviving "Angels of Bataan" lobbied to insure she received it.[18]

In 1947, Davison married Reverend Charles W. Jackson, who served as dean of Long Beach City College. They had originally met during her nursing studies in Pasadena.

WWII

Maude C. Davison graduated from Pasadena Hospital Training School for Nurses in 1917. She joined the Nurse Reserves of the United States Army Nurse Corps in 1918; she worked at Camp Fremont in Palo Alto, Letterman General Hospital, and at Fort Leavenworth. Canadian born, she finally became a U.S. citizen in 1920 and joined the regular Army Nurse Corps (ANC). She served in Germany from 1921 to 1922, assisting war casualties. In 1924 she became a first lieutenant. [19]

The Army deployed her to Fort Mills Station Hospital on Corregidor Island, Philippines, in 1939. They promoted her to captain in 1941 and chief nurse—all nurses in the Far East Command served under Davison. When the Japanese invaded the Philippines, after the December 1941 attack on Pearl Harbor, Davison organized civilian nurses to manage the casualties.

They evacuated the Army nurses from Manila to Bataan. Davison left for Bataan with the last of the American troops to coordinate nursing activities in the two jungle hospitals: Hospital #1 and Hospital #2. She had also directed nurses to set up the hospital on Corregidor in the Malinta Tunnel: she established eight wards in the underground hospital with one central hallway in lateral corridors, one hundred yards long. [20]

A strict disciplinarian, she required nurses to follow Army regulations to the letter, even in the Japanese-run camp. Camp conditions caused the death of 390 of the 3,785 captives. None of the nurses died. [21] When nurses arrived in the U.S. after their liberation, Davison, who normally weighed 135 pounds, weighed only 80. [22] She medically retired from the ANC in 1946.

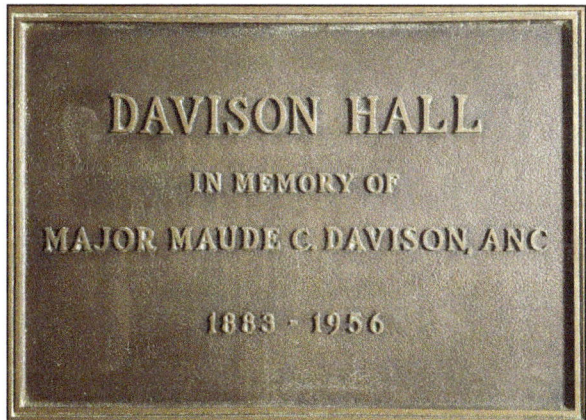

Figure 07.12. Plaque on the Memorial barracks, building 1002, Fort Sam Houston, San Antonio, Texas. On March 5, 1957, the ANC dedicated Davison Hall, a residence for women officers at Brooke Army Medical Center, Fort Sam Houston, Texas. (AMEDD)

Chapter Seven

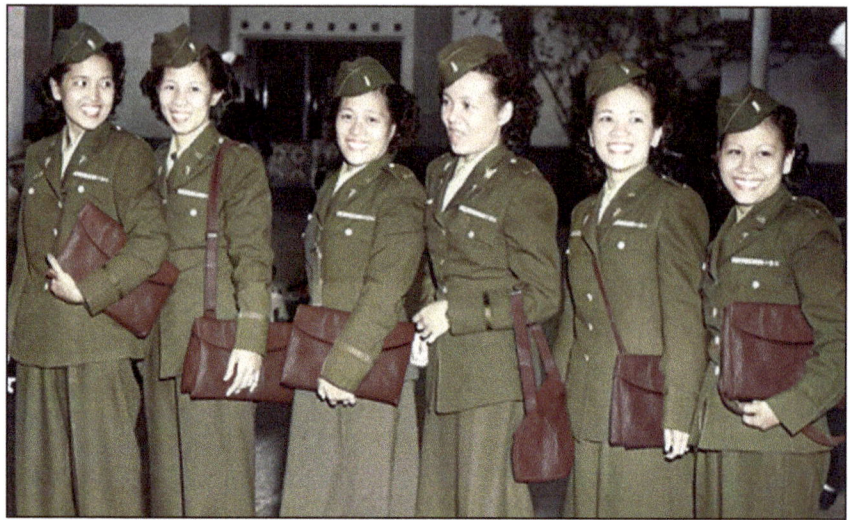

Figure 07.13. Six Filipino-American nurses arriving in Los Angeles after being released from a Japanese prison, August 8, 1945. C. (Department of Special Collections, Charles E. Young Research Library, UCLA)

According to POW nurse Lieutenant Josie Nesbit, twenty-five Filipino nurses were transported to Bataan via trucks on 24 December 1941. Filipino nurses who worked with the Army nurses were taken to Bilibid Prison. Two Filipino nurses, Maureen Davis and Betty Brian, were sent with the Americans because their husbands were American soldiers.

Little information was available about the POW Filipino American nurses. Lieutenant Gwendolyn Henshaw, interred at Santo Thomas, wrote a seven-part series in the *Los Angeles Times* on her internment while she recuperated at Birmingham Military Hospital in Van Nuys. She said, "At the time of surrender on Corregidor, about 9,000 patients were in the hospital with 58 American and 40 Filipino nurses. The Filipino nurses were separated from us."[23]

President Reagan proclaimed 9 April 1983 as National POW-MIA Day.[24] Lieutenant Edith Corns, a Los Angeles County Hospital graduate, reported that President Reagan invited sixty-two Filipino nurses to Washington, D.C., to be honored at the event.

Lieutenant Corns worked in the underground hospital in the Malinta Tunnel on Corregidor. "When Bataan fell, I could tell no help was coming," Lloyd said. "The prisoners' resiliency was one thing I think the Japanese never understood. When they cut down our rations, it would get us for a while, but we would bounce back, and I think that irritated them. We didn't take drastic action."[25]

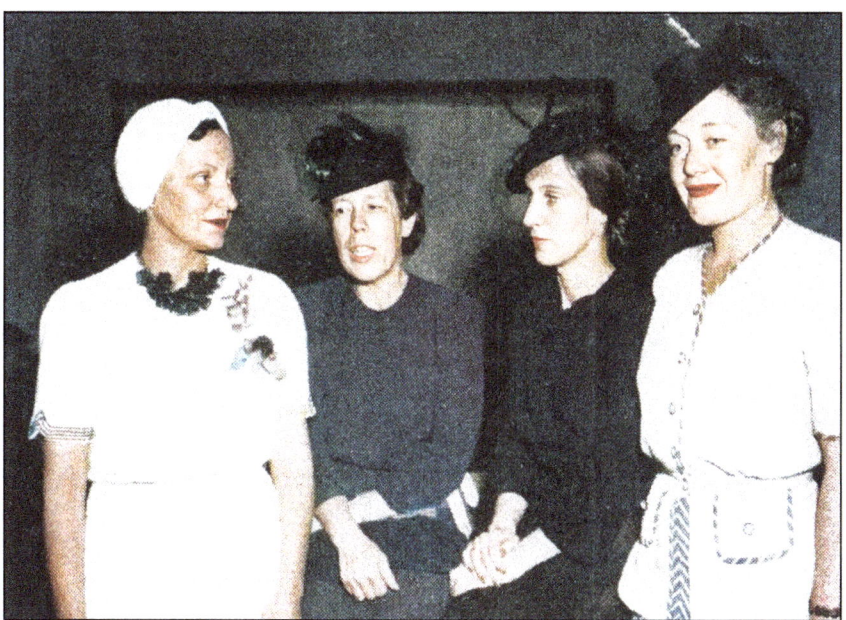

Figure 07.14. Lieutenant Doris Yetter, left, with three other POW nurses who served on Guam, after arriving home in 1945. C.

Los Angeles nurse Doris Yetter, USN, was one of five nurses the Japanese captured on Guam in 1942. The nurses lived in a prison camp in Zentsuji, Japan, with 300 male prisoners.[26] The Japanese didn't know how to manage female prisoners, so in June 1942 they exchanged them for Japanese prisoners.

Several nurses from the Los Angeles area were interred during WWII. Among them were Edith Corns, Verna Henson, Letha McHale, Gwendolyn Henshaw, Dorothy Still Danner, Doris Delancy, Doris Yetter, Edwina Todd, and Maude Davison.[27]

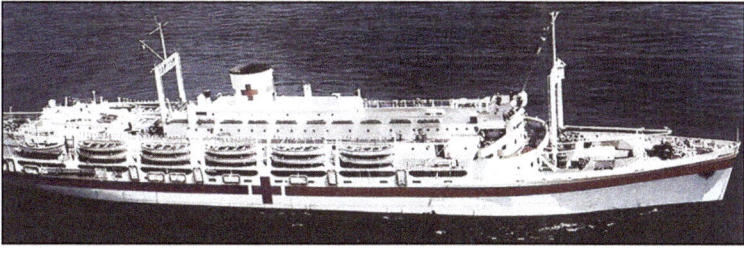

Figure 07.15. USS *Mercy* (A-H9) in San Pedro Bay, n.d. C. In 1943, the Navy converted the *Mercy* into a hospital ship in Los Angeles; Yetter sponsored and christened it. *Mercy* transported thousands from Leyte to New Guinea and from Saipan to Okinawa. *Mercy* returned to San Pedro in 1945.

Chapter Seven

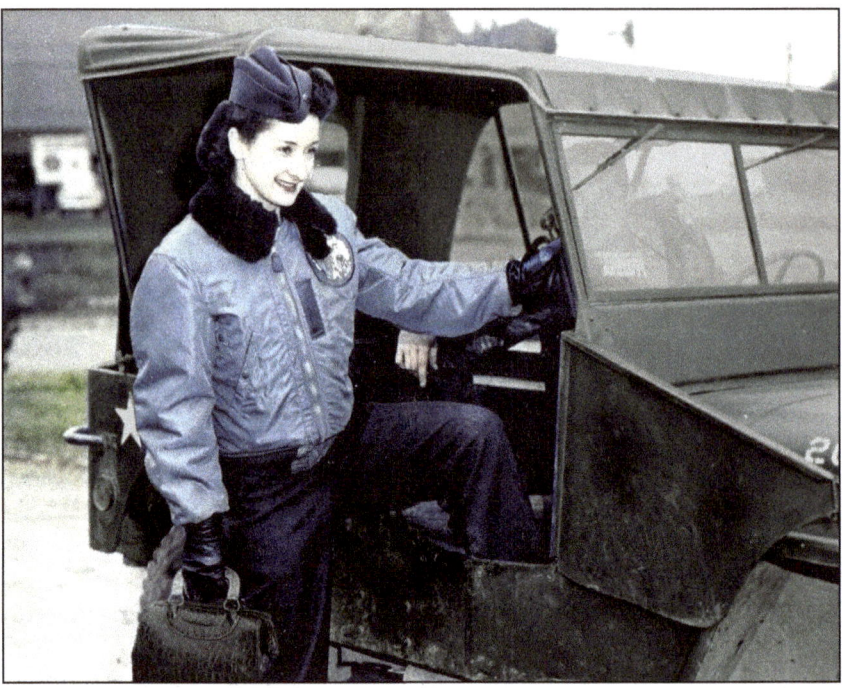

Figure 07.16. Lillian Kinkella Keil at Tachikawa Air Base during the Korean War, c. 1950. C. (U.S. Air Force)

In 1938, Lillian Kinkella Keil became a United Airlines stewardess. On a flight to Santa Barbara, in 1943, a passenger told Keil, "There's a war going on. You belong in the Air Force." The School of Evacuation at Bowman Fields accepted Keil; she became a pioneer flight nurse. More than one million patients were evacuated during World War II. Only four died en route.

Keil pulled frostbitten solders from B-17s and witnessed buzz bombs in London. She collected D-Day wounded from Normandy. She conducted 250 evacuation flights including twenty-three transatlantic flights.

In 1950, when the Korean War began, she rejoined the Air Force. Keil flew in 175 Korean air evacuations, logging 1,400 hours of flight time. She received nineteen medals for her service. When she returned home, she became a technical adviser for the 1953 Hollywood movie based on her life, *Flight Nurse*. In 1961 she generated one of the ten highest mail responses ever when she appeared on the popular television program "This Is Your Life." [28]

Following her flight career, she worked in the emergency room in her hometown of Covina, in Los Angeles County. In 2002, Covina dedicated the Lillian Kinkella Keil Post Office at 545 North Rimsdale Avenue. [29-31]

WWII

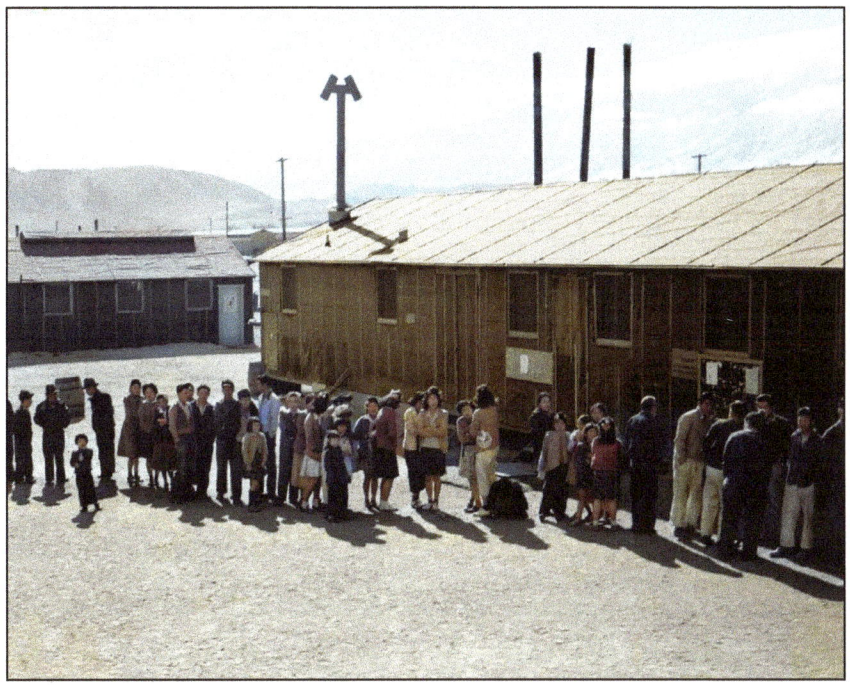

Figure 07.17. Internees wait in line at Manzanar Mess Hall, 1943. C.
Figure 07.18. Manzanar primary living quarters called barracks, 1943. C.

In 1942, Japanese American citizens and Japanese legal residents, from Los Angeles, were interred at Manzanar War Relocation Center in Owens Valley and other centers. The U.S. forcibly detained more than 110,000 men, women, and children in remote military-style camps due to the fear they would become Japanese sympathizers in the war. Ansel Adams, American's best-known photographer, volunteered to photograph the Manzanar War Center. He then donated all his images to the National Archive.[32]

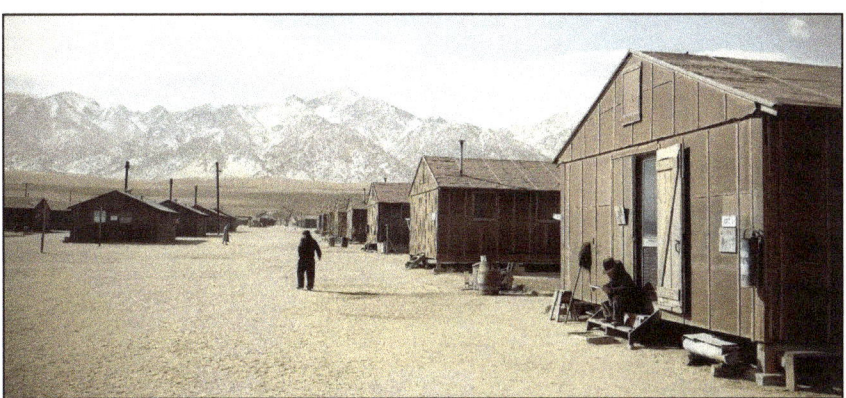

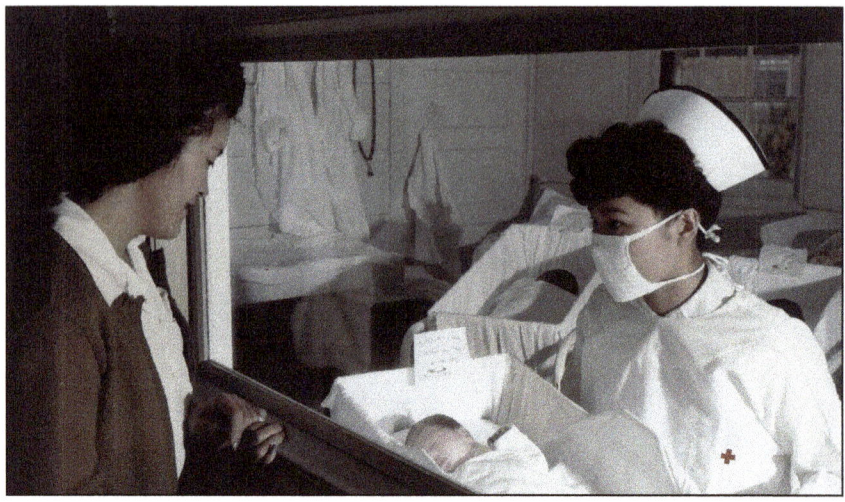

Figure 07.19. Nurse Aiko Hamaguchi (Ansel Adams' most photographed Manzanar resident), Frances Yokoyama, and her baby Fukomoto, 1943. C. Approximately 541 infants were born in Manzanar.

Hamaguchi was born in Long Beach; she lived in Los Angeles and Redondo Beach. She studied pre-nursing at Los Angeles City College and nurses training at Los Angeles General Hospital. She enjoyed reading, horseback riding, and tennis.

Figure 07.20. Nurses enjoying a bridge game in the Manzanar nurses quarters. Kazoko Nagahama, Aiko Hamaguchi, Chiye Yamanai, and Catherine Yamaguchi, left to right, 1943. C. Interred nurses worked in the camp hospital and clinics.

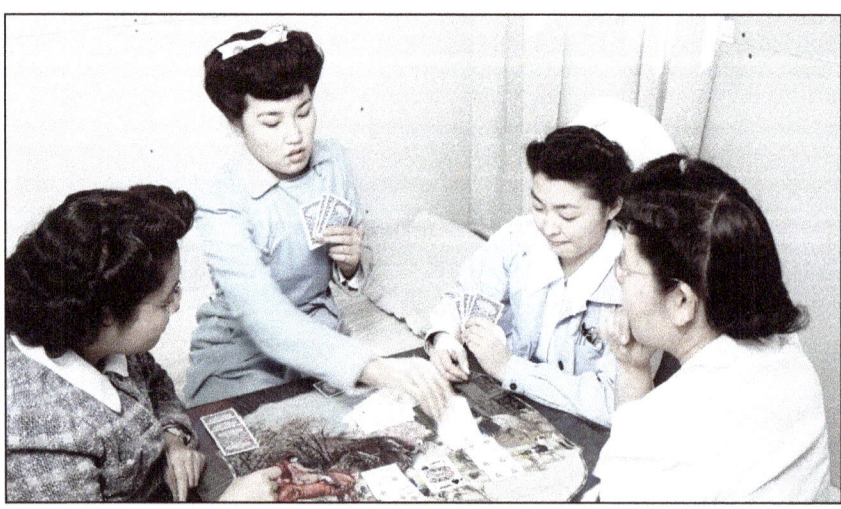

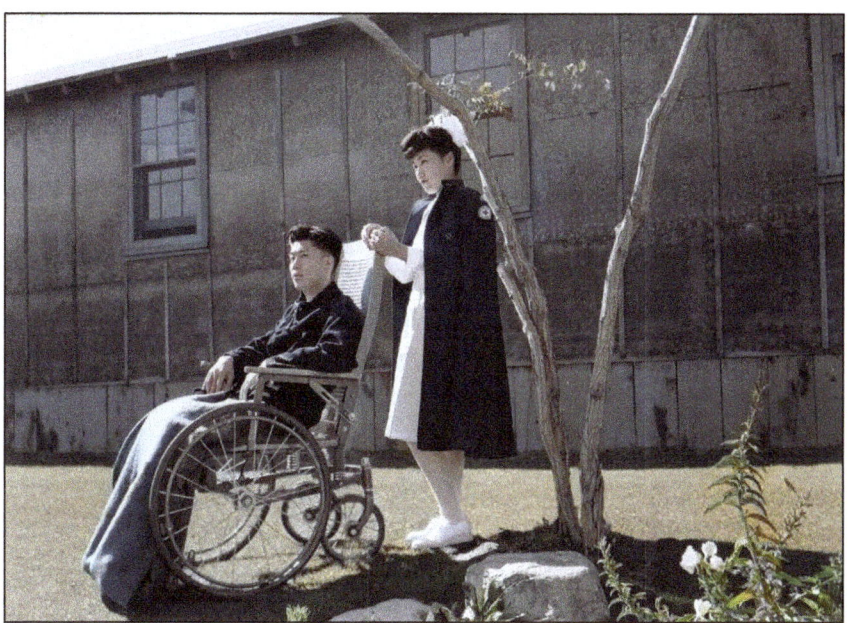

Figure 07.21. Aiko Hamaguchi tending to a patient Tom Kano, 1943, C. Hamaguchi told Ansel Adams that only after her evacuation did she realize she had enjoyed a false sense of security before the war. [33]

Some Manzanar residents found work and relocated to Midwestern or Eastern states. Hamaguchi found a position in a clinic in Detroit, left Manzanar, and became a public health nurse. The last internees evacuated in 1945. Former internees and others persuaded Congress of its historical importance; they established Manzanar as a National Historic Site on 3 March 1992.

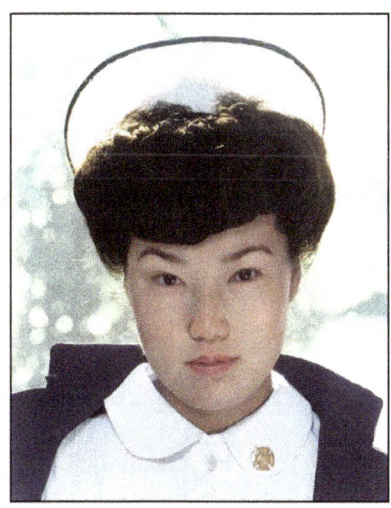

Figure 07.22. Aiko Hamaguchi at Manzanar, 1943. C. (Ansel Adams)

Most Japanese Americans interned in Manzanar lost their homes for "failure to pay taxes." Some had sold their businesses for pennies on the dollar and never recovered from the losses.

In 1988 Congress apologized, on behalf of the nation, for injustices inflicted on persons of Japanese ancestry. They authorized $20,000 payments to Japanese Americans who had suffered these injustices. [34]

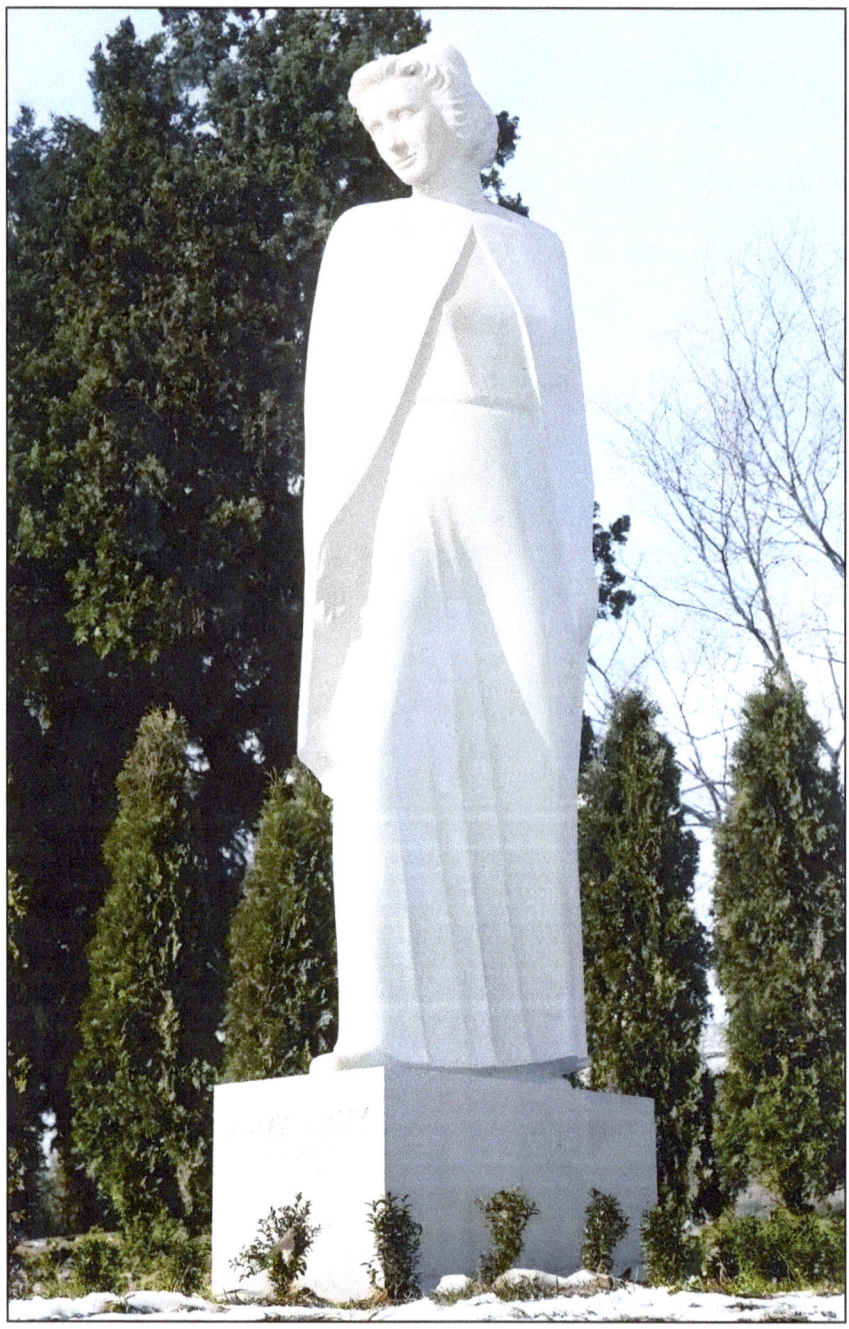

Figure 07.23. The *Nurses Memorial* at Arlington National Cemetery before the Navy Nurse Corps installed a bronze plaque over the carved inscription of Army and Navy Nurses, c. 1939. C. (National Archives)

WWII

Yoshiko Taigawa Traynor completed high school at Tule Lake Relocation Center. She decided to become a nurse; St. Barnabas welcomed her into their 1944 Cadet Nurse Corps. After graduation she tried to join the Navy, but they did not accept Japanese Americans. She didn't get angry; she just waited for the rules to change. In 1948 the rules did change, and Yoshiko was hired at Long Beach Naval Hospital as the only Japanese-American officer. She is buried in the nurses' section at Arlington National Cemetery. [35]

An eleven-foot statue, called the *Nurses Memorial*, stands at the top of the slope in Section 21 (the nurses section) of Arlington National Cemetery. The statue looks down the hill to a sea of white military nurses headstones.

Sculptor Frances Rich carved the eleven-foot-tall statue, made of Tennessee marble, in 1937. Rich became a special assistant to Mildred McAfee, Navy WAVES director. Rich left the service in 1946, ranked as a lieutenant commander. Although she wasn't Catholic or particularly religious, she was renowned for her sculptures of saints that adorned churches and museums along the West Coast of California. She also created various technical illustrations for airplane productions.

When the statue was originally installed in 1938, only a few words were carved on the base: Army and Navy Nurses. On July 13, 1970, Navy Captain Delores Cornelius, the deputy director of the Navy Nurse Corps, requested the authority to install a bronze plaque over the inscription on the base of the monument. On 20 November 1970, officials granted her the authority to place a 12-inch-by-18-inch bronze plaque over the carved inscription. [36]

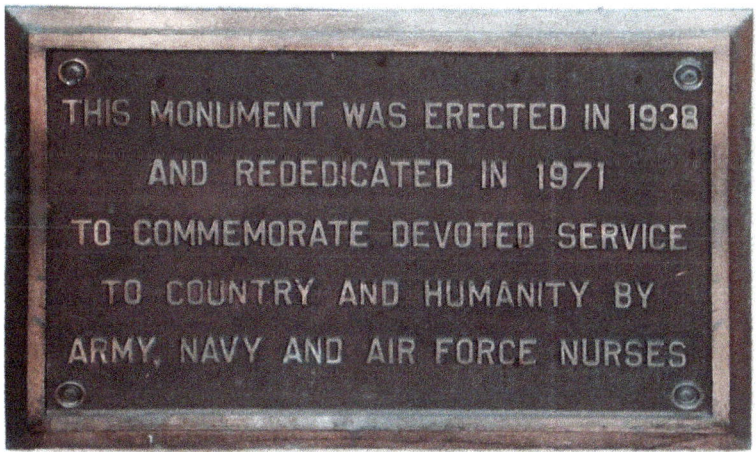

Figure 07.24. The bronze plaque installed at the base of the statue in 1970. The statue is considered a memorial to nurses in all branches of the service. It is sometimes called the *Spirit of Nursing*.

Chapter Seven

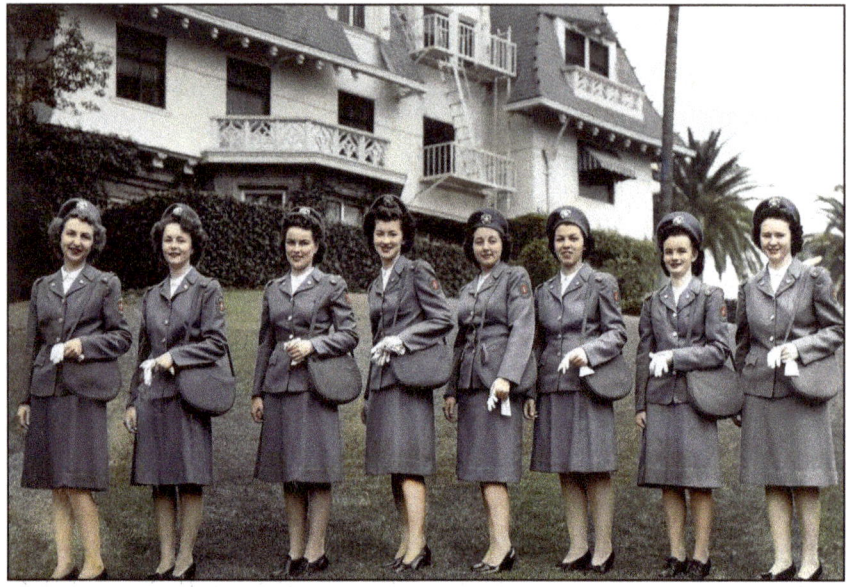

Figure 07.25. Good Samaritan Hospital Cadet Nurses at Lyman Stewart Mansion—the Senior Nurses' Home, 1945. C. (Good Samaritan Hospital)

United States hospitals faced critical shortages during the war because thousands of nurses were deployed overseas. This motivated Congress to pass the Bolton Act of 1943, which established the Cadet Nurse Corps (originally called the Victory Nurse Corps). The U.S. Public Health Service paid trainees' tuition, fees, and a monthly stipend upon enrollment in a school of nursing that met the prescribed standards.

They launched an aggressive recruitment campaign. The *Ladies' Home Journal, Mademoiselle, Cosmopolitan, Colliers, Harper's Bazaar,* and other magazines ran advertisements. Cadet Nurses were featured in movie newsreels, radio soap operas, and variety shows. Cities placed posters in areas frequented by high school girls. Training was accelerated: only 30 months instead of the traditional 36. Cadet Nurses signed a contract to work in a local hospital after graduation. Some joined the Army after completing their contracts. [37]

They issued Cadets two uniforms: a winter wool suit with a beret and a summer pinstriped suit with a large-brimmed hat. The Cadet Nurse uniforms, however, were mainly used for special occasions—students often shared uniforms. In the hospital, students wore their school uniforms with Cadet Nurse arm patches. The program ended in 1948. Graduates totaled 124,065 from all states. Eight Los Angeles hospitals participated: Good Samaritan, California, County General, Queen of Angels, St. Vincent's, White Memorial, Pasadena Hospital, and Glendale Sanitarium.

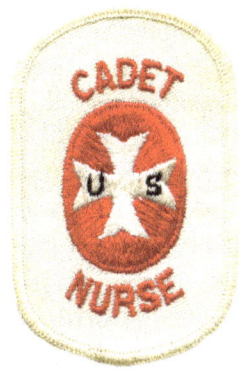 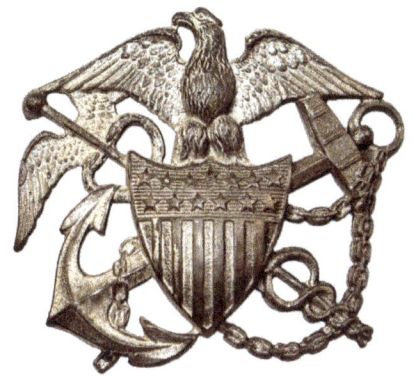

Figure 07.26. The Cadet Nurse Summer Uniform Patch & the Beret Pin.

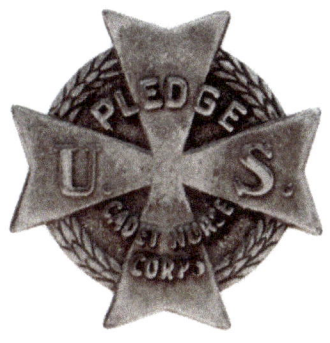

Figure 07.27. Cadet Nurse Corps Pledge Pin, 1943. The government initiated a Cadet Nurse Corps pledge program for high school juniors and seniors to attract and hold the attention of potentially qualified candidates.

During World War II, many American high schools participated in the High School Victory Corps to prepare for a war on the home front and the front lines. The schools provided juniors and seniors with an opportunity to learn a profession (military or civilian) by studying a special wartime program. They placed students who planned to become nurses in the Community Service Division; they studied fundamental courses required for nursing school, including first aid and home nursing. Daily physical education classes were required. The government phased out the Victory Corps program in June 1944. [38]

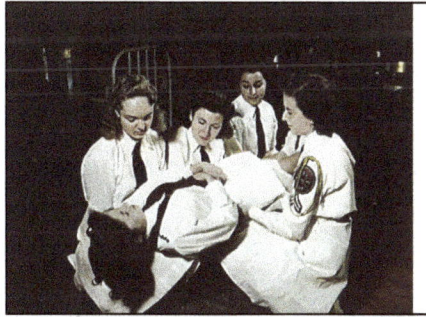 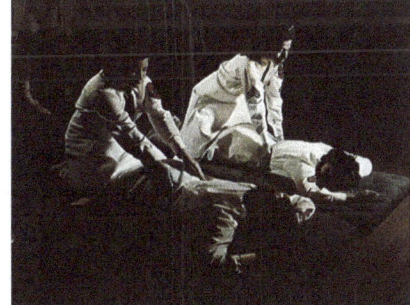

Figure 07.28. Victory Corps members at Roosevelt High School, Los Angeles, practiced first aid and artificial respiration on their classmates, 1944.

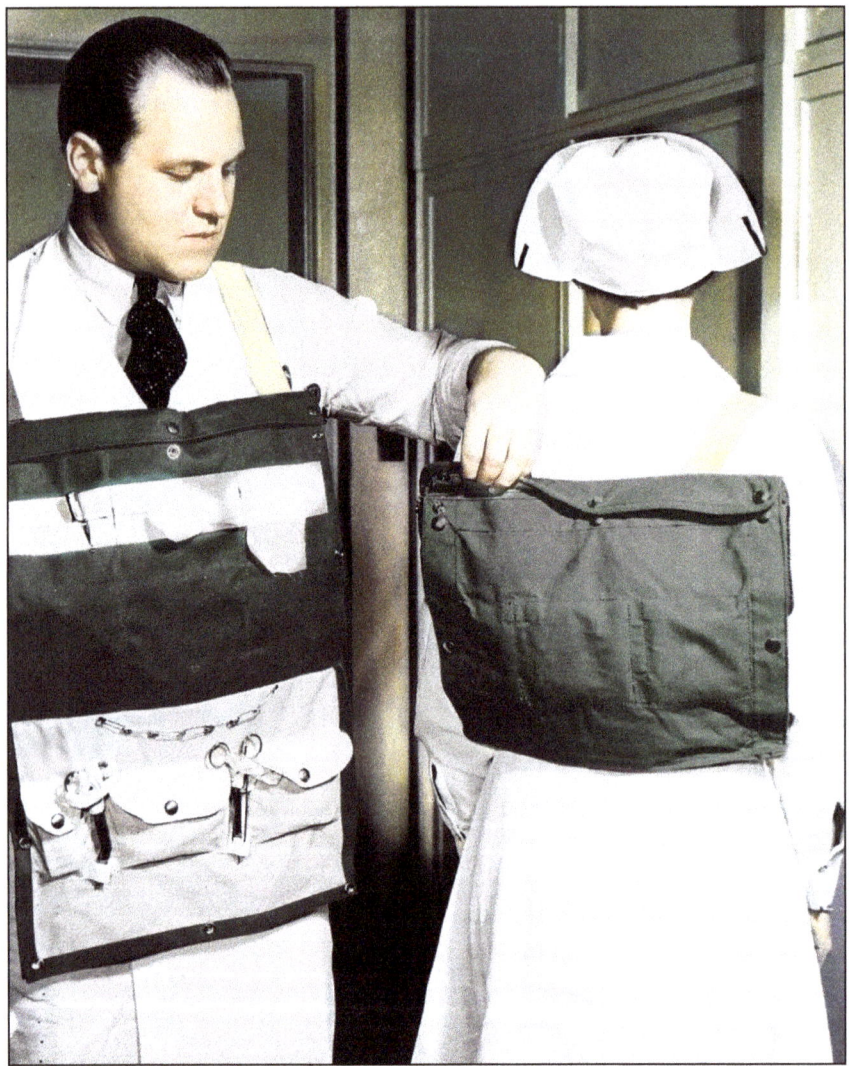

Figure 07.29. A doctor and nurse demonstrate the Campiglia kits, c. 1943. C. (Santa Monica Public Library)

Clementine Campiglia was chief of nurses at the Douglas Aircraft Company during World War II. She read several accounts of the difficulties doctors and nurses encountered while carrying first-aid materials to the scene of air attacks. She decided to design new kits. Her emergency kits were light, compact, and waterproof, yet they contained more than thirty items. The nurses kit weighed four pounds; the doctors kit weighed six. The kits were worn on the back and suspended with straps over the shoulders. At the scene, a doctor or nurse could turn the kit around, open it, and use it as an apron.[39]

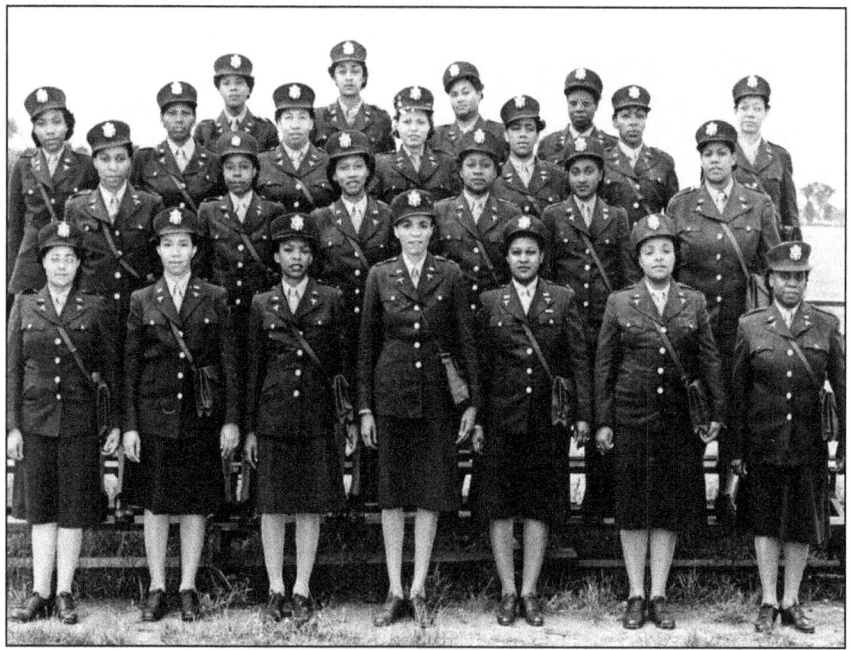

Figure 07.30. Twenty-four nurses who were part of the first contingent of Black nurses assigned to the European Theater of Operations as they landed in England on August 21, 1944, C. Second row, first on the left, is Arlayne Hall of Los Angeles. Benjamin Davis, the first Black brigadier general in the United States Army, greeted the nurses when they arrived.

Black nurses fought for the right to participate in World War II. In 1943, the Army Nurse Corps limited the number of Black nurses to 160. Black nurses were not allowed to treat White soldiers, and White nurses were not allowed to treat Black soldiers. Black nurses were greatly needed so wounded Black soldiers could receive expert care.

Approximately 2,000 Black student nurses were enrolled in the Cadet Nurse Corps program and hospital nursing schools. At the end of the war, about 500 Black nurses had served in Africa, England, Burma, and the Southwest Pacific; however, thousands had applied.

The National Association of Colored Graduate Nurses protested the racial policies in the Army Nurse Corps. An unfavorable public reaction forced the Army to drop its quota system in 1944.

By 1951, the National Association of Colored Graduate Nurses had dissolved into the American Nurses Association, which had extended its membership to all nurses regardless of race. [40]

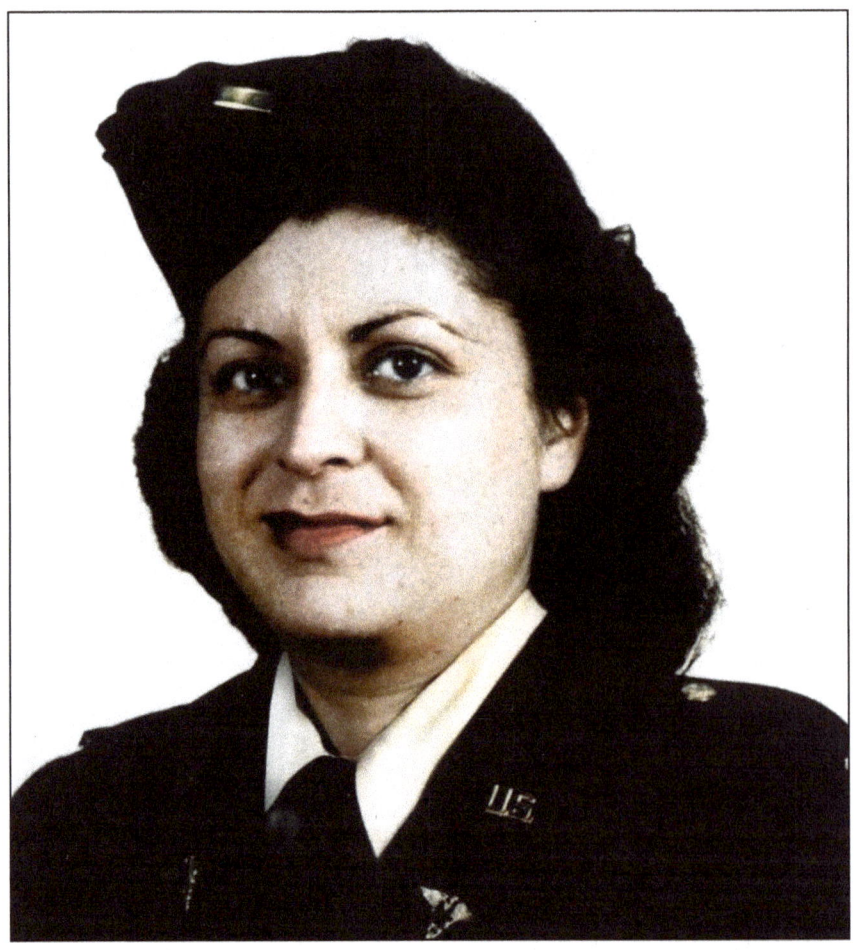

Figure 07.31. Carmen Salazar, Army Nurse Corps, c. 1945. C. (Courtesy of the Military Women's Memorial)

In April 1945, Los Angeles nurse Carmen Salazar joined the Army Nurse Corps. She was assigned to a hospital train unit at the Presidio in San Francisco. The unit transported thousands of wounded servicemen from Letterman General Hospital to hospitals across the United States.

Her patients included ex-prisoners of war from the Philippine Bataan Death March. The Japanese forced 75,000 American and Filipino prisoners of war to march from the Bataan Peninsula to prison camps. They were starved, mistreated, and many bayoneted to death. Between 7,000 and 10,000 POWs died during the march; 10,000 escaped into the jungle. Salazar said, "The soldiers were so grateful for the nursing care they received, and it made me feel that my work with the A.N.C. was very worthwhile." [41]

WWII

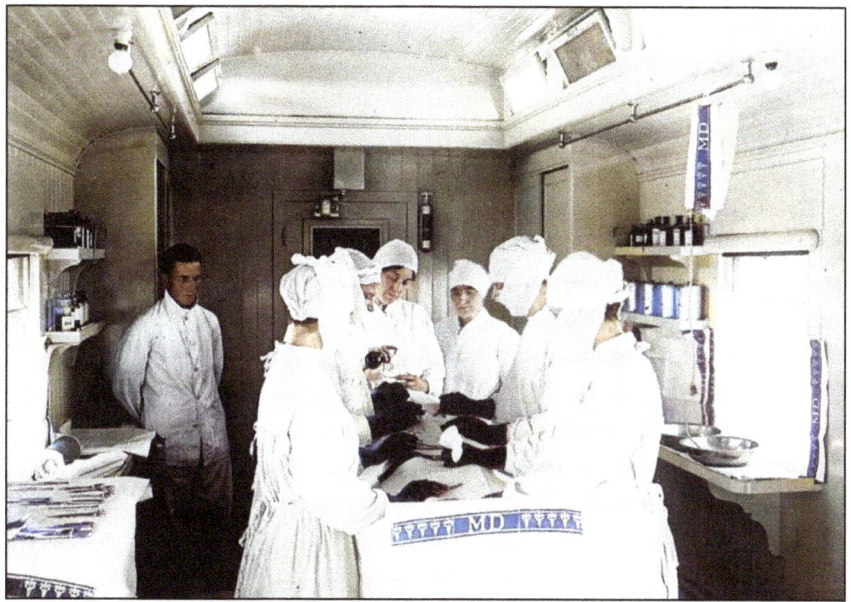

07.32. A Red Cross Railway Surgery Car, 1917. C.

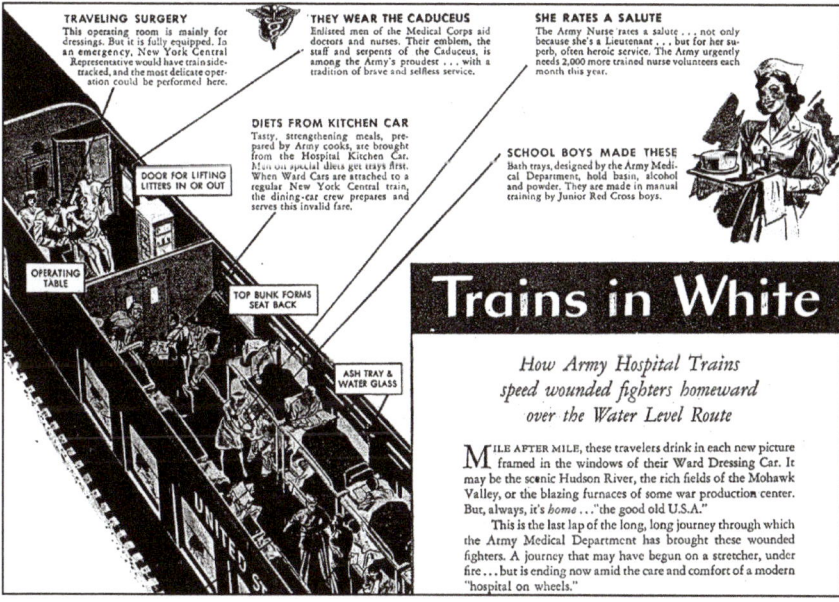

Figure 07.33. Advertisement for an Army Hospital Train in WWII, c. 1943. Each hospital army train contained a kitchen, surgery area, bunks for thirty-two patients, and sleeping areas for the crew. A captain of the Medical Corps commanded a train, assisted by five or six Army nurses and fifty to sixty Medical Enlisted men.

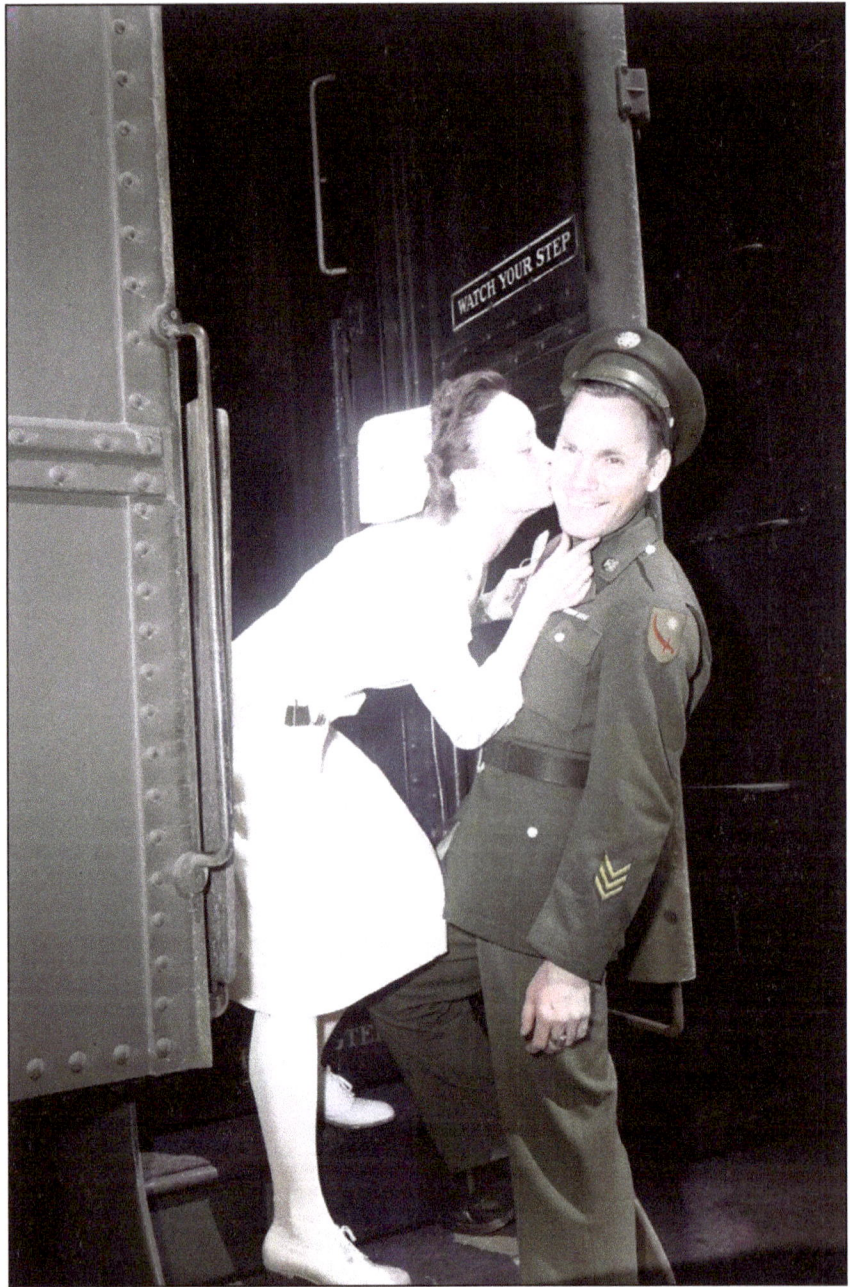

Figure 07.34. The arrival of a hospital train at the Birmingham Military Hospital in San Fernando Valley, 1944. C. Lieutenant Anne Wojick gives a farewell kiss to Private First Class Cecil Fleming. (Department of Special Collections, Charles E. Young Research Library, UCLA)

WWII

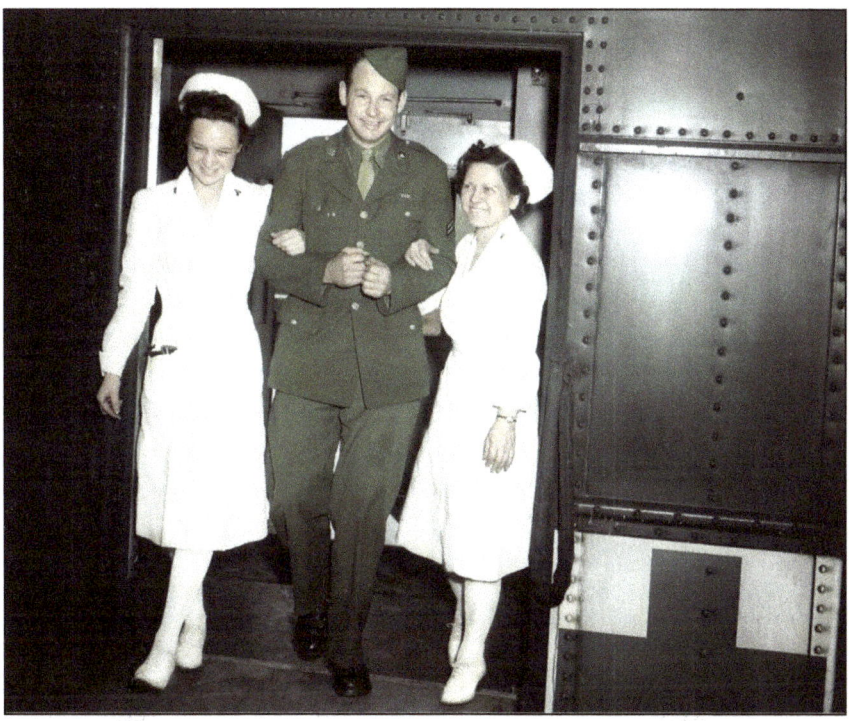

Figure 07.35. Lieutenant Anne Wojick, left, and Lieutenant Thekla Lennon, right, escort Corporal La Sueur from the hospital military train at Birmingham Military Hospital, May 17, 1944. C.

Figure 07.36. Birmingham Military Hospital, 1944. C. (Department of Special Collections, Charles E. Young Research Library, UCLA)

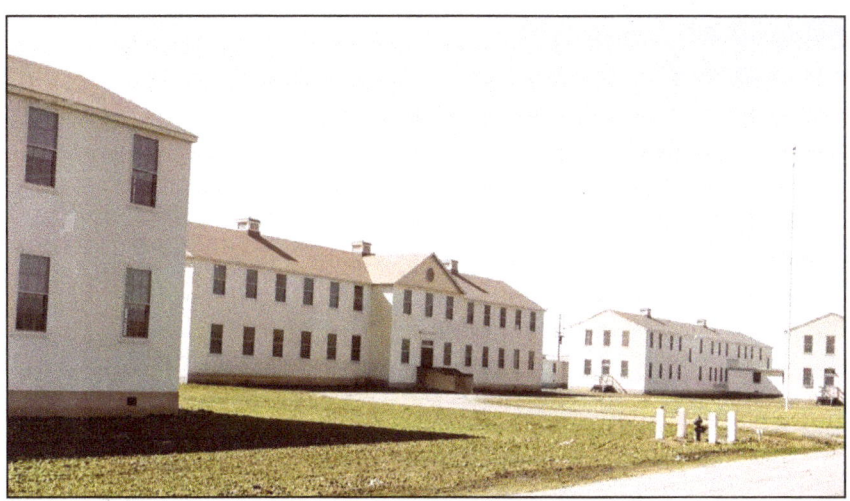

Chapter Seven

In 1943 the U.S. Government built Birmingham General Army Hospital in San Fernando Valley, on a 160-acre lima bean and carrot patch near Balboa Avenue and Van Owen Street in Van Nuys. The buildings housed soldiers returning from the European and Pacific theaters of war. Captain Elizabeth Fitch, the chief nurse, was the first to report for duty on 6 February 1944. The first group of wounded patients arrived on 29 February. A staff of 1,000 greeted them, including Army and civilian nurses. On 23 July, the hospital was still forty-three percent below the required quota of nurses. [42-43]

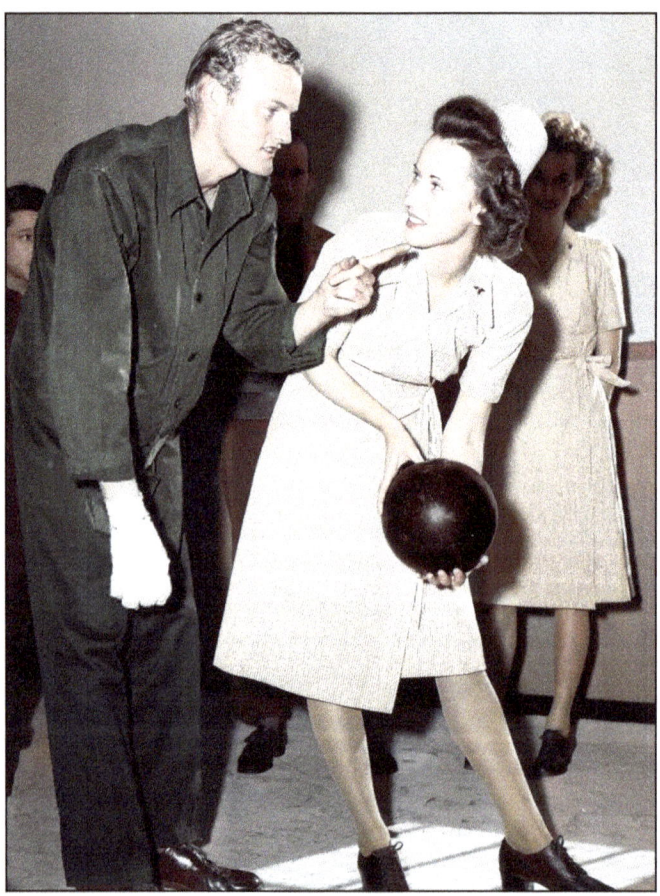

Figure 07.37. Birmingham Hospital Army nurse, in the bowling alley, wearing the brown and white seersucker field hospital uniform, n.d. C. (Dept. of Special Collections, Charles E. Young Research Library, UCLA)

Originally designed for nurses serving overseas, they extended the seersucker uniform to nurses serving in the U.S. in 1945. At first, nurses wore white uniforms, then switched to the seersucker, including the cap. Alice Turner said many nurses could not find stockings and often went bare-legged. [44]

WWII

Alice Sterling Turner was ten years old when the influenza of 1918 infected her entire family. They lived fifteen miles out in the county; only the most severe cases of pneumonia traveled to the twelve-bed hospital in Sweet Grass, Montana. Her brother was a patient. She visited him and thought it would be wonderful to help sick people, so at twenty-one she started nurses training in Great Falls.

Turner moved to Los Angeles in 1935 during the depression. She worked in a private hospital ten-hour shifts for thirty cents per hour. She was helping a doctor change a surgical dressing on 7 December 1941 when they heard the radio announcement about the attack on Pearl Harbor. She enlisted in the Army in 1942.

She joined, and two days later she was working in an Army hospital. The Army did not train nurses; they had to learn Army procedures on their own. She first went to Camp Stoneman and then to Birmingham Hospital in Van Nuys. She said the Navy soldiers were surprised to see nurses giving baths and treatments. They were used to corpsmen doing that job.

Turner said the Navy corpsmen were trained to care for patients, so the nurses just supervised them. The Army was different—the corpsmen could take temperatures but not much more. Some could not even count. Navy uniforms were prettier. She learned the Army's olive drab uniforms could look almost as beautiful as the Navy nurses blues if they tailored the drabs.

At first, the Army nurses earned ninety dollars a month; however, California Congressman Will Rodgers, Jr., felt it was a disgrace that military officers earned more than nurses when nurses had more training. He passed a bill, and nurses' wages were raised to one hundred fifty a month plus wardrobe and laundry.

The rooms in the wards at Birmingham were split: officers on one side and enlisted men on the other. The hospital also had a work camp for Italian prisoners. One day some men told Turner she treated a prisoner too nice. "No," she said, "he is a patient just like you. I come here to take care of patients, not to decide which ones have preference." After the war, she left the Army and worked for the telephone company in the first aid room.[45]

Many radio and movie stars visited patients at the hospital; Jack Benny broadcast his annual Christmas party from the hospital in 1944. Marlon Brando lived in Birmingham for one month to study for his role as a paraplegic veteran in the 1950 movie, *The Men*. After several years of activity, the United States government abandoned the grounds, and the buildings remained empty until it became the Birmingham Junior High School on 4 February 1953.[46]

Chapter Seven

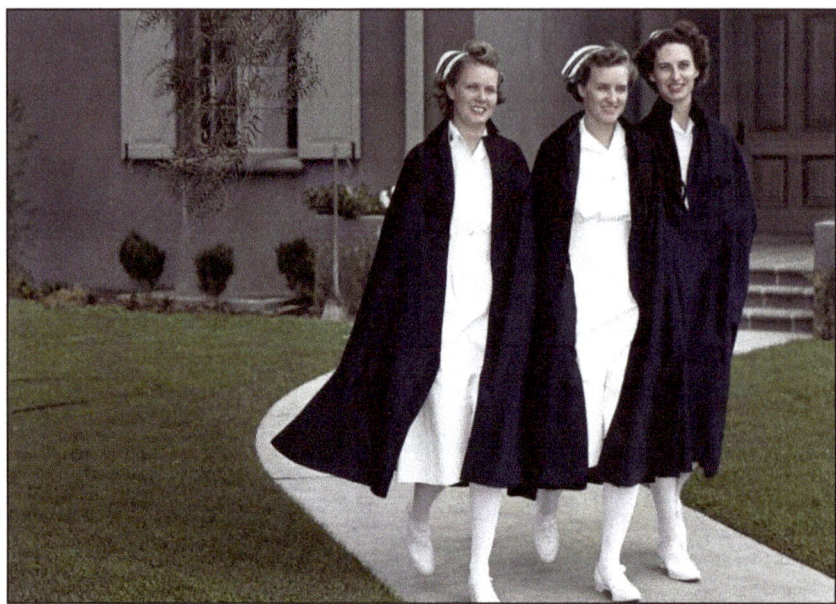

Figure 07.38. Ensigns Mavis Behrens, Helen Rhodes, and Dorothy Olsen, left to right, leave the nurses' quarters to report for duty. Olson joined the Navy Nurse Corps in 1943, and they assigned her to the eye, ear, nose, and throat department at Long Beach Naval Hospital. C. [47]

Figure 07.39. Olsen prepares an anesthesia cabinet for surgery, c. 1943. (Dept. of Special Collections, Charles E. Young Research Library, UCLA)

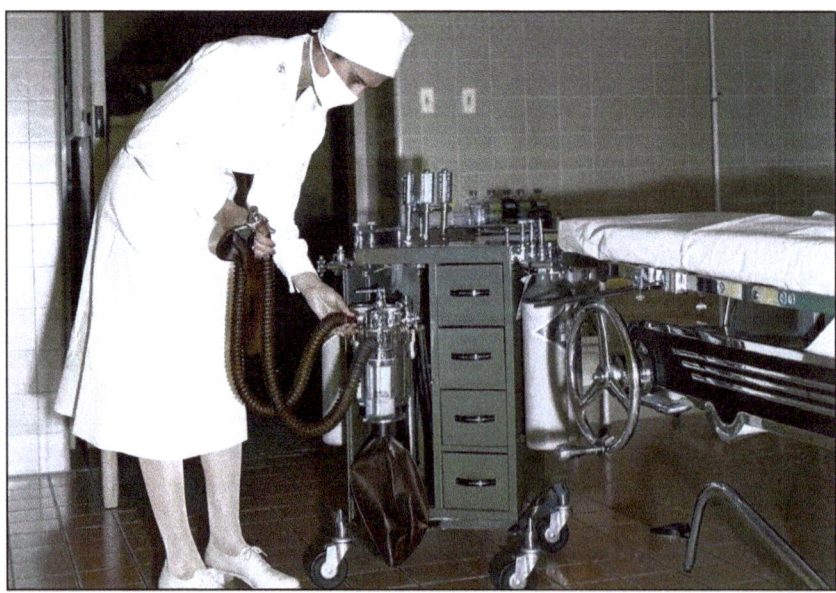

WWII

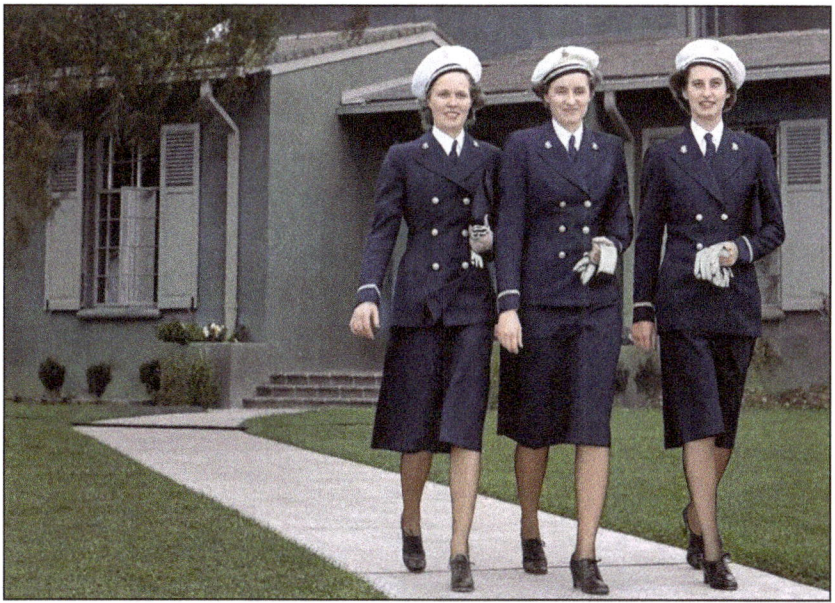

Figure 07.40. Ensigns Mavis Behrens, Helen Rhodes, and Dorothy Olsen head out on the town in their dress uniforms. C. Olsen worked a typical 7 a.m. to 3 p.m. shift; when she finished work, she returned to the nurses' quarters on the base. [48]

Figure 07.41. Olsen's off-duty activities included badminton, ping-pong, tennis, and bicycling. C. (Charles E. Young Research Library, UCLA)

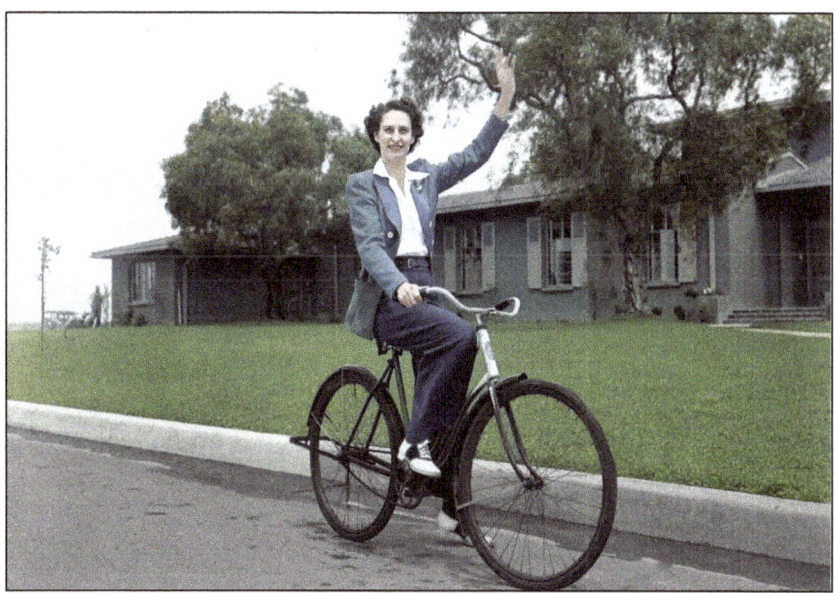

Chapter Seven

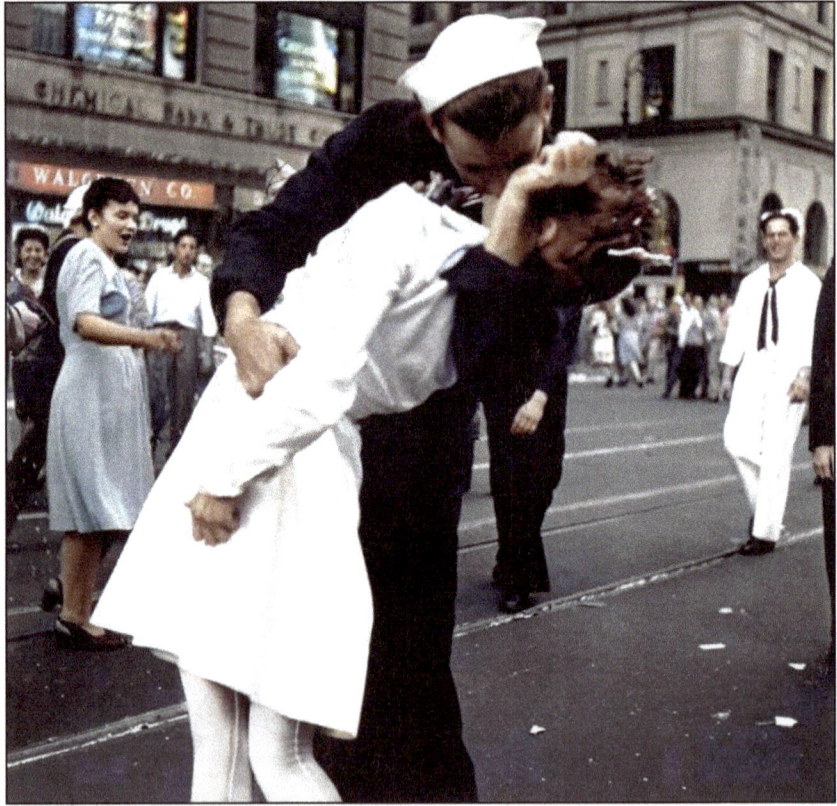

Figure 07.42. Edith Shain in the famous photograph often called "the Kiss" on V-J Day, August 14, 1945, (Photo by Lieutenant Victor Jorgensen). C.

When Edith Cullen Shain heard the radio say World War II ended, she ran to Times Square with a fellow nurse from Doctor's Hospital. "The men just grabbed women and kissed them," Shain said. "We didn't care because the men had almost died in the war." *Life* magazine sent photographer Alfred Eisenstaedt to document the celebration; his photograph made the cover of *Life*. Shain recognized herself, however, did not tell anyone. She moved to Los Angeles, worked briefly at Cedars of Lebanon Hospital, and then became a kindergarten teacher.[49]

In 1980, Eisenstaedt wrote an article for the *Los Angeles Times* about the photograph. Shain decided to reveal herself as the nurse. Other nurses also claimed the fame, but Eisenstaedt gave Shain a letter stating she was the nurse. The sailor's identity was never agreed upon, although many claimed that status too. *Time* declared the shot the most recognized photograph of the Twentieth Century.[50] Another photographer, Lieutenant Victor Jorgensen, squatted next to Eisenstaedt that same day and snapped his "Kiss" version.

Figure 07.43. *Unconditional Surrender* statue taken on its dedication day, February 10, 2007, in Mole Park, San Diego. Edith Shain (right) is pictured walking in front of an unknown man. Artist J. Seward Johnson created the 25-foot, 6,000 lb. statue of the kiss titled *Unconditional Surrender.* [51-52]

In 2005, New York unveiled a life-sized version of the statue in Times Square. Shain attended the Times Square dedication. [53] She said she reluctantly recreated the kiss with one of the men who claimed to be the sailor, even though she never believed it was him. [54]

Shain participated in many Los Angeles parades, dressed in whites, riding on a convertible. She served as Grand Marshall for the New York Veteran's Day Parade in 2008. President George Bush presented Shain with a proclamation that recognized her as a symbol of world peace. Celebrities always lined up to take their photo with her. [55]

Figure 07.44. Edith Shain riding on a convertible in Washington, D.C., at the National Memorial Day Parade, May 26, 2008. (Courtesy of D. B. King)

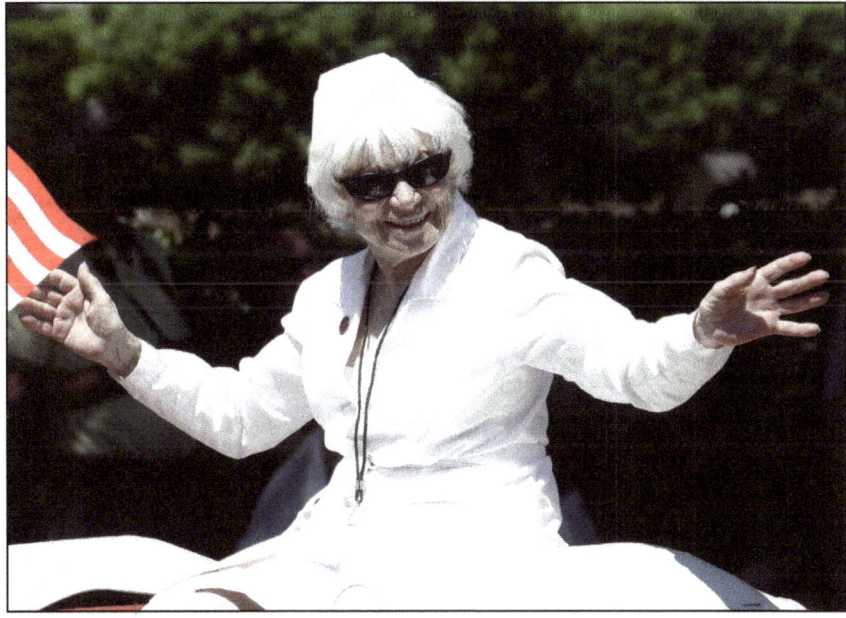

Everything but the Utility Sink

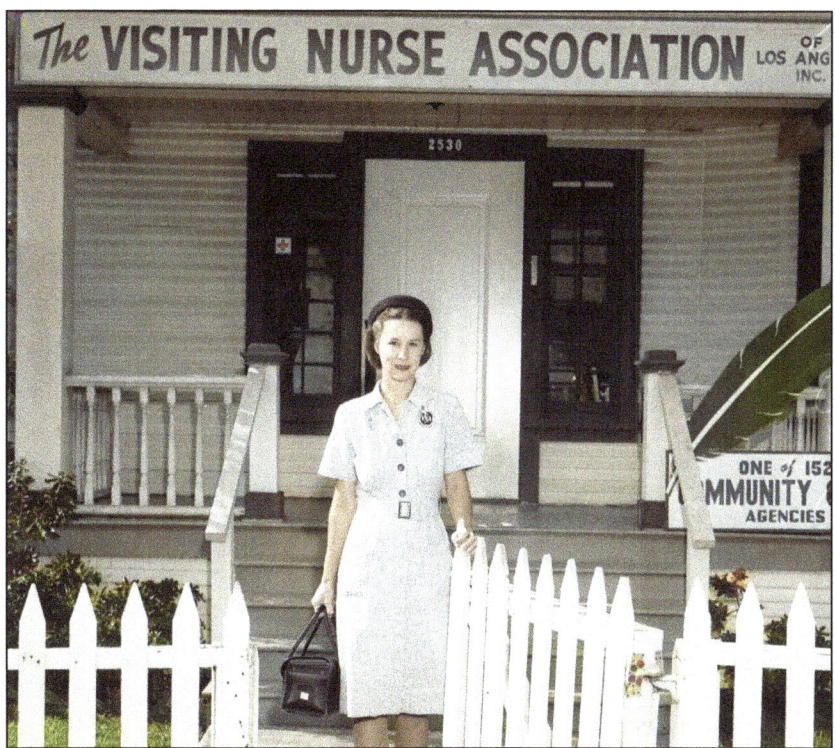

Figure 08.01. Visiting nurse Florence Peters, leaving the second VNA location at 2530 W 8th Street, October 1946. C. (Charles E. Young Research Library)

Philadelphia established the Visiting Nurse Association (VNA) in 1880. Los Angeles, however, did not start their VNA until 1940.[1] The Los Angeles Department of Public Health visited indigent patients, but the middle class also needed home care—few middle-class people could pay for private nurses.

On 1 March 1940, a group organized an association with funds from the Community Chest (later called the United Way) and private groups. Patients contributed $1.50, or a partial payment, for a one-hour VNA visit. Only three public health nurses covered the Los Angeles territory initially (Chicago employed 141 nurses and Boston 150).[2]

The Los Angeles boundaries included Hoover Boulevard to the east, Santa Monica City limits to the west, Vernon Avenue to the south, and Franklin Avenue to the north. The original VNA office building was at 660 South Western Avenue; Elizabeth Hill was the first director.[3]

Chapter Eight

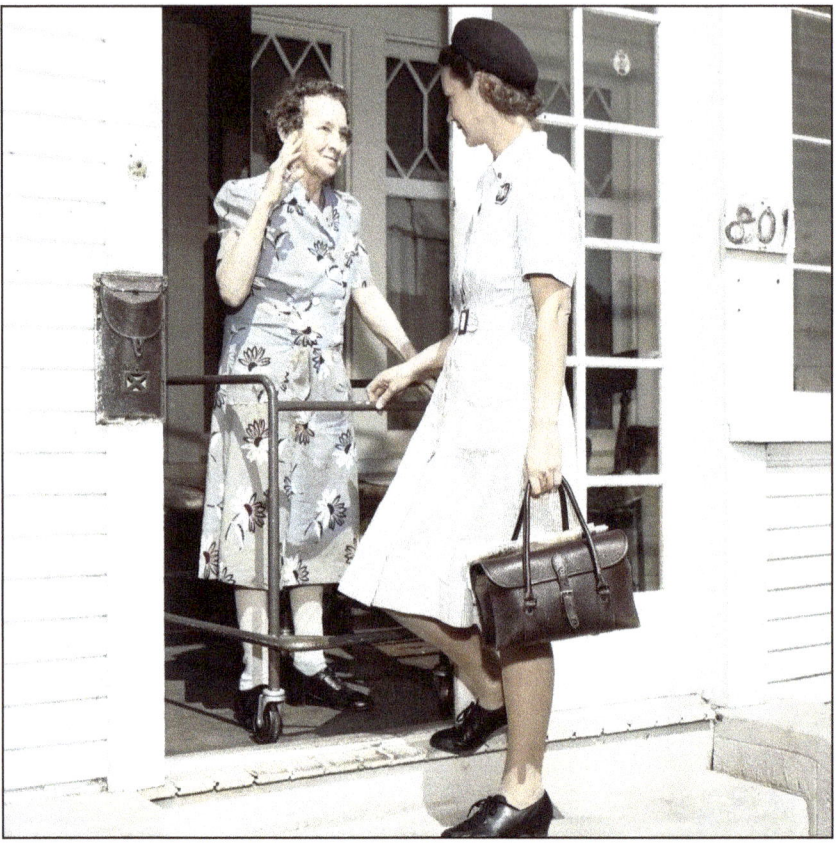

Figure 08.02. Florence Peters of the VNA visited a patient on her route in October 1946. C. (Courtesy of Charles E. Young Research Library, UCLA)

World War II caused additional needs: civilian patients were discharged early as the wounded occupied most hospital beds. In 1943, the service expanded to provide nurses for industrial plants. *Los Angeles Times* reporter Zeanette Moore followed Florence Peters on her route one day in October 1946.

She reported that Peters bathed a cancer patient, changed a colostomy pouch, cared for a tuberculosis patient, administered injections for anemia, and bathed newborns. The charge for each should have been $1.80; however, the nurse charged most twenty-five cents or less.[4] That year, twenty-six nurses visited approximately 4,760 patients per month.[5]

In 1983, when the HIV/AIDS epidemic emerged, VNA nurses were the primary hospice caregivers for patients with AIDS. They cared for 20,000 housebound patients annually. The Los Angeles VNA merged with Sun Healthcare Group in 1997, and Sun Healthcare disbanded.[6]

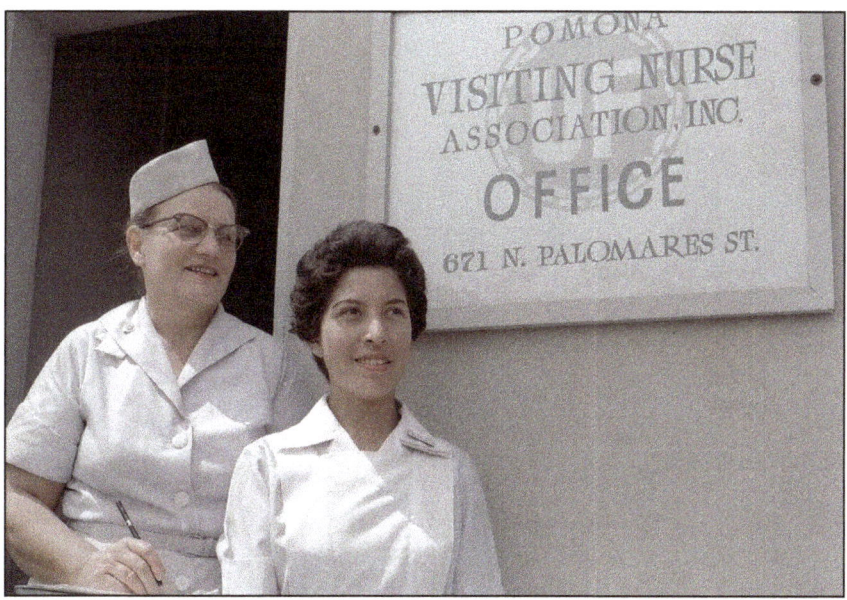

Figure 08.03. Mount San Antonio College School of Nursing student and instructor at the Visiting Nurse Association Office, in the Assistance League buildings in Pomona, 1958.[7] C. 08.04 Mount San Antonio College School of Nursing students and their instructor conduct VNA rounds, 1958. C. (Mount San Antonio College Digital History)

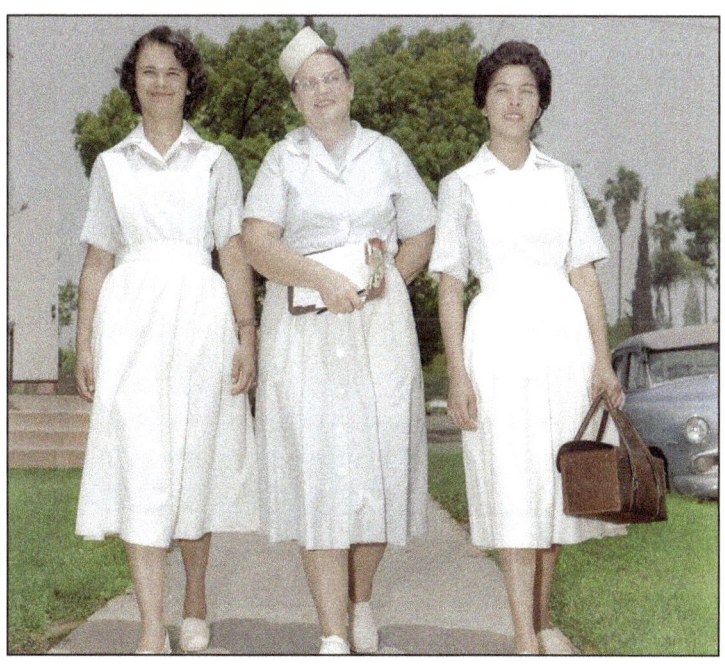

Chapter Eight

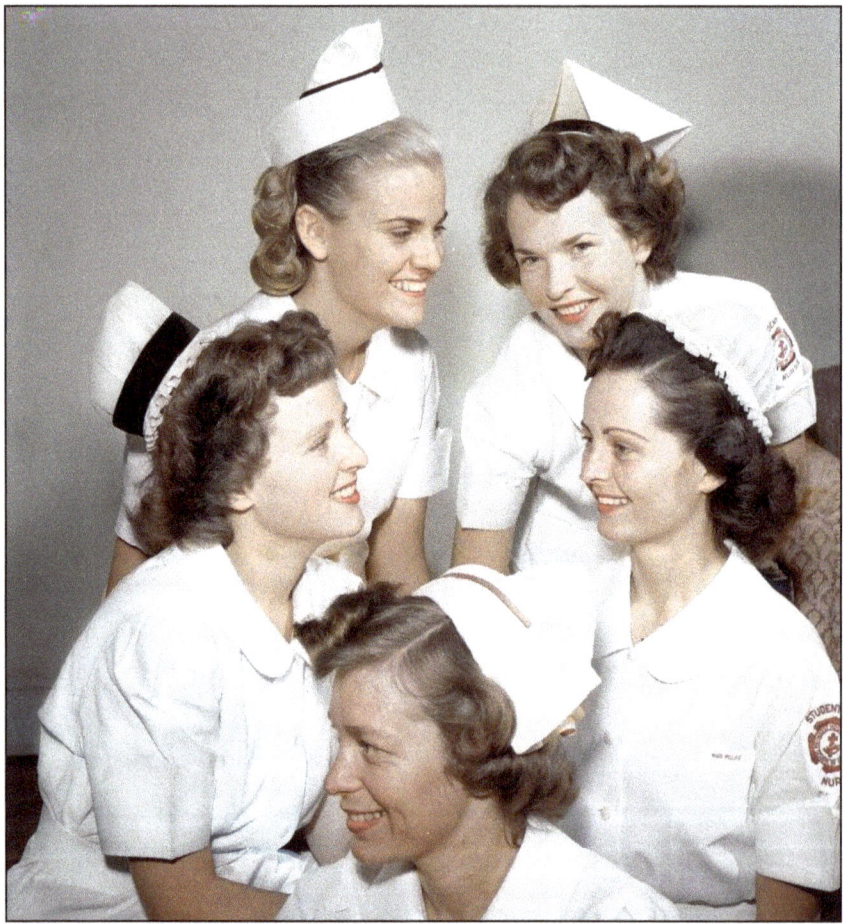

Figure 08.05. Student nurses from Methodist Hospital on Hope Street model caps of nurses who worked at the hospital, 1947. C. The hospital employed graduate nurses from 129 different schools of nursing with 129 unique caps. C. (Dept. of Special Collections, Charles E. Young Research Library, UCLA)

No one knows the exact impetus that created the idea for nurses to wear caps: references are not definitive. Most women in Nightingale's era wore hats to hold their long hair, so wearing a cap was commonplace. The Daughters of Charity nurses adopted their cornette from the hat local French women wore.[8] Early nurses wore caps to protect their hair in unsanitary conditions.

The use of caps began to wane in the 1970s with the feminist movement. Nurse leaders insisted that other professionals didn't wear caps. Why should nurses? Caps also distanced male nurses from the overall group since they did not wear them. Most U.S. schools had eliminated caps by the 1980s. Early nurses spoke of appreciation for their caps; many nurses in the 1970s did not.

Everything but the Utility Sink

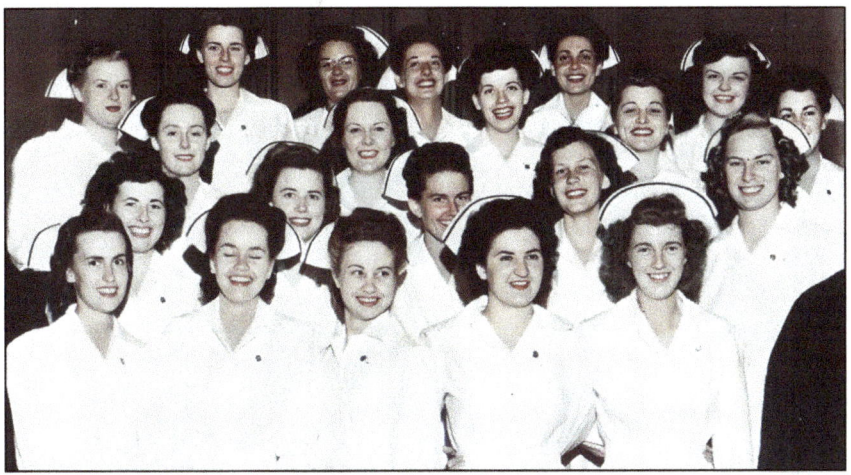

Figure 08.06. The first class of graduates at Hollywood Presbyterian Hospital School of Nursing, 1947. C. Listed in alphabetical order: M. Abramoff, L. Albercht, B. Beckes, B. Blue, E. Cowie, H. Elson, B. Faughnder, M. Grana, B. Heyne, D. Johnson, S. Lee, L. Lucas, P. McMurry, A. Morris, J. Peterson, J. Size, B. Stearns, T. Taylor, D. Tulless, A. West, D. Zeider, D. Zwolinski. [9]

Figure 08.07. Ruth Fiedler, first director of nursing at Hollywood Presbyterian School of Nursing, 1944. C. Fiedler received a Bachelor of Arts from UCLA in 1928 and graduated from Bishop Johnson School of Nursing in 1933. [10]

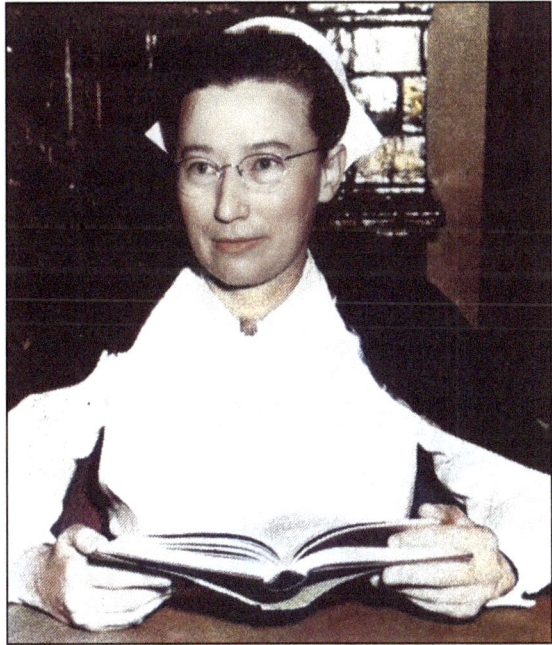

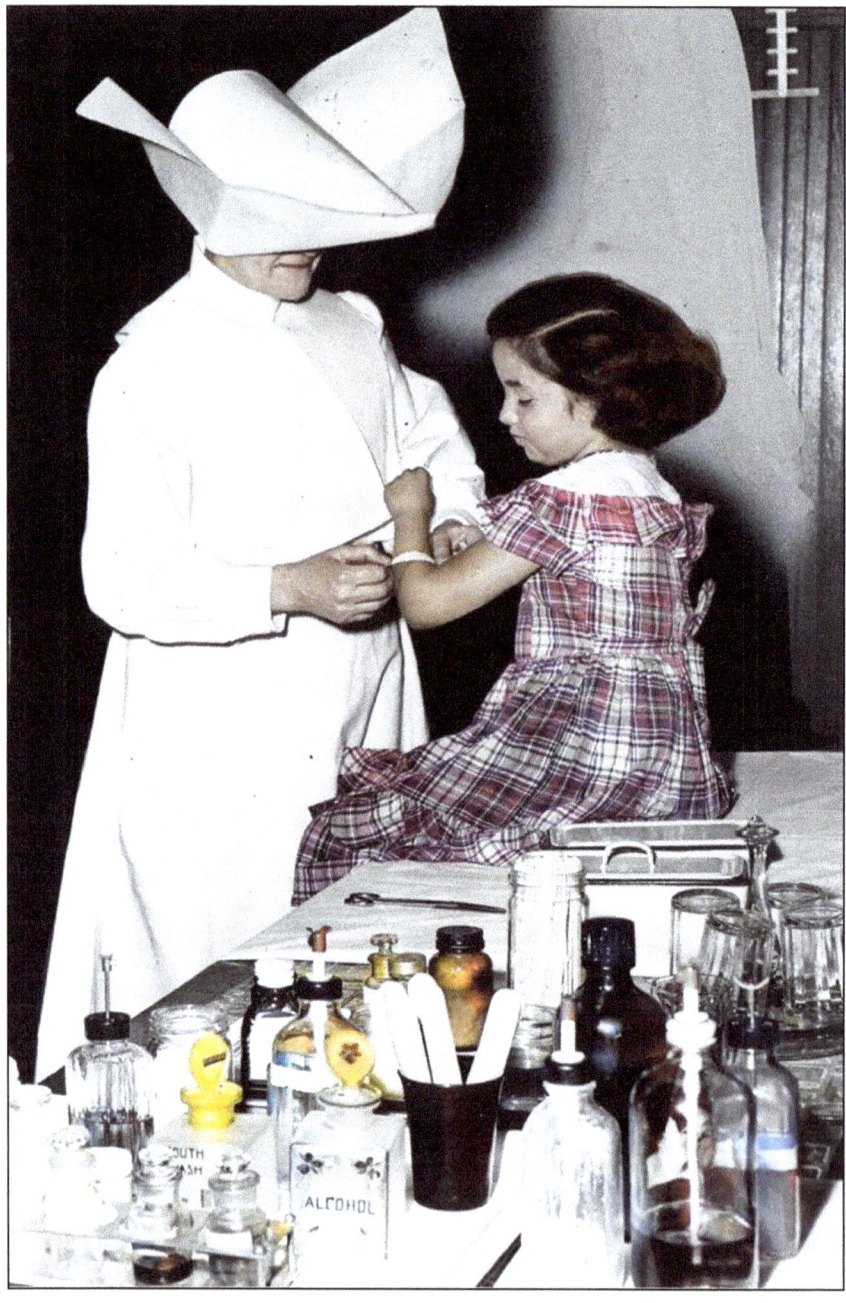

Figure 08.08. Sister Esther, Daughter of Charity, attends to a patient at the Los Angeles Orphanage on August 15, 1950. C. At the forefront is an array of containers, including two look-alike bottles—one labeled mouthwash and the other alcohol. (University of Southern California Archives)

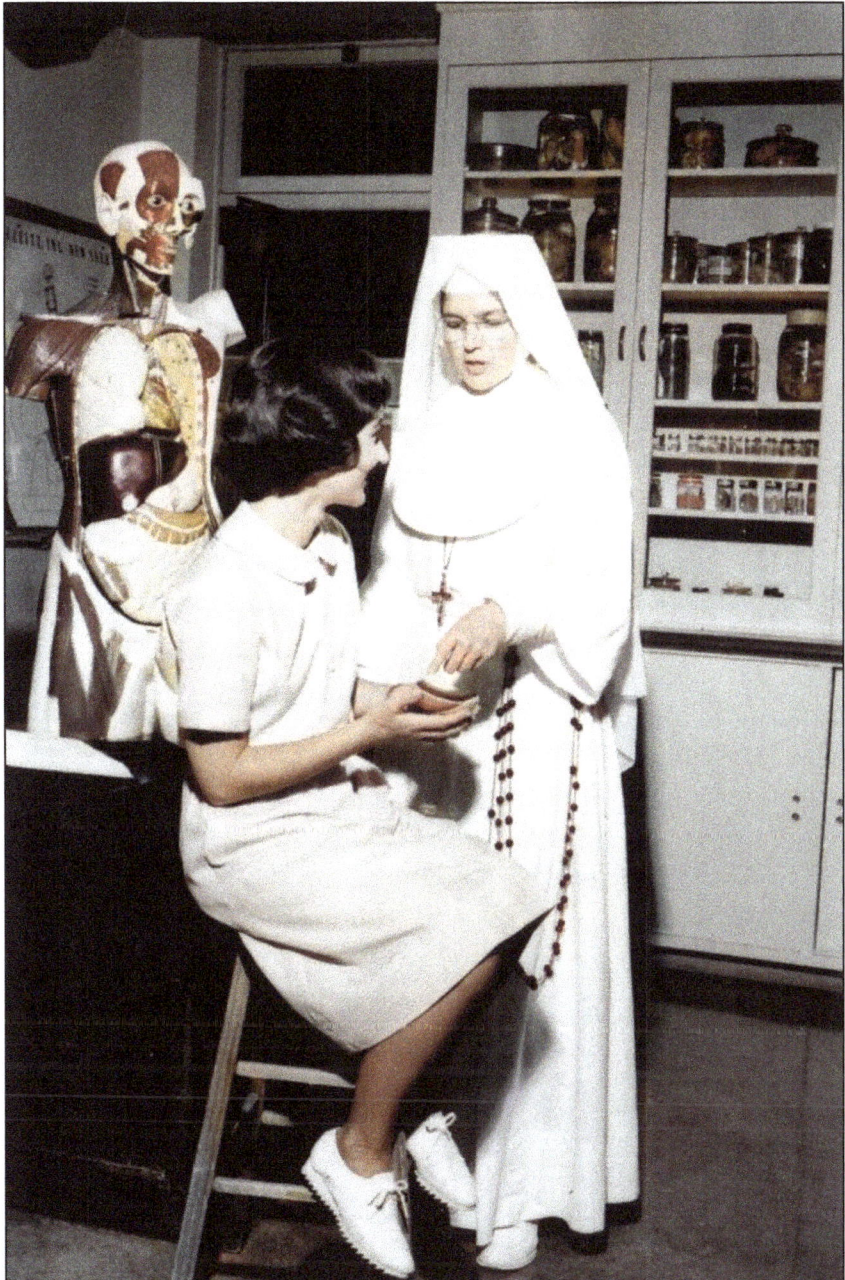

Figure 08.09. Sister Mary Stevens of St. Joseph of Carondelet, wearing a white nurse's habit, instructs a nursing student in the lab at Mount St. Mary's College. C. In the cabinet are various bottles of pathological specimens, presumably used in scientific studies. (Mount St. Mary's College)

Chapter Eight

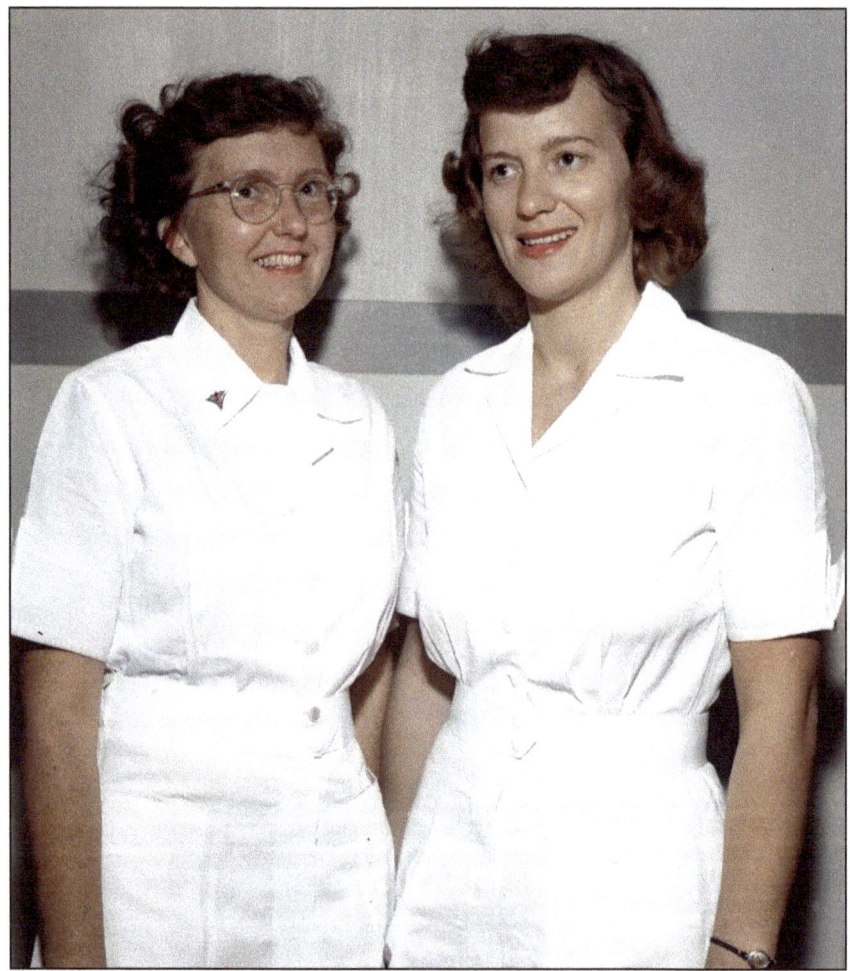

Figure 08.10. Florence Slater, left, and Ann Harmon, of Wadsworth Veterans Hospital in Sawtelle (West Los Angeles), received two of the twelve Warm Springs Foundation scholarships granted to nurses in 1947. C. (Department of Special Collections, Charles E. Young Research Library, UCLA)

The Warm Springs Foundation, part of President Roosevelt's initiative, offered scholarships for advanced polio training. They assisted disabled polio patients using hydrotherapy and psychological treatments and provided social support that general hospitals did not offer.[11]

Both nurses served as lieutenants in the Army Nurse Corps during World War II. Slater attended the Army School of Nursing at Walter Reed Hospital in Washington, D.C. Harmon received her nurse's training at Fitzsimons General Hospital in Denver, Colorado.[12]

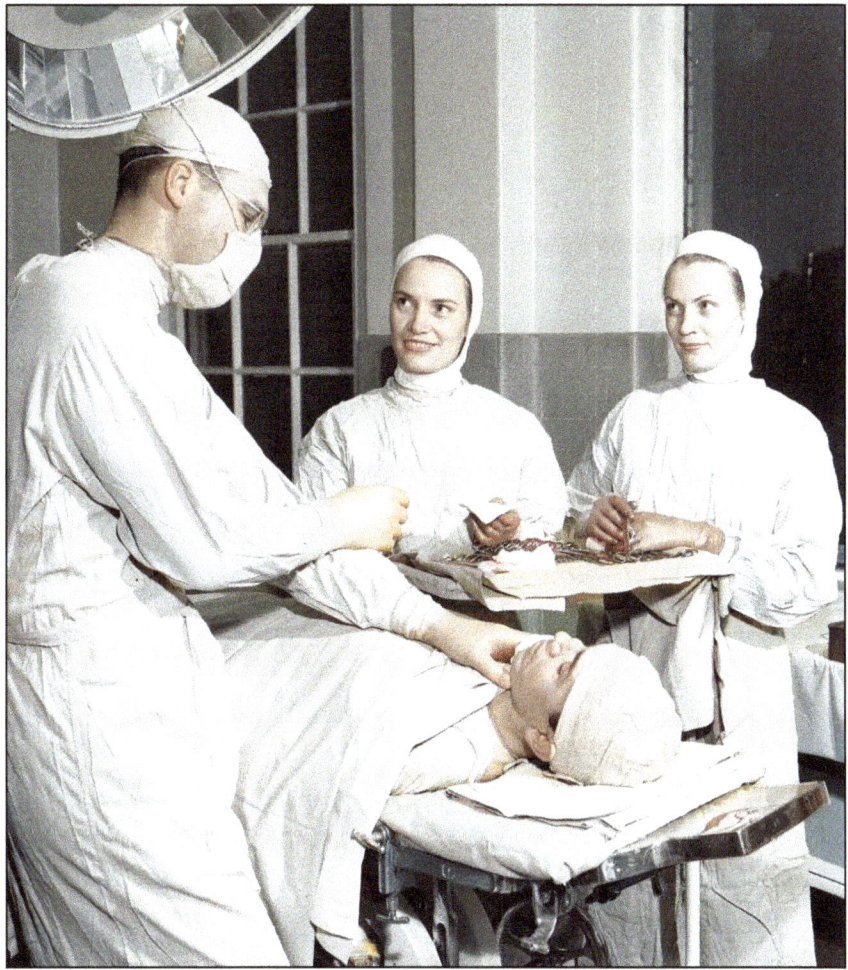

Figure 08.11. Surgeon Ralph M. Milliken, Ramon Garcia (posing as a patient), Thelma Trammel, and Zelma Trammel, left to right. C. (Department of Special Collections, Charles E. Young Research Library, UCLA)

Zelma and Thelma Trammel wanted to join the Navy in 1944, after they had graduated from Baptist State Hospital in Little Rock, Arkansas. Unfortunately, the Navy could not assure them they wouldn't be separated. Wadsworth Veterans Hospital in Sawtelle assured them they could work side by side. The twins had been inseparable their entire lives.

Chief Nurse Fern Long said the twins were ambitious and conscientious. They lived together in Sawtelle and worked on the same surgical floor. Zelma said they would stay together the rest of their lives. "We just like to be together," Thelma said, "and I guess we always will."[13]

Chapter Eight

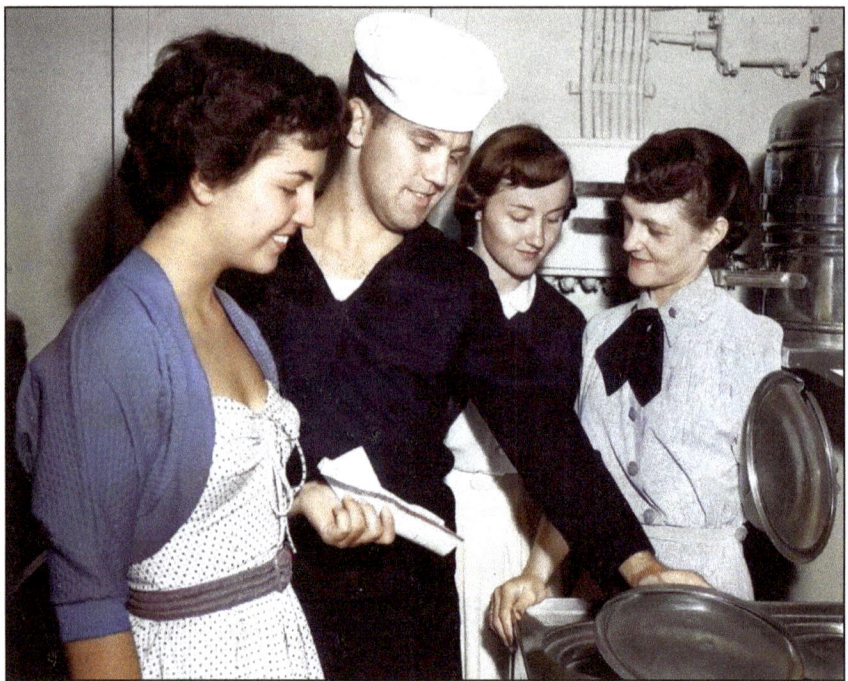

Figure 08.12. Student nurses Ann Robertson and Peggy Herbst view the galley with Wayne and Lieutenant Anna Kaes, left to right, n.d. C.

On 14 May 1952, several hundred student nurses from Los Angeles and Orange County previewed the life of a Navy nurse at sea when they attended an open house aboard the Navy hospital ship, the USS *Repose*, in the Long Beach Harbor. This day marked the 44th anniversary of the establishment of the Navy Nurse Corps. The *Repose*, called "The Angel of the Orient," evacuated more than 11,000 wounded from Korea. The ship could handle 1,000 patients in many sick bays.

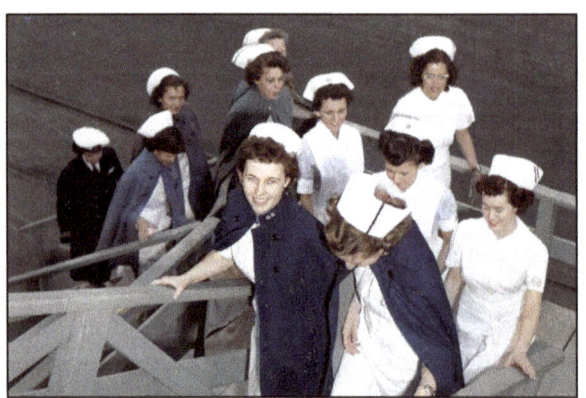

Figure 08.13. Student nurses walk up the gangway to the ship, n.d. C.

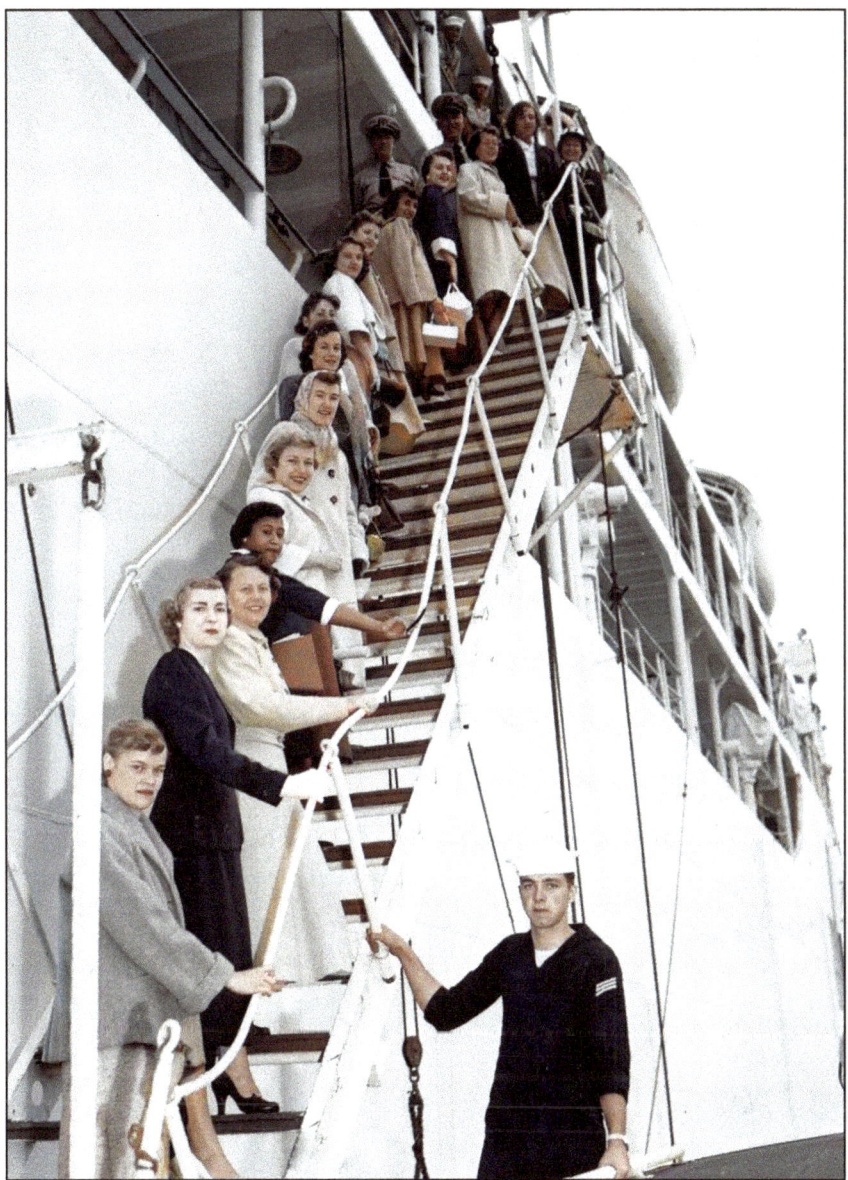

Figure 08.14. Student nurses from more than a dozen Los Angeles hospitals trooped up the gangway of the USS *Consolation* Navy Hospital Ship for a preview of the facilities, May 10, 1954. C.

Los Angeles nurse and former WWII POW, Captain Edwina Todd, had been the commander of this ship during the Korean War—the first woman appointed as a commander of a Navy hospital ship. (Photos from the Department of Special Collections, Charles Young Research Library, UCLA)

Chapter Eight

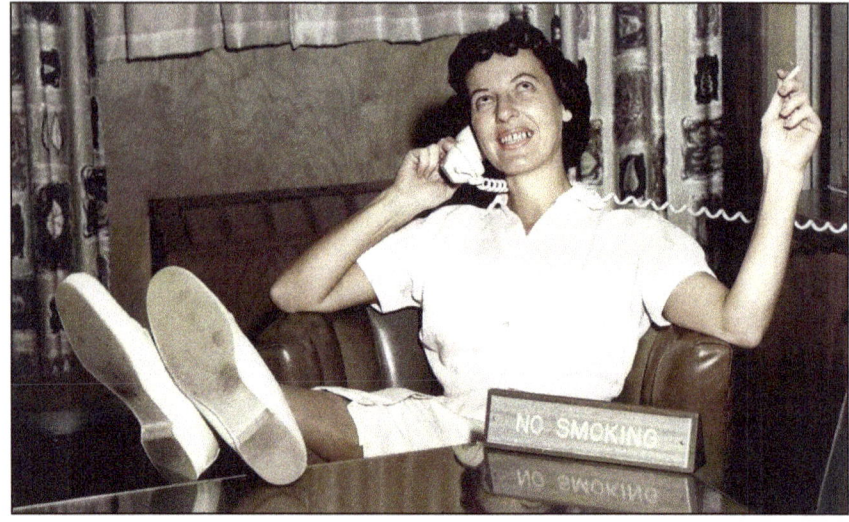

Figure 08.15. Glendale Hospital nurse, Gloria Hopkins, smokes in jest, but in the 1940s and 1950s, nurses and doctors advertised cigarettes, emphasizing health properties of smoking they believed to be accurate then, n.d. C.

Figure 08.16. Cleo Hood, a nurse at West Hollywood Emergency Hospital, smoking at the wheel of the car, June 26, 1942. C. She said she would not smoke on the street but believed, "it was all right in a car if the wind was not blowing so hard to make it dangerous." (Courtesy of Shades of L.A. Archives/Los Angeles Public Library)

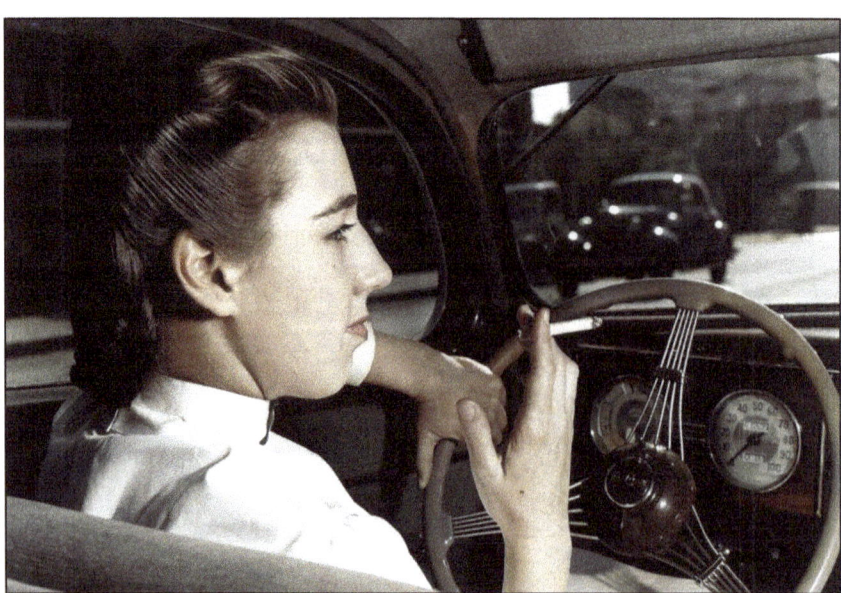

Figure 08.17. The Santa Fe Coast Line Hospital, in Boyle Heights, East Los Angeles, 1955. C.

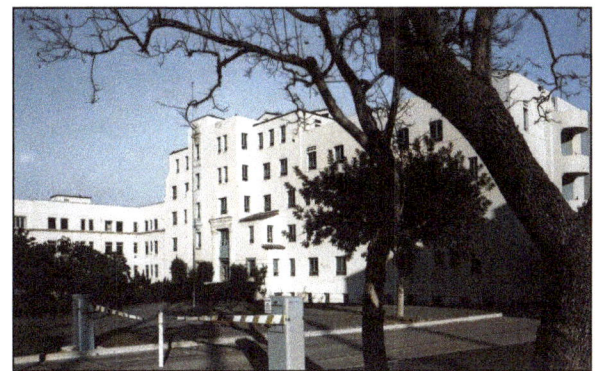

The building was built in 1937 on the site of the original 1905 building, which burned down.

The current building became the Linda Vista Hospital in 1937. It ceased business in 1991. The empty structure was used as a filming location for TV shows and movies: *Moonlight, ER, Charm School, Dexter, Ghost Adventures, the Colony, Outbreak, End of Days,* and *Pearl Harbor.* Rock bands shot videos inside: Garbage's "Bleed Like Me" and Duran Duran's "Falling Down." The National Register of Historic Places added the building in January 2006. [14]

In 2013 the new owner converted the nurses dormitory to 23 senior apartments. He also converted the laboratories and patient rooms using funds from L.A.'s Housing Department's Neighborhood Stabilization Program. [15]

Figure 08.18. Ann Care working at the nurses' station desk in Linda Vista while Barbara Bustin flips open a metal chart from the chart room rack, c. 1950s. C. (Courtesy of Kansas Historical Society)

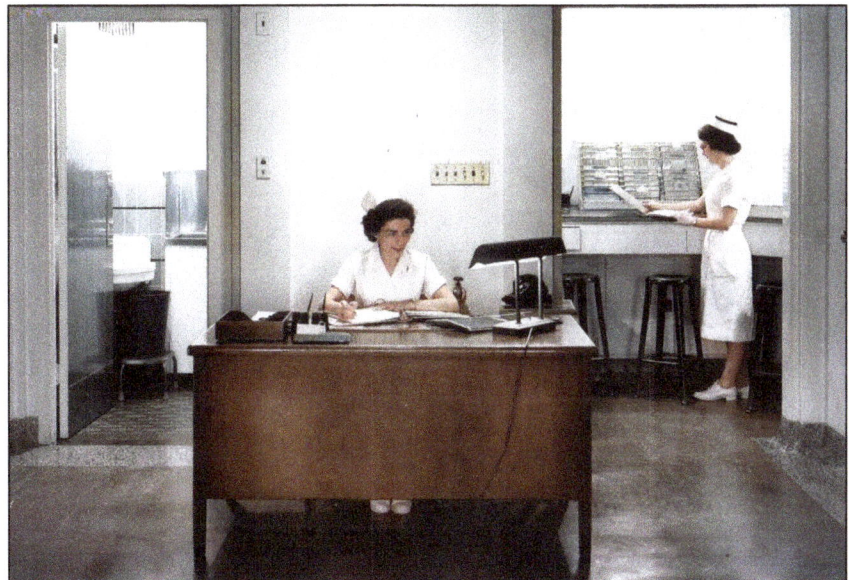

Chapter Eight

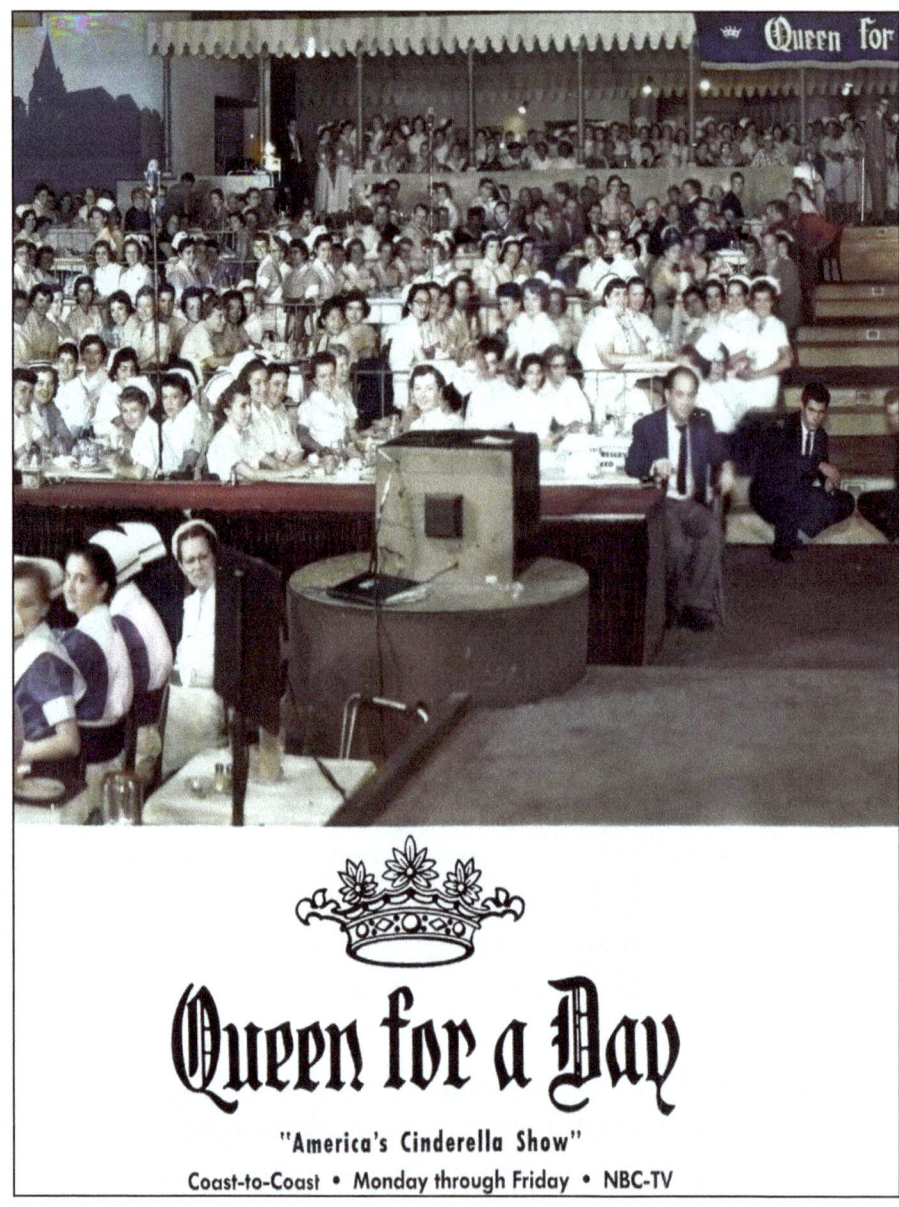

Figure 08.19. Los Angeles nurses during a Nurses Show on September 27, 1956. C. "Queen for a Day" began as a radio show in 1947. It moved to television, 1956–1964, and broadcast from the Moulin Rouge near Sunset and Vine Streets. Each week, the show featured one special group as both audience members and contestants. The show invited four women to tell their sad stories of need. Contestants made requests: a refrigerator, a wedding dress, or equipment for a local nursing home were among the requests.[16]

Everything but the Utility Sink

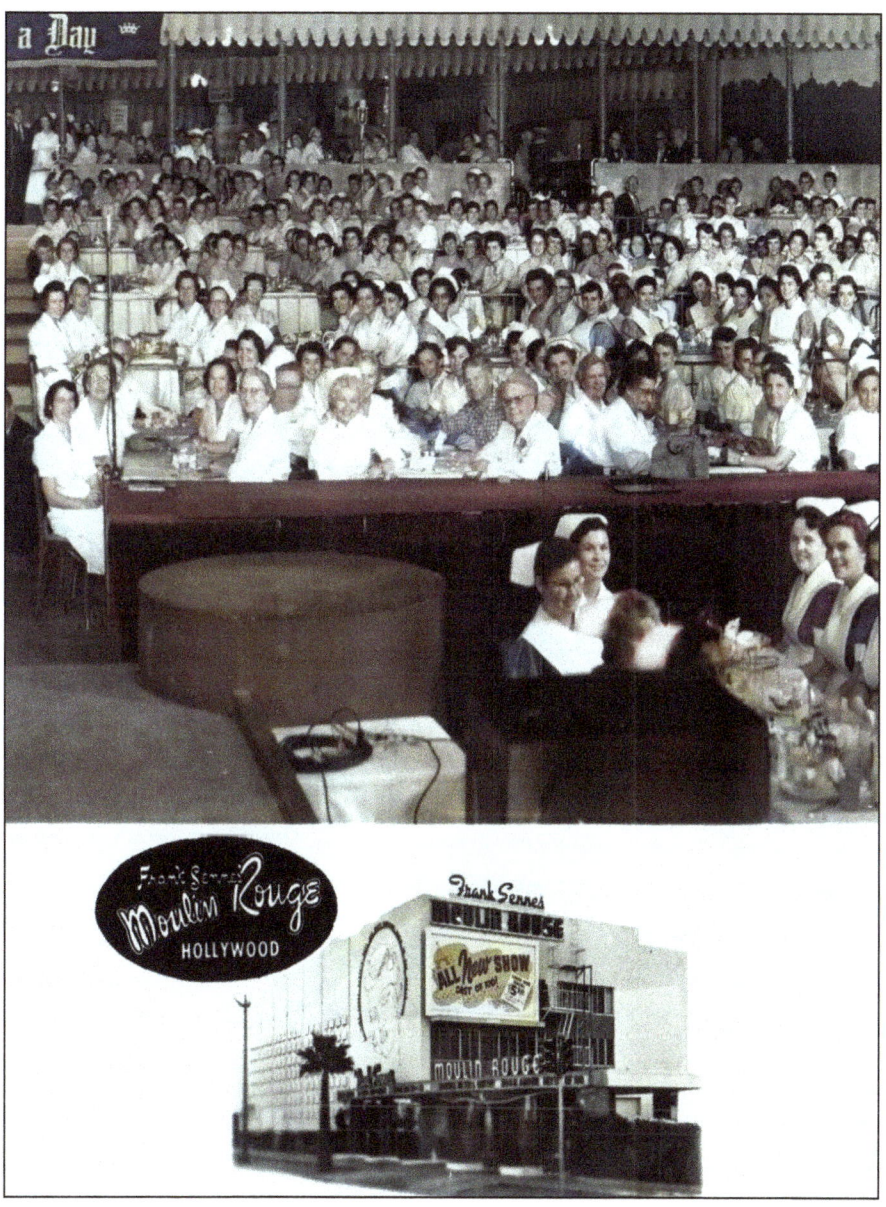

The audience applauded each contestant. An applause meter registered the winner. Tears and contestants' dire circumstances helped win the audience's sympathy. The band played "Pomp and Circumstance" as the host, Jack Bailey, draped the winner in a red velvet robe. He placed a crown on her head, presented her with a bouquet of roses, and announced her "Queen for a Day." She was granted her request, a night on the town, and other prizes. Courtesy of Queen for a Day)

Chapter Eight

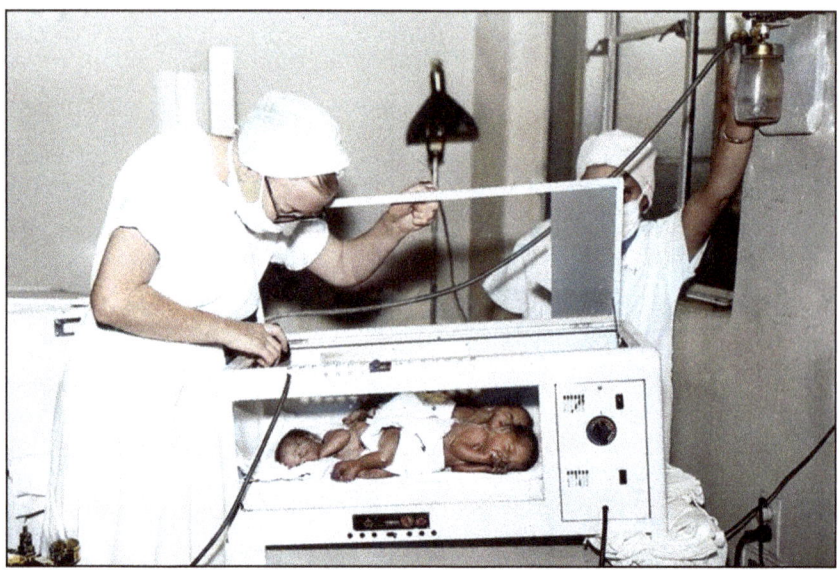

Figure 08.20. Gladys Barnes, left, and Carol Darlington administered blow-by oxygen to a set of triplets at County General Hospital on October 9, 1951. C. All three shared one incubator, no longer allowed due to infection control.

In 1949, County General Hospital trained ten nurses to care for their premature infants in a room called the T.L.C. (tender loving care) room—the first neonatal class in Los Angeles. The hospital remodeled the nursery to include a separate room for incubators. Anyone who entered the room had to wear masks and gowns.[17] (Charles E. Young Research Library, UCLA)

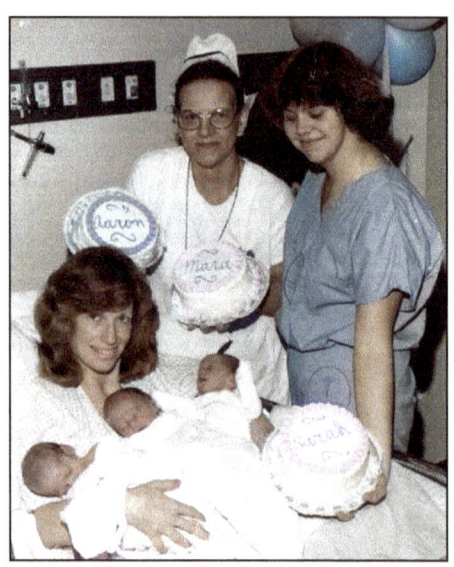

Figure 08.21. Three cakes with the names of Aaron, Mara, and Sarah are for the Leap Day triplets born February 29, 1980. (Courtesy of Cedars-Sinai Medical Center)

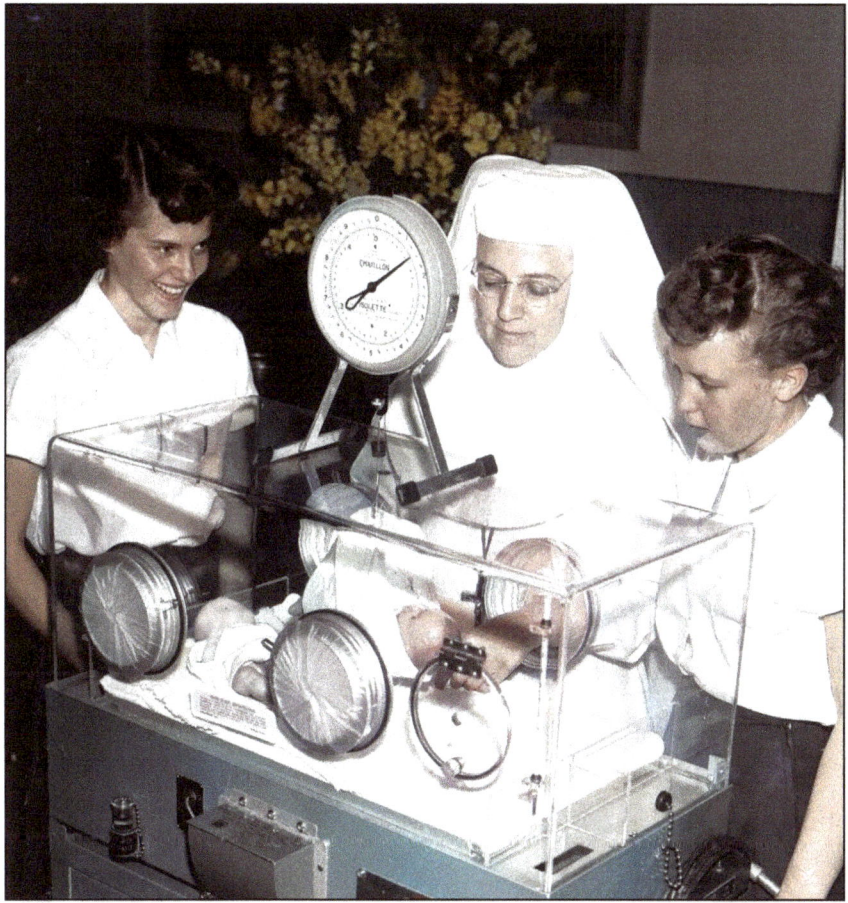

Figure 08.22. Sister Leo Paul demonstrated an Isolette (with a newborn doll) to students Myrna Finn, left, and Jo Anne Brozik on May 14, 1953. C.

St. Luke's Hospital, in Pasadena, hosted Youth Day during National Hospital Week, designed to attract youth to a career in nursing. The campaign hosted high school and junior college students. Two hundred students from five schools toured the hospital. The *Los Angeles Times* reported 6,000 hospitals in the U.S. held similar disaster drills for Hospital Week in May 1956.

Exhibits included a surgery setup, a pediatric ward, an X-ray machine, a laboratory equipment display, and a demonstration of the newest device: the Isolette. The Isolette functioned as an incubator, isolation room, and pressurized oxygen tent with ports for nurses to reach inside. A built-in scale allowed nurses to weigh infants without removing them. Heated Isolettes are still used, but oxygen is not pressurized, and they are not for isolation.[18] (Dept. of Special Collections, Charles E. Young Research Library, UCLA).

Chapter Eight

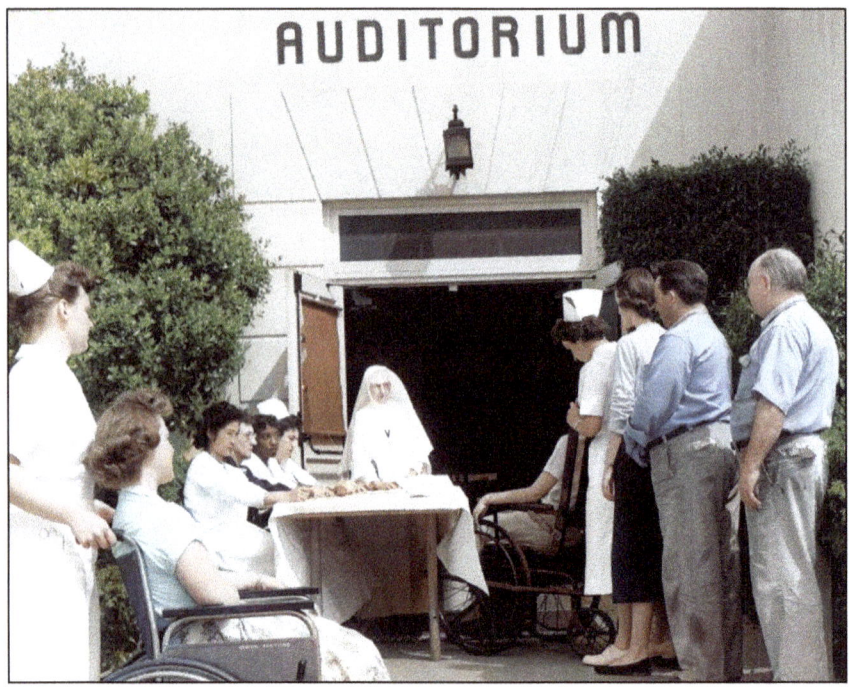

Figure 08.23. Nurses showed they could expand from the normal 500 patients to 1,500 using the corridors and the auditorium, May 6, 1956. C.

Figure 08.24. During Hospital Week, nurses at Queen of Angels Hospital conducted a training drill to demonstrate that the hospital could triple its capacity during a disaster, May 1956. C. (Photos courtesy of the Department of Special Collections, Charles E. Young Research Library, UCLA)

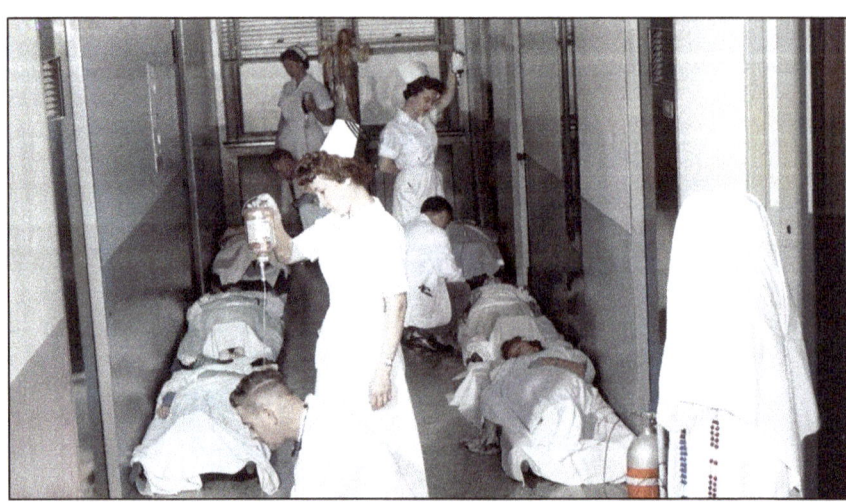

Everything but the Utility Sink

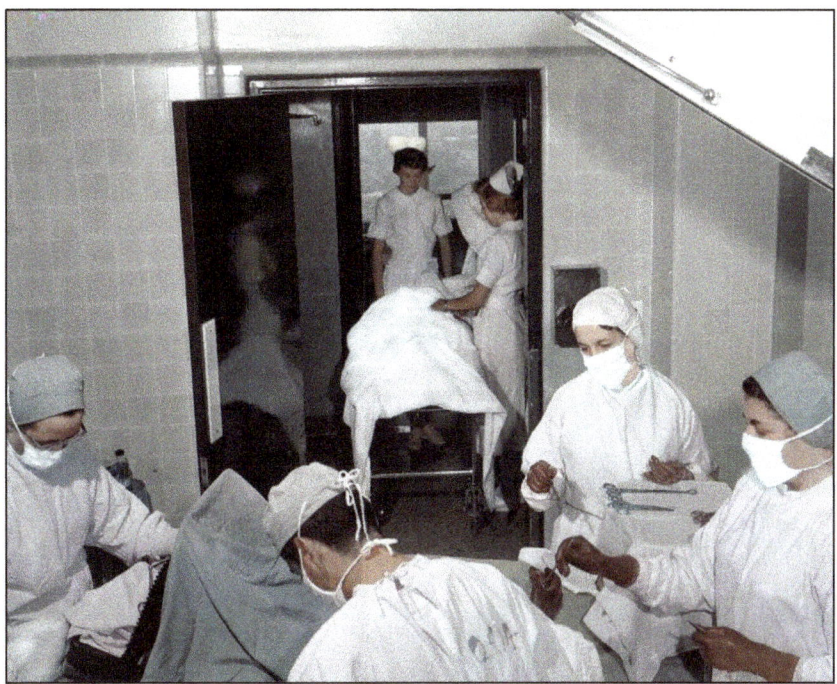

Figure 08.25. Student nurses at Queen of Angels Hospital practiced using improvised operating quarters, May 6, 1956. C.

Figure 08.26. California Hospital students set up a phone center, May 1956. C. In 1974 President Nixon proclaimed a National Nurse Week. In 1982, Congress passed a resolution and President Reagan signed May 6 as the day. In 1990, the ANA extended it to include Nightingale's birthday: May 6-12. [19]

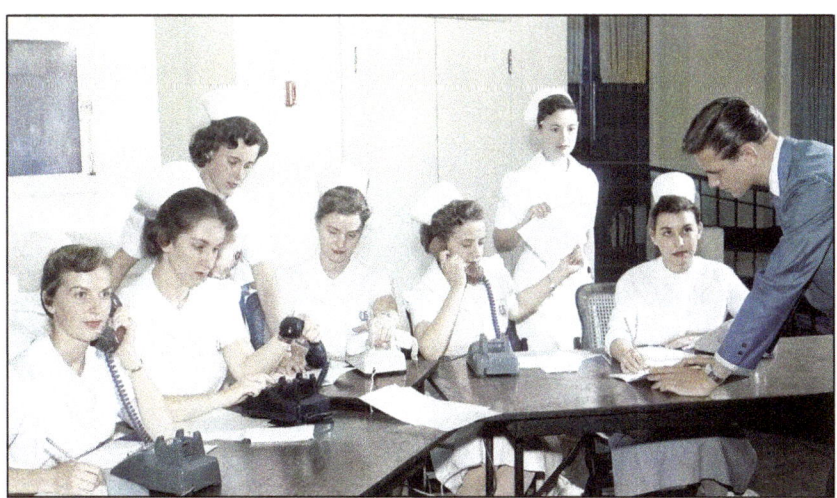

Chapter Eight

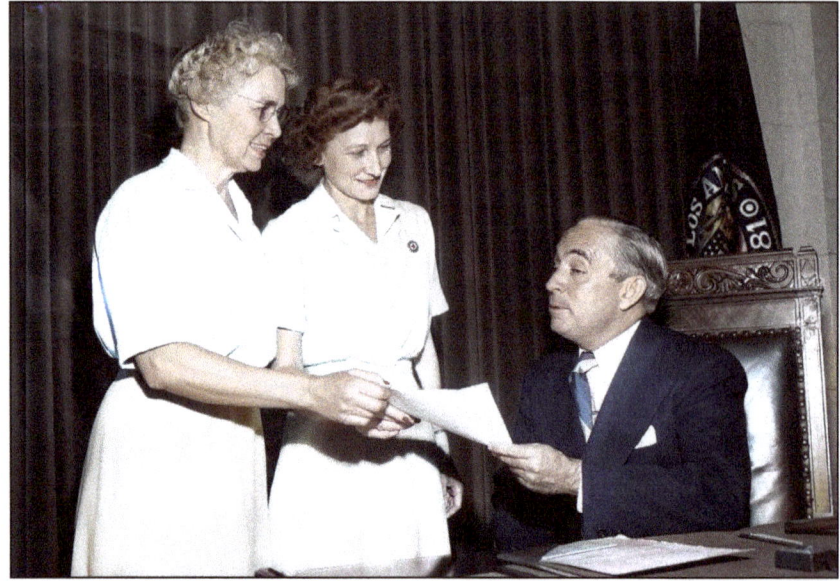

Figure 08.27. Public health nurses Lona Peterson, left, and Dorthea Hansen show Los Angeles City Council President Harold Henry, the original 1897 health resolution—an agreement that Los Angeles would pay the first salary in the U.S. for a public health nurse, December 24, 1947. C. Eighty-two public health nurses celebrated the 50th anniversary of this accomplishment.

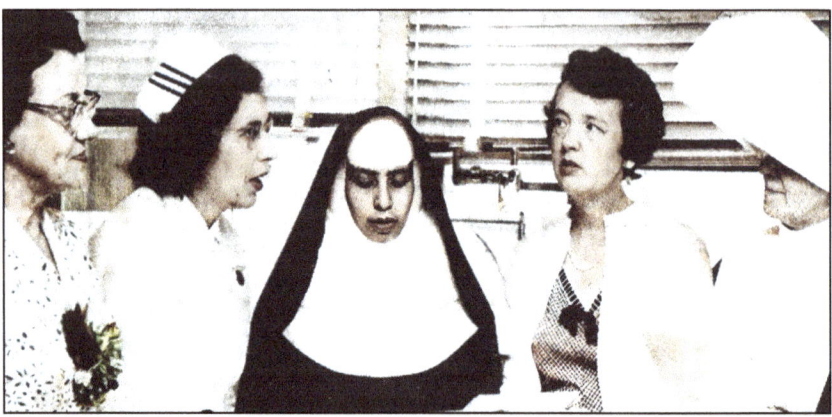

Figure 08.28. Dean Lulu Hassenplug of UCLA School of Nursing, Mary Patterson of Cedars of Lebanon Hospital, Sister Mary Carmelita of Mercy Hospital in San Diego, Eleanor Lambertson from Columbia University, and Sister Gregory of St. Vincent's Hospital, July 1955. C. Fifty nurses from six Western states assembled at Cedars of Lebanon Hospital for a two-week extension course designed to teach leadership methods to administrative nurses. (Special Collections, Louise M. Darling Biomedical Library, UCLA)

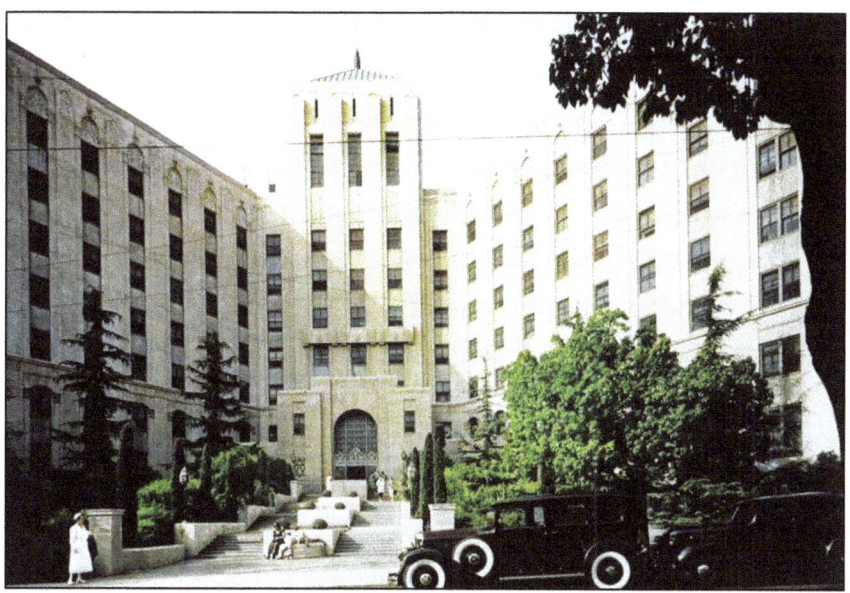

Figure 08.29. A nurse stands in front of the Cedars of Lebanon Hospital, on Franklin Boulevard, c. 1939. C. In 1961, Cedars of Lebanon Hospital merged with Mt. Sinai Hospital to become Cedars-Sinai Medical Center.[20] The Church of Scientology purchased the building in 1976. (University of Southern California Archives)

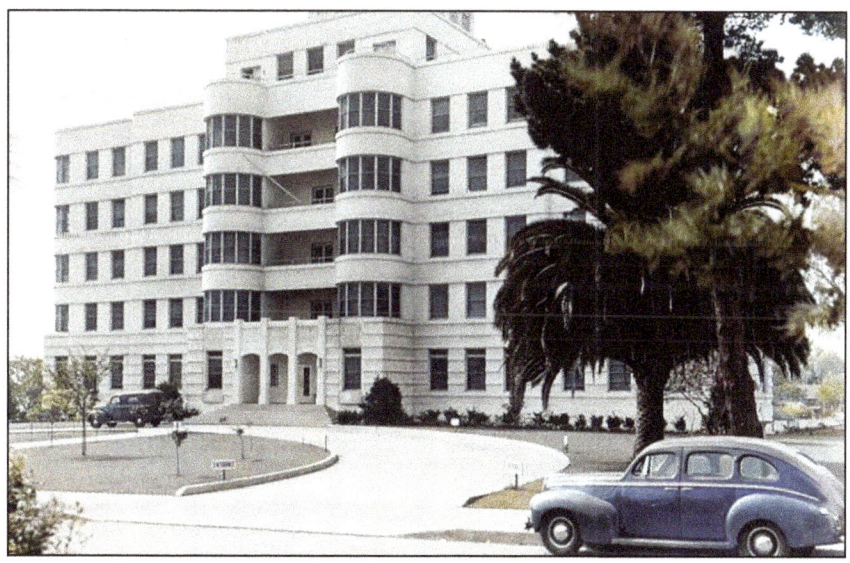

Figure 08.30. St. John's Hospital in Santa Monica, c. 1947. C. (Courtesy of Santa Monica Public Library)

Chapter Eight

Mary Tomassini was such a conscientious nurse that ICU doctors told her patients, "If your nurse is Big Red, you will not be dead." Big Red, named for her hair, cared for many famous people during her career: Natalie Wood, Robert Wagner, Julie Andrews, Johnny Carson, Bing Crosby, and Jane Mansfield, to name a few. Walt Disney once sketched Tomassini's portrait.

When Angela Lansbury's husband was hospitalized, all the nurses feared her. They assigned Tomassini to the job. When Lansbury disagreed with Tomassini's care of her husband, Tomassini told her, "This is my show. Go to your room." Years later Tomassini met Lansbury again. She still remembered the redheaded nurse who sent her to her room.

Tomassini had wanted to become a nurse since she received her first toy nurse's kit at the age of five. She graduated in 1958. She worked the night shift in the intensive care unit at St. John's Hospital in Santa Monica, starting in 1960. She continued to work there until after her 50th anniversary in 2011. [21]

After retirement, she continued her friendship with the staff, especially at Christmas when she filled her two-story house with Santas, 1,800 lights, and a giant stuffed bear sitting in a bathtub. After fifty years of collecting, she never took them down. "My husband thinks I'm crazy," she said.

Her annual holiday parties were as much of a legend as she was. Guests brought unique decorations. One St. Nick dispensed Santa-imprinted toilet paper in the bathroom. And, yes, he sang "Jingle Bell Rock." She opened her house to children's parties the hospital had organized. [22]

Figure 08.31. Tomassini, left, with a fellow probie nurse and favorite nursing instructor at St. Michaels School of Nursing, Toronto, Canada, 1955, C. The book was a frequently used textbook in the fifties, *Nursing Arts*, by Montag and Filson. When they took this photograph, Tomassini had been in the program only a few months and hadn't yet received her coveted nurse cap.

Figure 08.32. Mary Tomassini taking the blood pressure of a patient who had frostbite (congelatio), 1957. C. He was smiling because his hands had just been released from his thighs—as a treatment for frostbite in the 1950s, they attached the patient's hands to his thighs by wrapping a large dressing around them. His hands gently warmed, but he was not allowed to move his hands for several weeks. The student nurses fed him all of his meals.

Tomassini was wearing the blue-striped uniform of a junior nurse. Her cap was plain white. At her school, they awarded nurses a black stripe for their caps during the final six months of their senior year; nurses attached the stripe with white pearl stick pins. Tomassini lost the cap, yet managed to keep the black stripe and stick pins. [23] (Photos courtesy of Mary Tomassini)

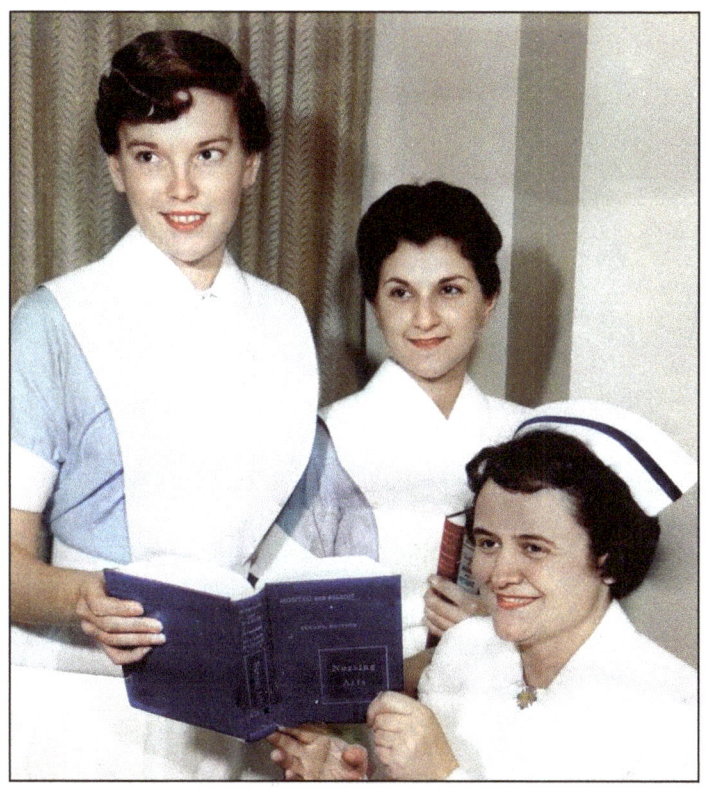

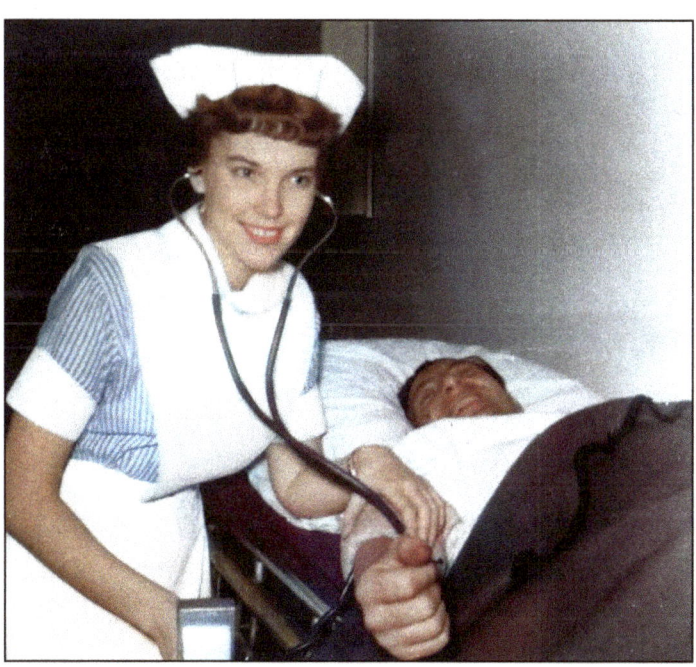

Chapter Eight

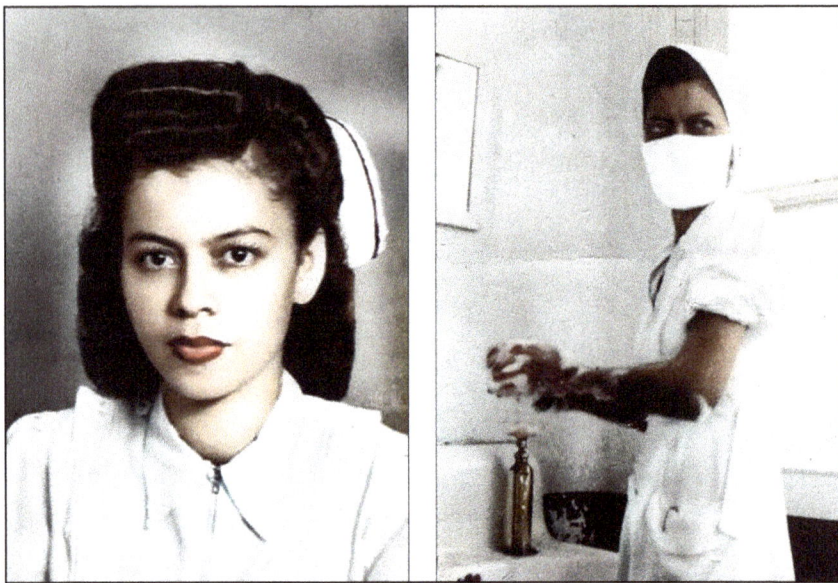

Figure 08.33. Rosa Silva working in Nicaragua after graduating from nursing school in Managua, 1956. C. (Courtesy of Darren William Smith)

Rosa Martina Silva was born in Managua, Nicaragua. She worked for an oil company treating the workers injured on oil platforms. She also worked as a nurse in the Canal Zone in Panama before moving to Los Angeles in 1958. When Silva and her children visited her home in Managua on 23 December 1972, a massive earthquake leveled five square miles of the city. Of the 400,000 people living in Managua, 20,000 were killed and 250,000 became homeless. The stench of burning flesh filled the air, and smoke obscured the stars. Silva's family held Christmas Day looters off with a knife and two pistols. Everyone fled the city as there was no water, electricity, or gas.

Silva returned to Los Angeles. Still, she could not forget the suffering she had seen. Whenever she opened a refrigerator filled with food or took a warm bath, she felt a stab in her heart. [24]

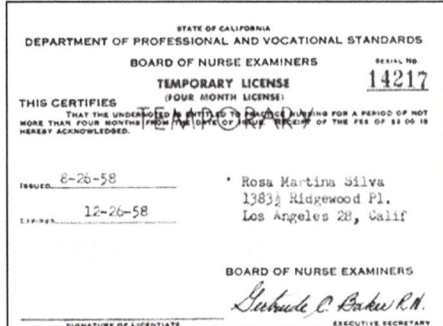

Figure 08.34. Rosa Martina Silva's 1958 temporary license from the Board of Nurse Examiners in California. The permit cost $2.00.

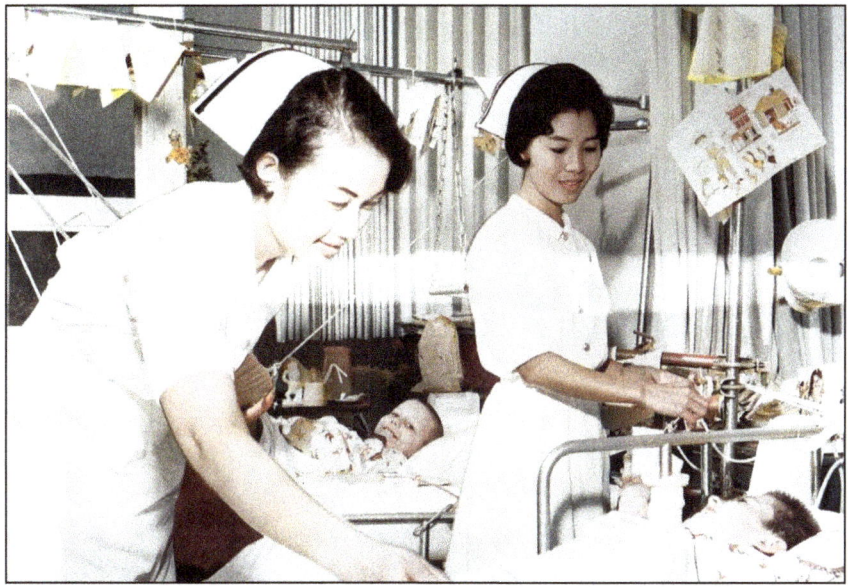

Figure 08.35. Nurses Vichitra Pimsarn, left, and Suvannee Quitraku, at Arcadia Methodist Hospital, the year they arrived in Los Angeles, 1966. C. (Courtesy of the Department of Special Collections, Charles E. Young Research Library, UCLA)

Vichitra Pimsarn and Suvannee Quitraku had wanted to immigrate to the United States since 1958. The International Rotary Club of Los Angeles, a non-religious, non-political service organization, helped them with the difficult paperwork to secure nursing licenses in California and found staff positions for them at the Arcadia Methodist Hospital in 1964.[25]

Coworkers at Methodist Hospital had difficulty pronouncing the Thai names. Quitraku adopted the nickname Noi, which meant small, as she was five feet tall and 90 pounds. Pimsarn chose Mam, meaning too big, because Thailand standards considered Pimsarn's height of five feet five inches and weight of 125 pounds as large.

Pimsarn and Quitraku attended Therapud Nursing College and the Women's Hospital of Midwifery in Bangkok. Therapud Nursing College and the Women's Hospital of Midwifery became the Boromarajonani College of Nursing. The original school was established in Bangkok to address the shortage of nurses during World War II.[26]

The 100-year-old nursing profession in Thailand evolved from a hospital-based, apprentice training model to the development of doctoral programs taught by doctoral-level nurses.[27]

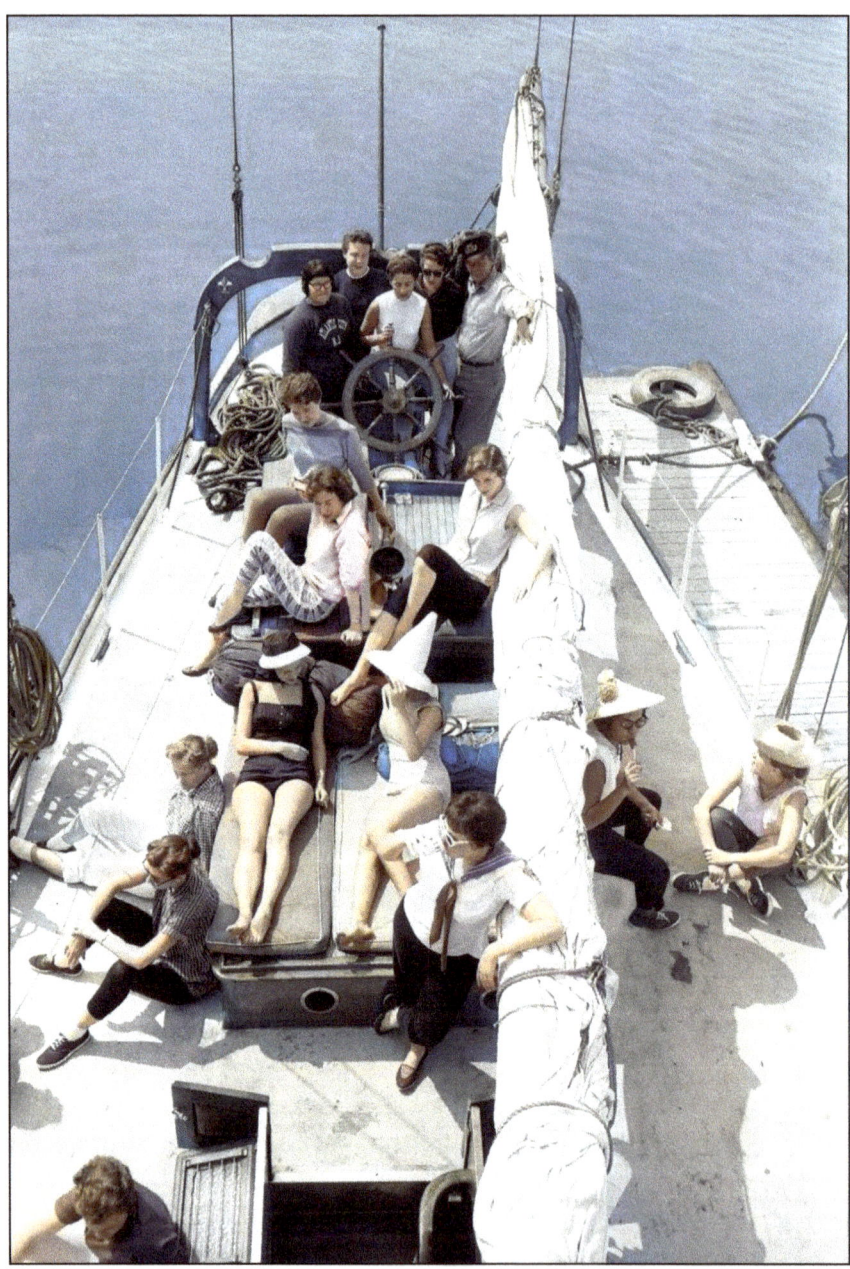

Figure 08.36. Captain Herb Rebeau gave nursing students a steering lesson, August 1, 1958. C. Kathleen DeLeury and Barbara Gjerset, the student class presidents for County General Hospital, planned a two-day celebration trip to Catalina Island for their graduating class aboard the *Cynthia*—a 90-foot sailing vessel. (Charles E. Young Research Library, UCLA)

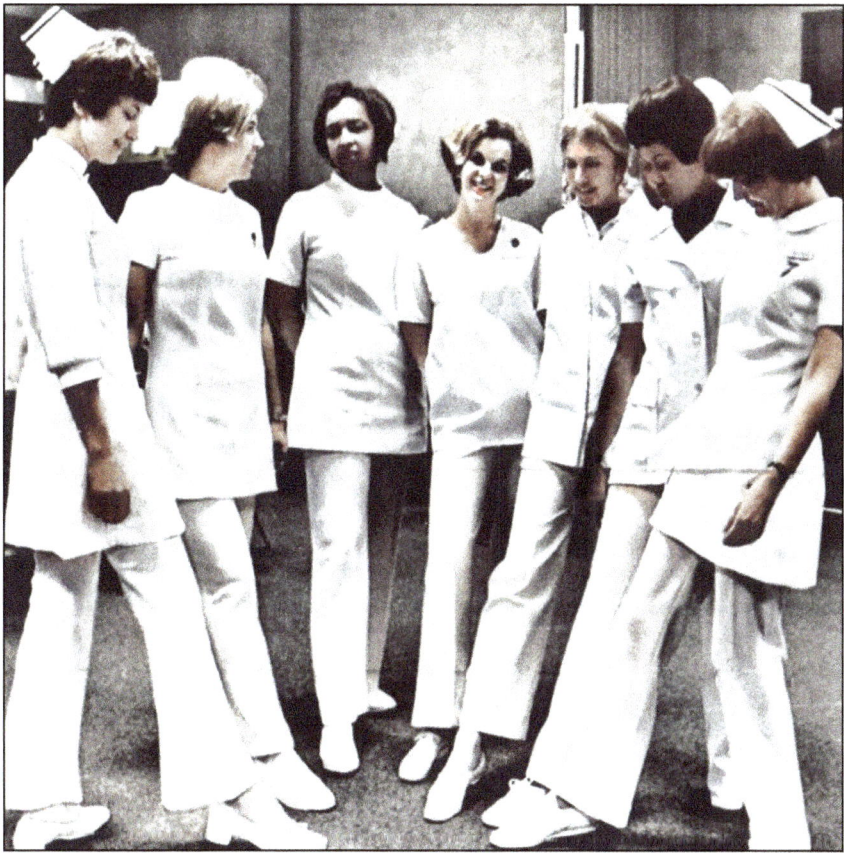

Figure 08.37. Queen of Angels Hospital nurses showed off their newly won right to wear pants, June 1970. C. (Charles Young Research Library, UCLA)

In the 1970s, the Queen of Angels nurses petitioned the administration for the right to wear pants and won. Various newspapers reported, "Fashion is Catching Up With the Women in White." Vanderbilt Hospital said a Chicago hospital started the trend in June 1970—the same month the Queen of Angels pants-rights began. Were the Queen of Angels nurses actually the first? [28]

Nursing schools in the 70s still required dresses. That would soon change. Nurses argued pantsuits were functional because nurses bent and lifted. More men entered nursing, and pants further standardized the look. Pale colors replaced white as the colors were easier to clean and less glaring.

By the 1960s, surgical staff used green scrubs. In the 1980s, ICU and ER nurses wore scrubs too. By the 2000s, many hospital employees, even non-medical, were issued scrub uniforms; departments assigned designated colors. In 2024 some nurses, especially pediatric nurses, switched to street clothes.

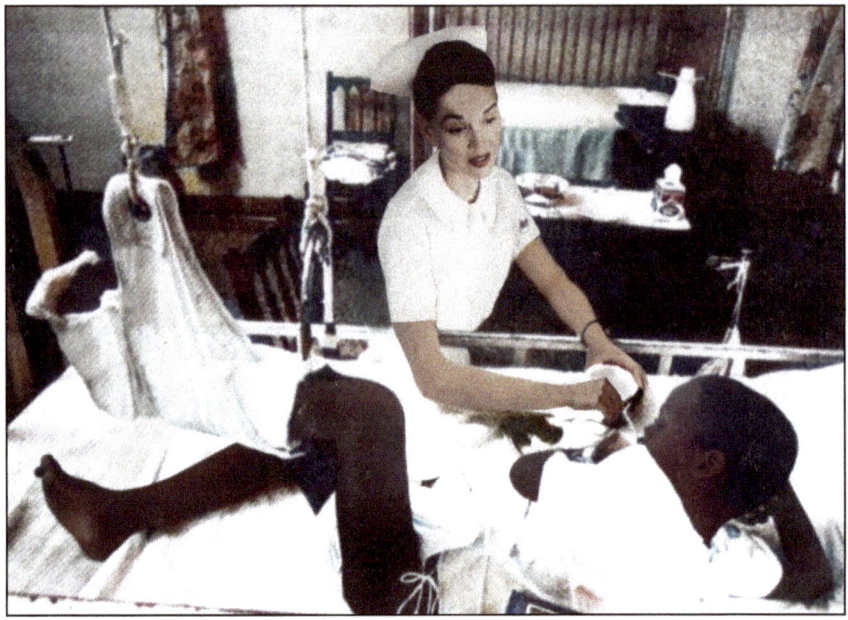

08.38. Student Nurse Kathryn Crosby at Queen of Angels Hospital feeding a child with his leg in traction, c. 1963. C. Her training included typical hospital work in wards and surgery. (Bing Crosby Enterprises, Inc.)

Kathryn Grant Crosby worked as an actress in Hollywood; however, the study of nursing intrigued her. She said, "Many of life's hurdles are met in hospitals; it seemed the perfect place to learn. People are born, have medical emergencies, give birth, and die in the hospital. Everything but get married." She applied to Queen of Angels Nursing School in Hollywood.

She met singer Bing Crosby while making the movie *White Christmas,* and their courtship began. They decided to marry. Various issues delayed the wedding, so she continued with her plan to become a nurse.[29] She received her acceptance into Queen of Angels School of Nursing only a few days before her impromptu Las Vegas wedding in 1957. By this time, the nuns allowed married students into the program, and Crosby was still interested. She started school in early 1958.

Crosby told *Look* magazine that Bing said she would never finish school. Marriage, the birth of three children, and several film appearances slowed her progress; however, she graduated in December of 1963. After graduation, she volunteered to administer injections in the doctor's office at her winter home in Las Cruces, New Mexico. Bing's mother lived with them, and she was proud to say when her mother-in-law became ill, they did not require a private nurse. Crosby cared for her.[30]

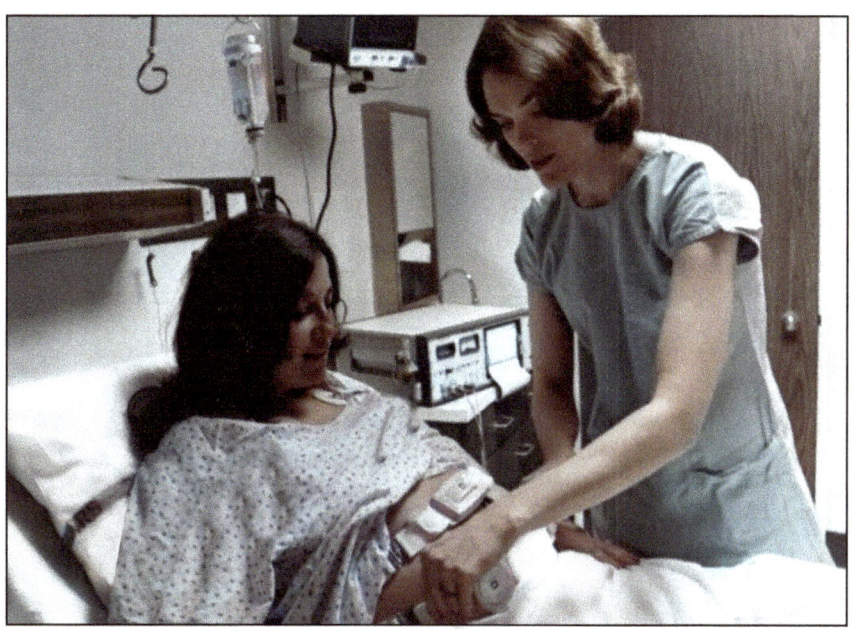

08.39. Nurse Pat Clinton checking a fetal heart-rate monitor at Mt. Sinai Hospital, in Los Angeles, March 21, 1976. C. Hammacher and Hewlett-Packard produced the first electronic fetal heart monitor in 1968 (HP-8020), named the Babysitter.[31] (Special Collections, Charles E. Young Research Library, UCLA)

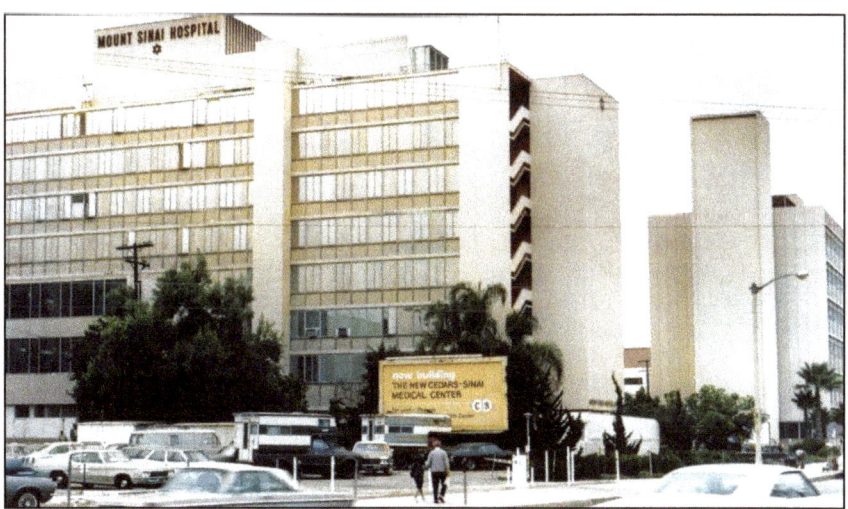

08.40. Mt. Sinai Hospital, on Beverly Boulevard, c. 1975. C. The sign said, "Now building the new Cedars-Sinai Medical Center." The new building opened on April 3, 1976, at the same location. (Cedars-Sinai Medical Center)

Chapter Eight

"Man, woman, birth, death, infinity," marked the opening of the 1960s medical television drama, *Ben Casey*. Doctor Ben Casey was a handsome resident neurosurgeon at County General Hospital who reported to the brilliant, wild-haired Doctor David Zorba, chief of neurosurgery.

Alice Rodriguez—a staff nurse and 1951 graduate of Los Angeles County General Hospital School of Nursing—played a surgical nurse on the show for seven episodes. They filmed the show at County General, and they often used County Hospital nurses in scenes.

Rodriguez checked all scenes involving nurses because correct surgical procedures took years to learn. She would step into camera range during operating room scenes. Nurse Rodriguez said actresses couldn't possibly duplicate the "precise sterile techniques drummed into us nurses until they become automatic." Her notes saved precious time. [32] Rodriguez also acted as a nurse in a 1969 episode of *Marcus Welby* and in the 1974 television movie, *Dr. Max*.

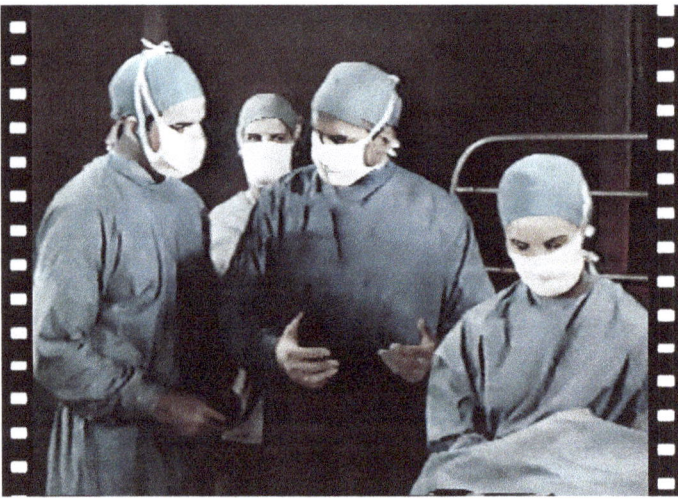

Figure 08.41. A still from the episode, "I Remember a Lemon Tree," 1961. C. Actor Vince Edwards, left, played Ben Casey; George C. Scott, center played Karl Anders; and Alice Rodriquez, RN, right, played the surgical nurse. Anders had just screamed at the nurse because he thought she gave him the wrong size gloves. Casey stepped in and calmed him. Anders was irritable because he had been pilfering morphine, and he needed his fix. [33]

At the end of the episode, Anders suddenly died while Casey sat on his hospital bed talking to him. Casey never called for help or tried to resuscitate Anders—he just took his pulse, covered him with a sheet, and walked out. End of scene. [34]

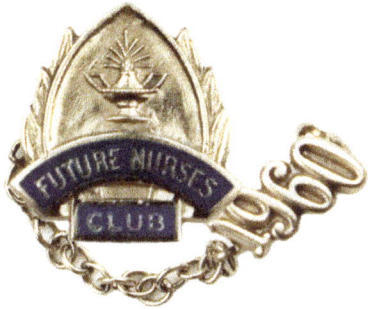 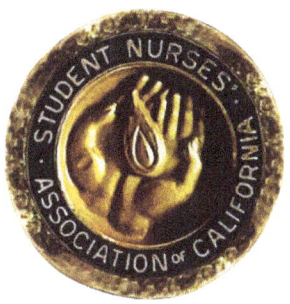

Figure 08.42. A 1960 Future Nurses Club pin, left, and a Student Nurses Association of California pin, right, 2009.

The National Student Nurses Association (NSNA) was established in 1952. By 1960, eighty-seven percent of student nurses belonged to the NSNA. Dues were fifty cents. The top echelon of the American Nurses Association (ANA) mentored NSNA leaders. NSNA members became involved in social issues. They were effective recruiters and established high school clubs called Future Nurses of America.

The local clubs chose famous monikers: Daughters of Florence Nightingale, Clara Barton League, Future White Caps, and Nursettes of Tomorrow. They initiated a nationwide project named "Breakthrough to Nursing" and secured scholarships. Los Angeles was one of the first areas included in the scholarship project. Members of the Future Nurses Club encouraged minorities, including men and Native Americans, to become nurses. [35]

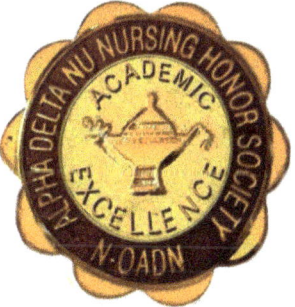

Figure 08.43. Alpha Delta Nu Nursing Honor Society pin, 2024.

The Organization for Associate Degree Nursing (OADN) began in 1984 as the only organization advocating for the Associate in Nursing at the national level. The Alpha Delta Nu Nursing Honor Society acknowledged the academic excellence of students in ADN programs. In 2024, 181 Alpha Delta Nu college chapters existed in the United States.

The organization also established the Academy of Associate Degree Nursing (AADN) to honor individuals who model dedication to ADN education. [36]

Chapter Eight

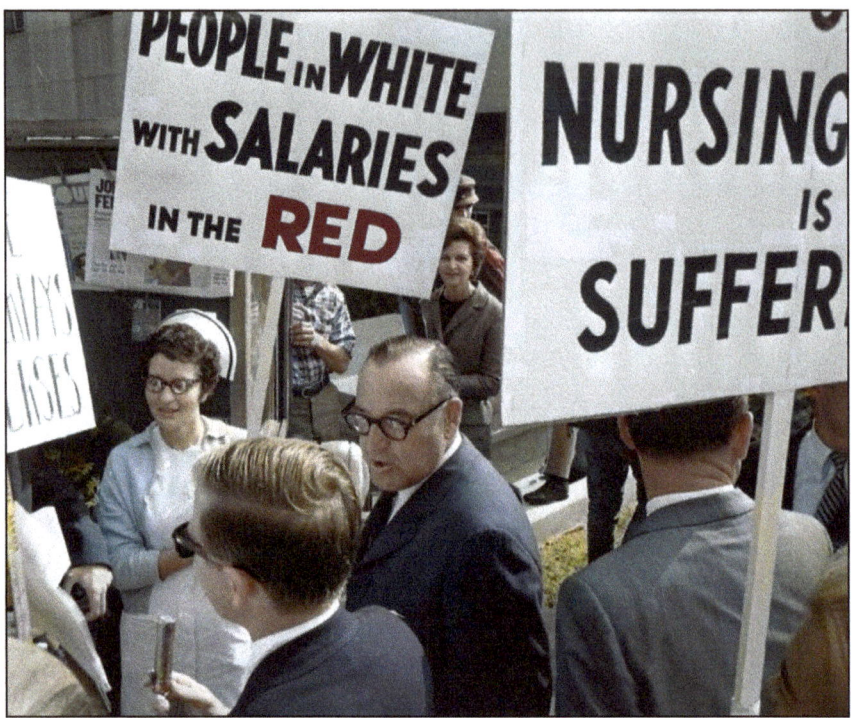

Figure 08.44. State-employed Los Angeles nurses participated in a statewide campaign for higher pay at the Civic Center in downtown Los Angeles, October 14, 1966. C. (Department of Special Collections, Charles E. Young Research Library, UCLA)

When the crowd heard Governor Edmund Brown was leaving the Hall of Administration at 500 West Temple Street, the group surrounded him and demanded he renew the promise to secure them a pay raise. One of the nurses told him there was a discussion of a walkout at UCLA Hospital. "Now don't do that, girls," Brown said. "Have confidence in the Gov."

In the previous year, nurses in San Francisco had received a twenty-five percent increase after they threatened mass resignations. Nurses in private hospitals also received similar increases in pay. Another picketing nurse told Brown the salary for a state-employed graduate nurse was $505 to $585 per month. The same nurse had seen an advertisement in the paper from Cedars of Lebanon Hospital, offering new graduates $660 to $780.

Nurses demanded a pay scale of $644 to $783 per month. Governor Brown told the nurses that, if reelected, he would do everything in his power to meet their demands. The following month voters elected Ronald Reagan as Governor of California.[37]

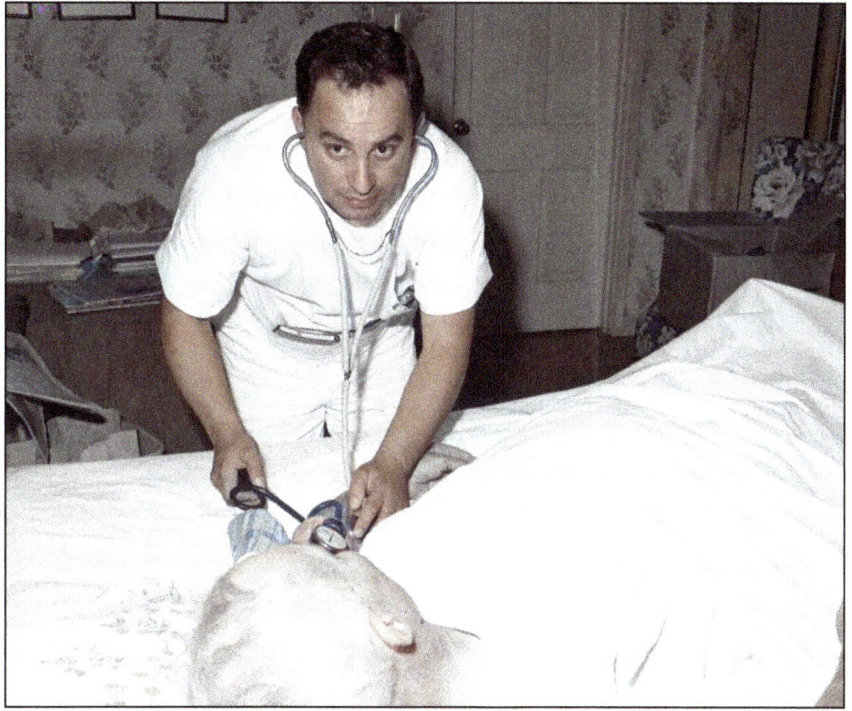

Figure 08.45. Nurse Tony Assinesi, August 29, 1965. C. (Department of Special Collections, Charles E. Young Research Library, UCLA)

Tony Assinesi said about his profession, "You watch over life and you live with death." He cared for the rich and poor and watched them die. He witnessed friends and relatives watching their loved ones die. Assinesi was originally a salesman, but he had to stop working to care for his sick child born with a congenital defect.

Assinesi's first child died on September 5, 1960. His wife learned she was pregnant again the day after the baby's funeral; his second child was four at the time of this photo.

This experience made Assinesi decide to become a nurse. His wife, also a nurse, wanted him to become a doctor—Assinesi thought he would make a better nurse than a doctor. He had no illusions about what people thought about male nurses. "But when someone jokes about my manhood, I give it right back to them," he said. Assinesi graduated from nursing school in 1960 and worked at Lincoln Heights Jail and Central Receiving Hospital.

He told his patients, "You've got to think of yourself before it's too late. Don't wait too long to get your fun out of life—you may not be around to do it." [38]

Figure 08.46. SAINTs, the first mature adult nursing students in the U.S. Betty Armstrong, Mary Lou Trinity, and Werner Heidelberg, left to right, 1968. C. (Special Collections, Charles E. Young Research Library, UCLA)

In January 1968, Queen of Angels School of Nursing began the first U.S. program to train mature adults as registered nurses. The SAINTs program (selected adults in nurse training) enrolled seven students in the first year. The youngest was 37 years of age and the oldest 51. At that time, most training programs for nurses had an age limit of 35. Betty Armstrong commuted 320 miles from China Lake for the pilot program. [39]

Figure 08.47. Inactive registered nurses during a retraining/refresher course. Left to right standing: F. Harris, L. Schlesinger, U. Coffin, M. Beach, and instructor, C. Reinhardt. Left to right seated: I. Wester and I. Kofsky, October 1967. (Courtesy of Hollywood Presbyterian Medical Center)

During the 1970s, widespread reports emerged concerning the shortage of RNs to staff the nation's hospitals and nursing homes. To help alleviate the shortage, Hollywood Presbyterian Hospital joined Valley College to retrain inactive registered nurses who had not practiced for many years. Twelve nurses joined the pilot class in 1976. [40]

Everything but the Utility Sink

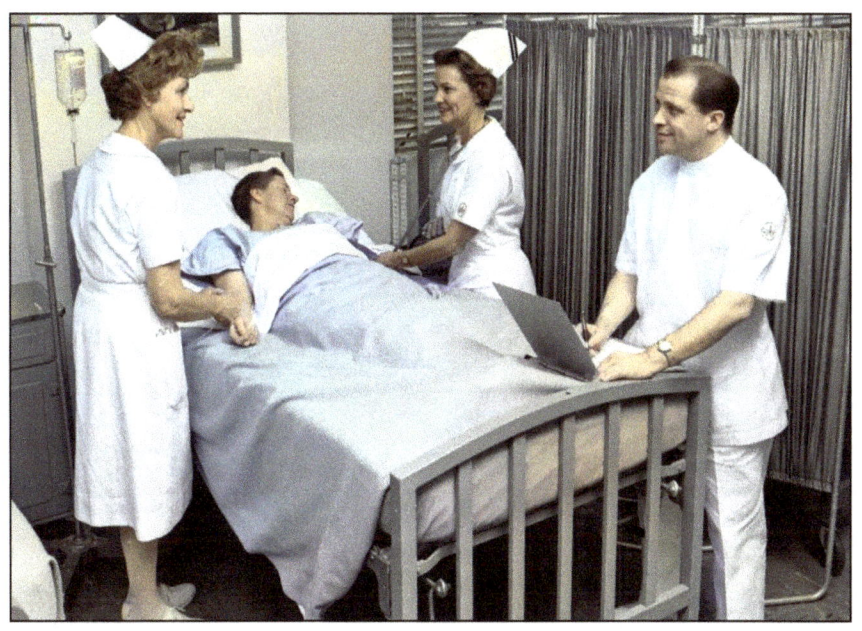

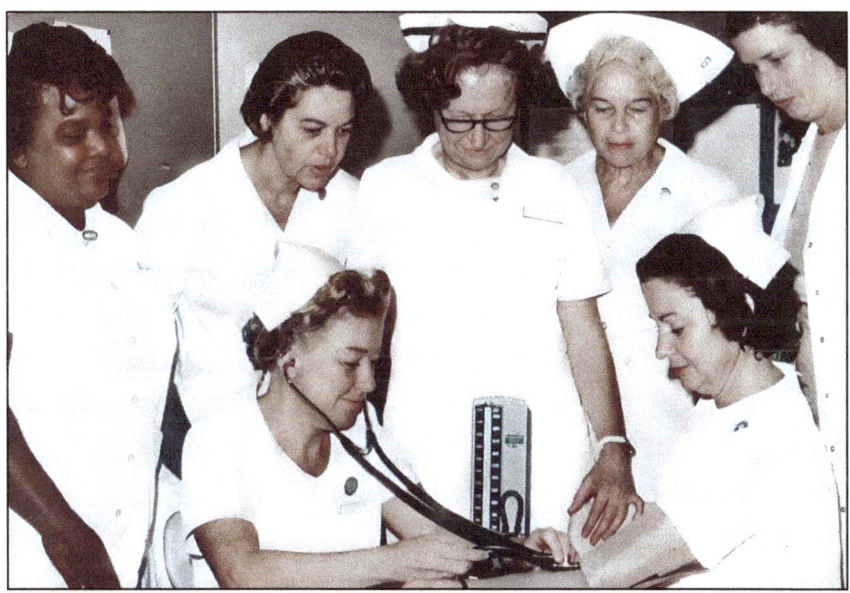

Figure 08.48. Student Nurse Robert Messerly during his training at Good Samaritan Hospital, May 1971.

When Robert Messerly started nursing school, he was a twenty-five-year-old married man with an economics degree from UCLA and two children. He switched careers after a brief experience as a hospital orderly.

He was the only male student in his class at California State University, Los Angeles. They assigned him to a separate locker room. He could not partner with other female students to practice his nursing skills; he had to use mannequins. His three-year-old daughter must not have noticed anything unusual, though, because Messerly said his daughter told people she wanted to be a nurse like her daddy. [41]

Figure 08.49. Student nurse Lynn Loufek caring for an infant at Childrens Hospital in Los Angeles. (Courtesy of the Department of Special Collections, Charles E. Young Research Library, UCLA)

Lynn Loufek didn't think it necessary to correct the baby's mother when she asked, "How's my baby, doctor?" He knew he was not a stereotypical nursing student; he was male. Loufek, an ex-army operating room technician, had worked in broadcasting and as a psychiatric tech. "But jobs were tight, pay and chance for advancements were lousy," Loufek said. "Nursing is better." [42]

Everything but the Utility Sink

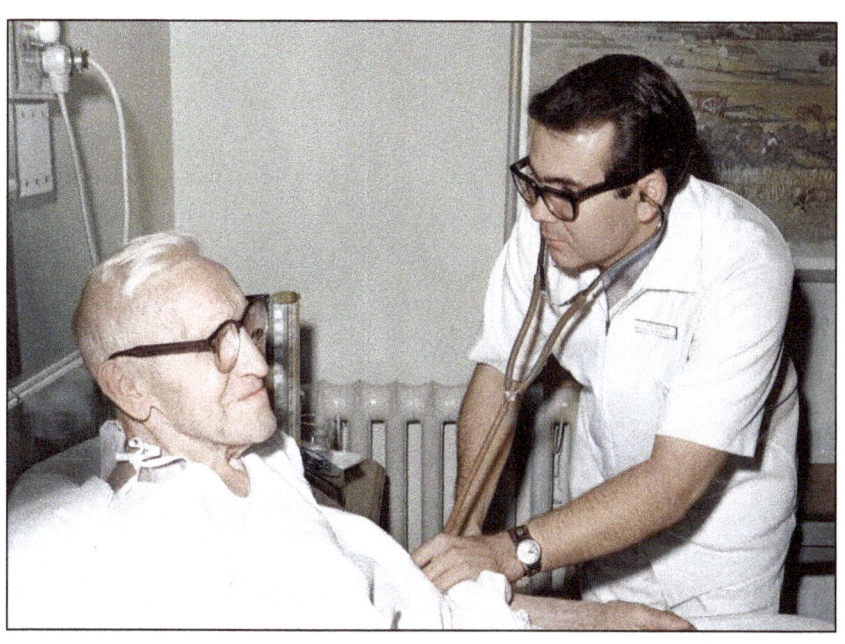

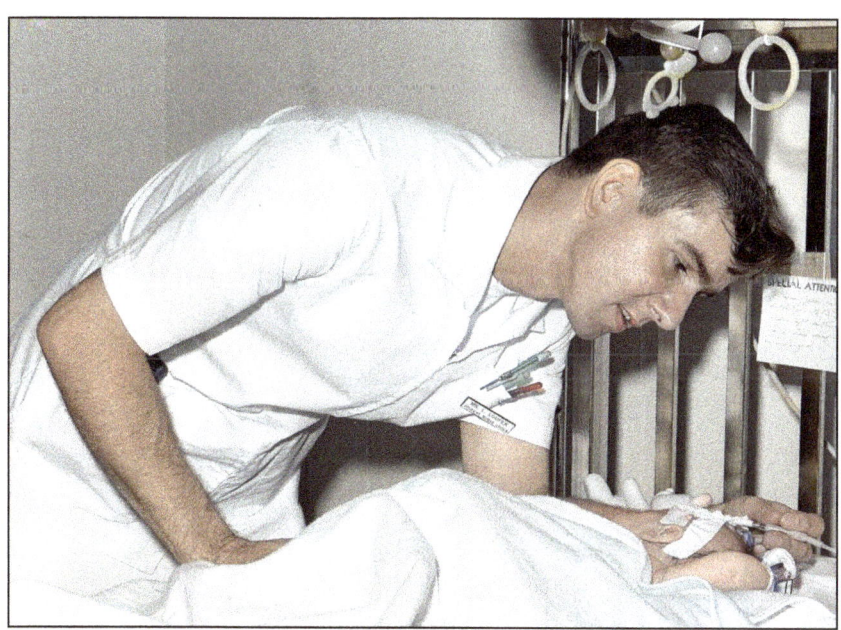

Chapter Eight

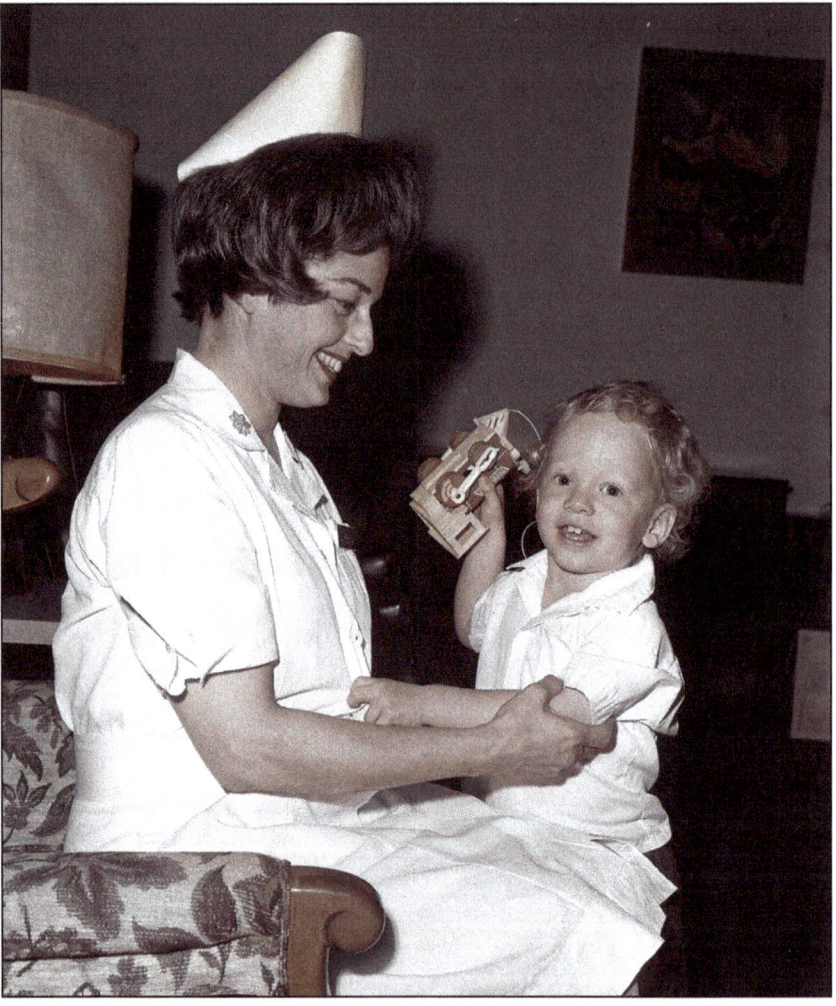

Figure 08.50. Major Lorraine R. Johnson with her two-year-old son after winning her federal lawsuit, July 12, 1970. C.

When Major Lorraine R. Johnson gave birth in 1968, the Army Reserve Nurse Corps discharged her immediately. She had been a commissioned officer for ten years and had only eight years to qualify for retirement. The Army invoked regulations 135 to 175: Any female officer who became a parent, step-parent, foster parent, or guardian of a child under the age of 18 would be discharged. Men were not subject to the same regulations.

She filed a suit in federal court that charged the decision violated federal and executive orders banning sex discrimination. The Army had never been sued for this. Several years later, she won her case and was reinstated.[43]

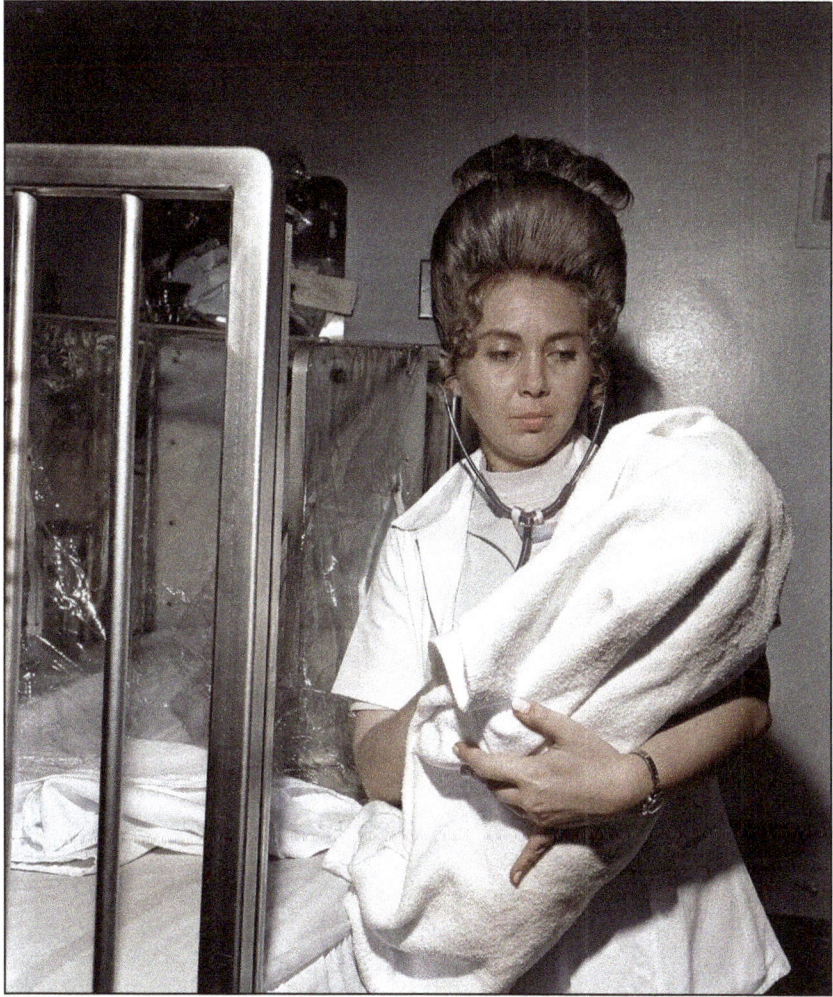

Figure 08.51. Doctor/Nurse Ruth Stupak during her internship at County-USC Medical Center, 1970. C. (Images courtesy of Special Collections, Charles E. Young Research Library, UCLA)

In June of 1970, Ruth Stupak was one of only 600 women in the United States who received a medical degree. She was the only nurse with a dual MD/RN degree in California and only one of three in the United States. At graduation she ranked in the upper fourth of her class at the University of California, Irvine.

She had worked for five years as a nurse in Los Angeles before entering medical school. Stupak said she had an advantage over her doctor colleagues because she understood the role of a nurse.[44]

Chapter Eight

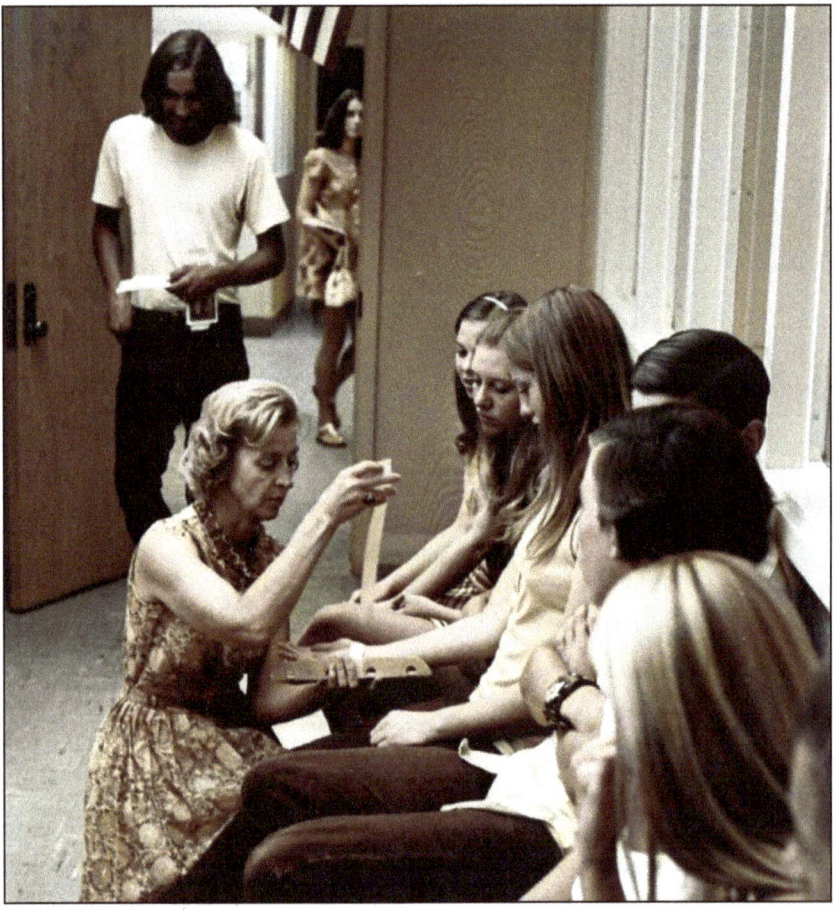

Figure 08.52. School nurse Audrey Hedlund tapes a student's sprained wrist while other teenagers wait in line, May 11, 1972. C.

Audrey Hedlund managed the health emergencies of 2,000 students at Grover Cleveland High School in Reseda. She attended to sprained wrists from pole vaulting, strains, and blistered feet. Drug use, pregnancy, and sexually transmitted infections were more serious issues she commonly faced. School nurses were required to have a Bachelor of Nursing degree, an earned state credential for school nurses, and several years of RN experience. Hedlund feared that less-qualified paraprofessionals might replace school nurses because of the decreased budget.

Nurses were paid the same salary schedule as teachers—$759 to $1,433 a month—yet nurses were usually the first to lose their jobs during a budget crisis. The State Department of Education had a teacher-student ratio; they did not have a nurse-student ratio.[45]

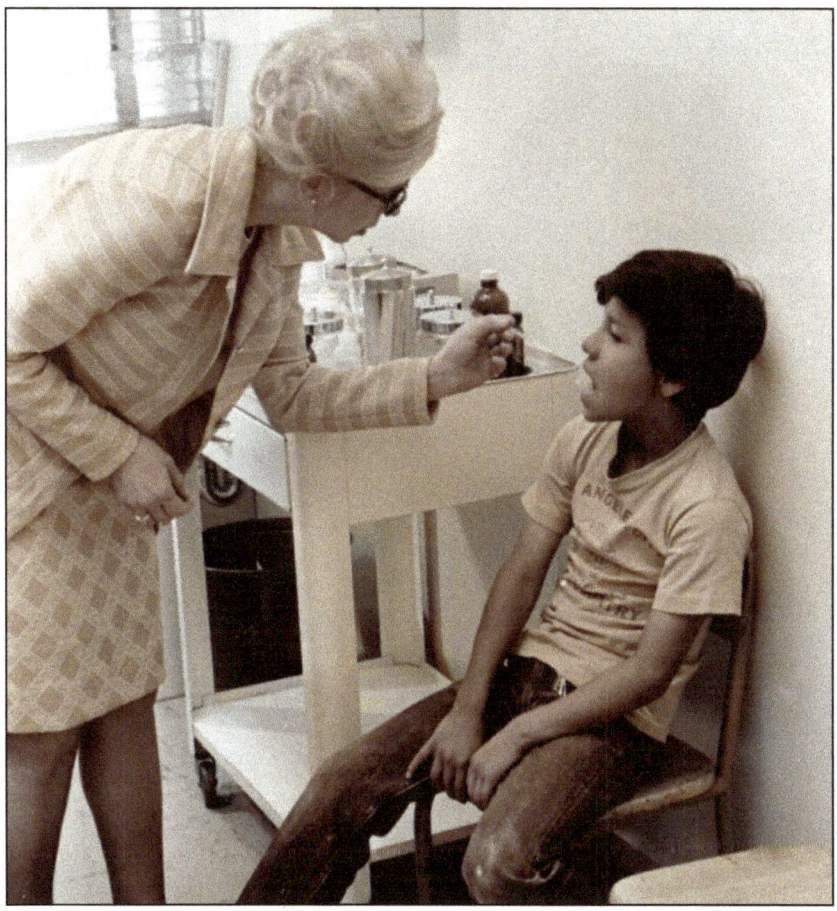

Figure 08.53. School nurse Nina Melching taking the temperature of a fifth-grade student, May 11, 1972. C. (Images courtesy of the Department of Special Collections, Charles E. Young Research Library, UCLA)

In 1972, the *Los Angeles Times* reported that the city planned to ask 127 of the 361 school nurses to turn in their thermometers. The reporter, Lynn Lilliston, spent two days with school nurses to investigate whether schools needed a nurse or if the nurses were merely a frill.

By 9 a.m. Melching had already seen a steady flow of students through her door at Murchison Elementary School. She had treated stomachaches, sore throats, and a lacerated lip, among other problems. During the post-recess lull, Melching visited the classrooms to examine students for possible contagious diseases such as mumps and impetigo. She then spoke to a mother who had questions about her incontinent child. Next, she treated several bruises with ice packs—all before noon.[46]

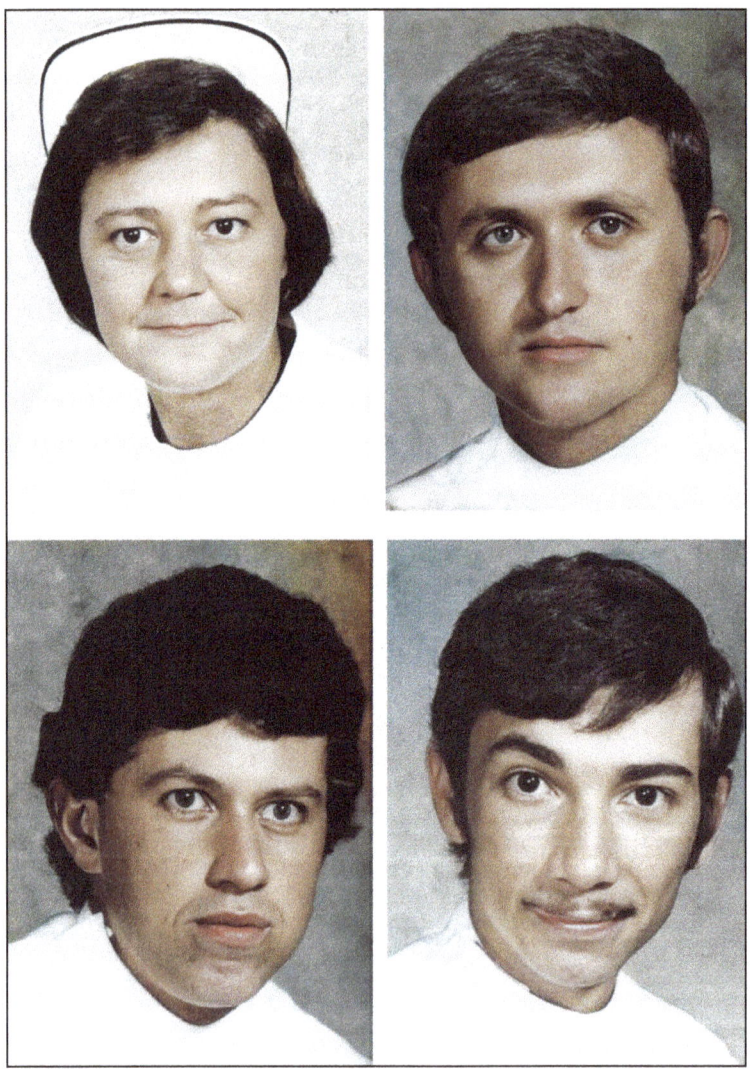

Figure 08.54. Four graduates, former medical corpsmen, from the Los Angeles area: Barbara Dixon from Santa Monica, Andy Roach from Chatsworth, Nicholas Vainas from Santa Ana, and Michael Robertson from Hollywood, 1972. C. (Courtesy of Hollywood Presbyterian Medical Center)

Four former medical corpsmen (two Army and two Navy) graduated from a special eighteen-month accelerated program at Hollywood Presbyterian Hospital School of Nursing in 1972. Students were given advanced credit for their service experience. The medical corpsmen were sought particularly for emergency and critical care assignments. All four passed their state board examinations and intended to obtain Bachelor of Science degrees.[47]

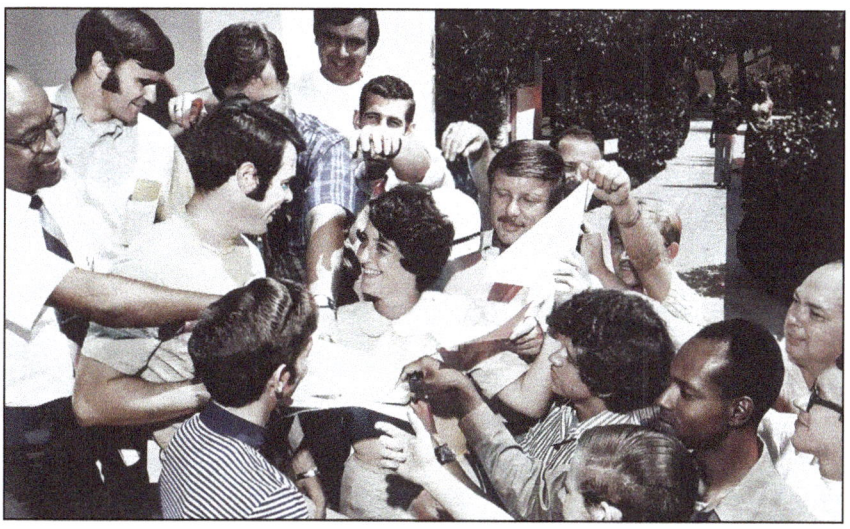

Figure 08.55. Male student nurses during registration and training, 1972. C. Sixteen men transferred into the junior class at Hollywood Presbyterian Hospital School of Nursing in 1972—thirteen were former corpsmen. This year was the first year men were admitted into a regular program. [48]

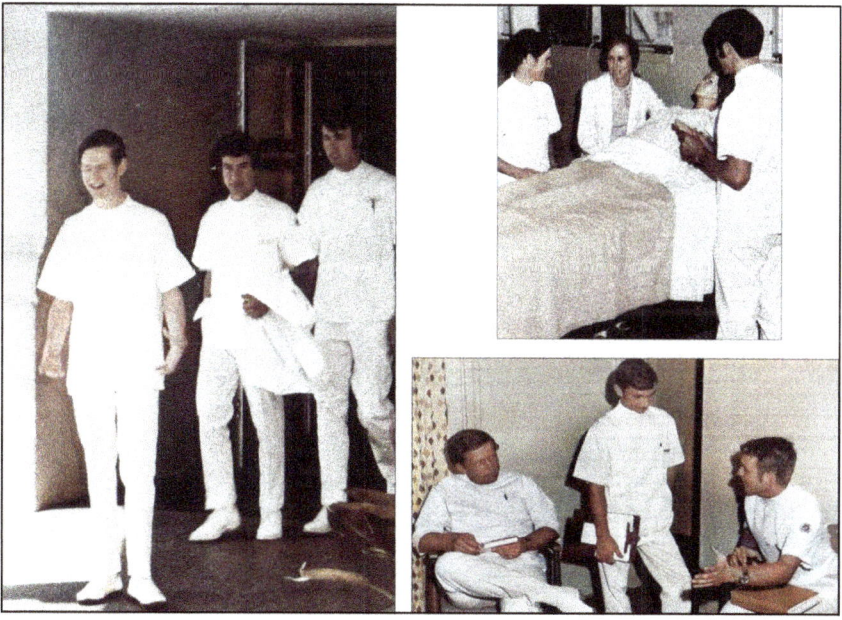

Chapter Eight

Figure 08.56. Nurse Adeline Brown waves to the crowd in front of California Hospital, December 6, 1974. C. (Images courtesy of the Department of Special Collections, Charles E. Young Research Library, UCLA)

California Hospital gave Brown a ticker-tape parade down a block on Hope Street to commemorate her forty-five years of service. Employees presented her with forty-five roses and a 215-foot scroll with 900 signatures. [49]

Figure 08.57. Surgeon John C. Jones kisses Marie G. Brotherton during a reception held in her honor, January 11, 1975. C.

Nurse Brotherton retired from Childrens Hospital in Los Angeles after forty-eight years of service. She worked with Jones when he performed the first recorded heart surgery at Childrens Hospital in 1939: a ligation of a patent ductus arteriosus. [50]

Jones performed another unique surgery in 1956, which involved an eight-year-old boy who had two, instead of one, superior vena cavas; this finding surprised the surgeons during the operation as they had never encountered a double vena cava. The vena cava carries deoxygenated blood from the upper body to the heart. The boy's extra vena cava disturbed the normal heart circulation. The surgery required the surgeons to decrease the boy's body temperature from 98.6 to 88 degrees for ten minutes to create a bloodless surgical field. Ten days after the surgery, the boy walked around smiling and said he wanted to be a football player. [51-52]

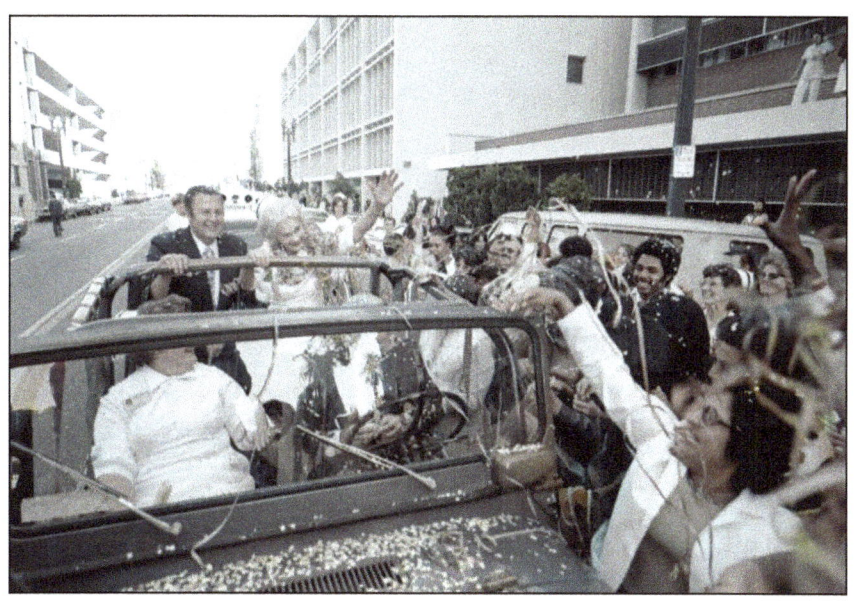

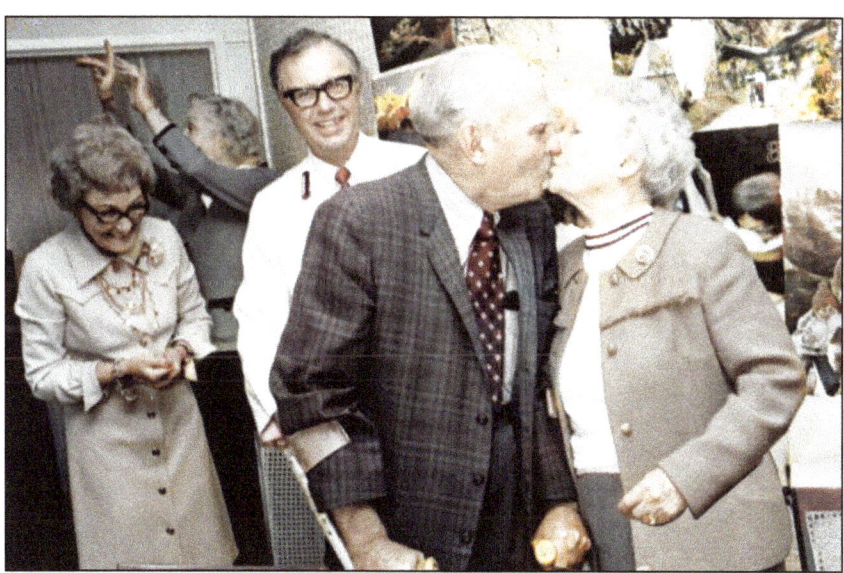

Chapter Eight

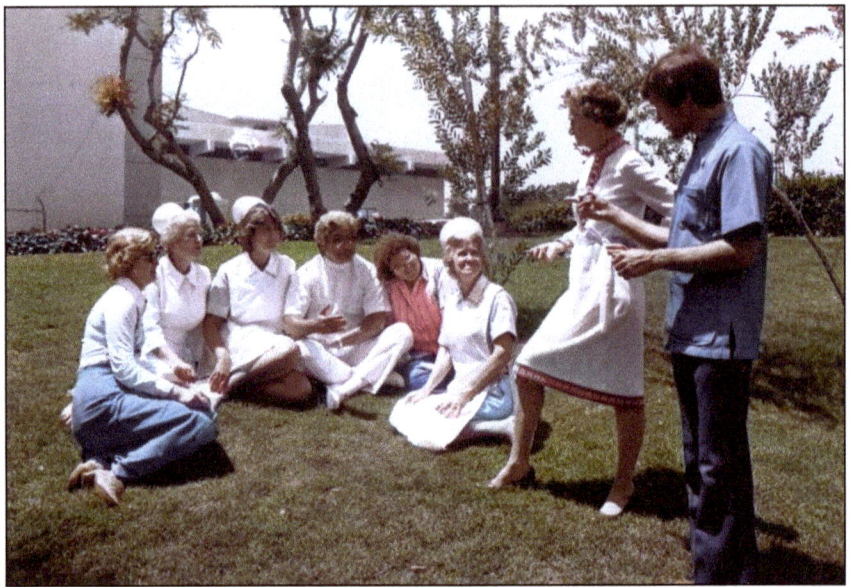

Figure 08.58. Ronnie Fisher, RN, talking with the deaf vocational nursing class at Los Angeles Trade Technical College. Seated, left to right, are the assistant instructor, Katherine Carlson, and the students Charlotte Friedman, Adrianne Riley, Koni Battad, Lana Swearington, and Genevieve Baldwin. Ronnie Fisher and the interpreter, Darryl Allen, are standing, June 27, 1976. C. (Special Collections, Charles E. Young Research Library, UCLA)

When Ronnie Fisher decided to develop a nurse's aide training program for the deaf in 1974, state agencies told her it was against the law. It was not. She found two hospitals that allowed her students to train in the facilities, and eight students completed the course.

In 1975 she developed a licensed vocational nurse program for the deaf at Los Angeles Trade Technical College. Fisher had taught nursing at the college for eighteen years. Her biggest hurdle was the lectures, not the clinicals; the technical lectures were difficult for the interpreter to translate into sign language. Four women and one man completed the required 1,500 hours of classroom lectures and hospital skills. deaf nurses adapted to clinical situations as needed. One technique they used was to back out of a room while keeping their eyes on the patient, in case the patient needed something else. However, they mostly functioned the same as hearing nurses would. They read lips when needed. Patients generally accepted them.[53]

Frank Hochman, the first deaf physician in the United States, spoke at the students' graduation ceremony. He told the students that hearing people should not decide what is best for deaf people.[54]

Everything but the Utility Sink

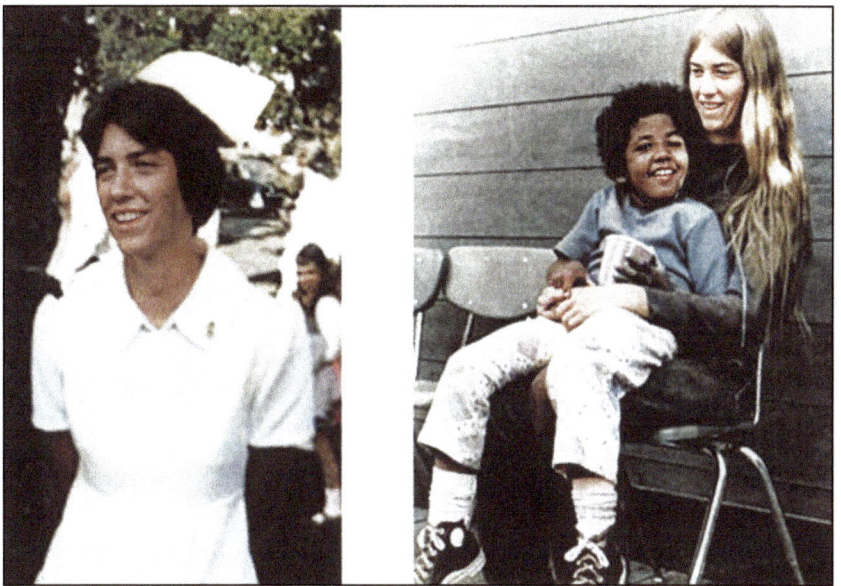

Figure 08.59. Annie Moore at her 1975 nursing school graduation and at Jonestown with one of the children. C. (Courtesy of Jonestown Institute)

Jim Jones opened the Peoples Temple in Los Angeles in 1972. A registered nurse, Annie Moore, joined the church. The members moved to Guyana in South America in 1977 and started a religious utopia called Jonestown.

Family of several Jonestown members who lived in the U.S. reported to their congressman that it was a dangerous cult. On November 18, 1978, Congressman Leo Ryan and four others flew to Guyana to investigate.

When they tried to leave and take several members, a Jonestown militia assassinated Ryan and the others on the tarmac. Jones then instructed the nine-hundred-member group to commit mass suicide with potassium cyanide punch and feed it to their children. A few escaped and survived.

Moore was Jones' personal nurse. Her body was found in Jones's cabin doorway near a gun and her suicide note. Only Jones and Moore died from gunshots. One theory said she shot him first, so he would not have to drink cyanide, and then she shot herself.

Her 651-word suicide letter detailed love for Jones and Jonestown. She said the children were intelligent and happy. The seniors had dignity, respect, and gardens. Few were sick, and when they were, they were given the best care. She signed it, "We died because you wouldn't let us live in peace!" [55] The survivors told a different story of exhaustion, hunger, and coercion. [56]

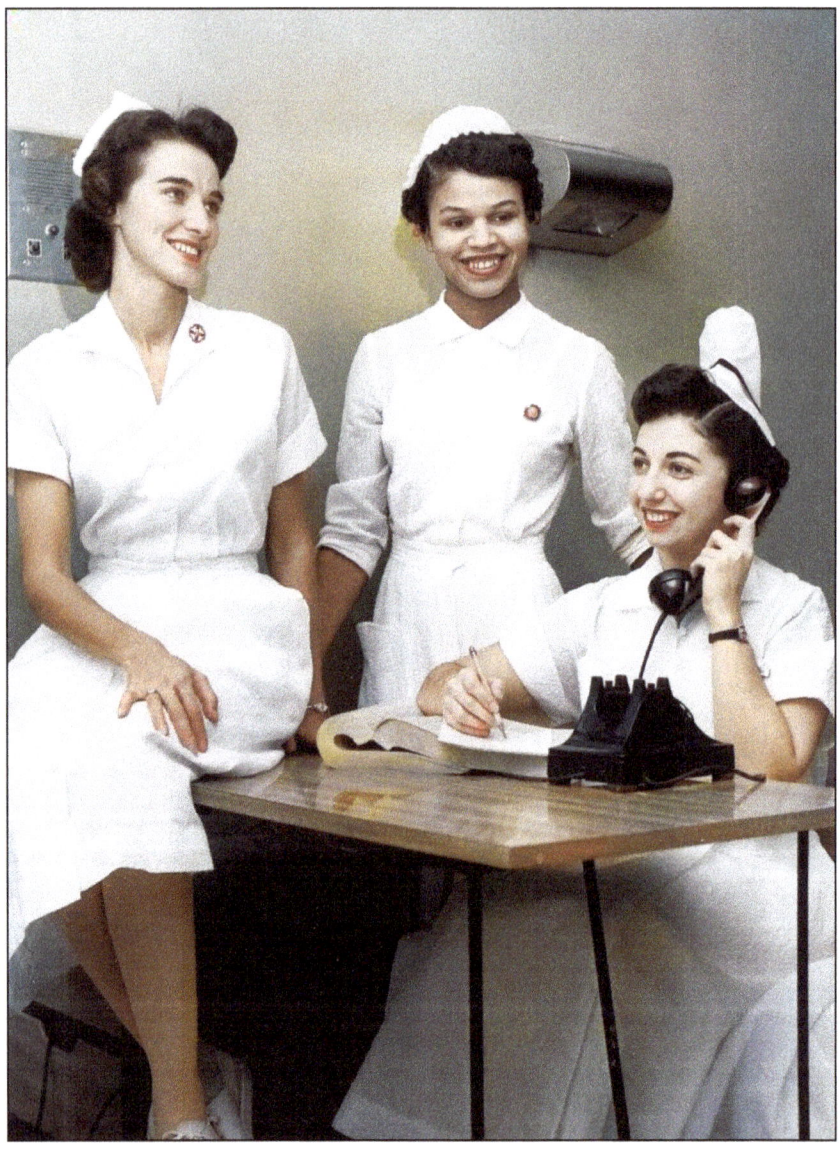

Figure 08.60. Nurses Madeleine Lauasseur, Eva Bowser, and Sylvia Ramnich, in Los Angeles, 1940s. C.

A nurse talking on the phone and writing was a staged nursing photographic theme for decades. Bowser is wearing a graduate pin from the Bellevue School of Nursing. Bellevue Hospital in New York was one of the first three American hospitals to start a training school utilizing Florence Nightingale's principles. The other two were the Connecticut Training School and Boston Training School. All three schools opened in 1873.

Everything but the Utility Sink

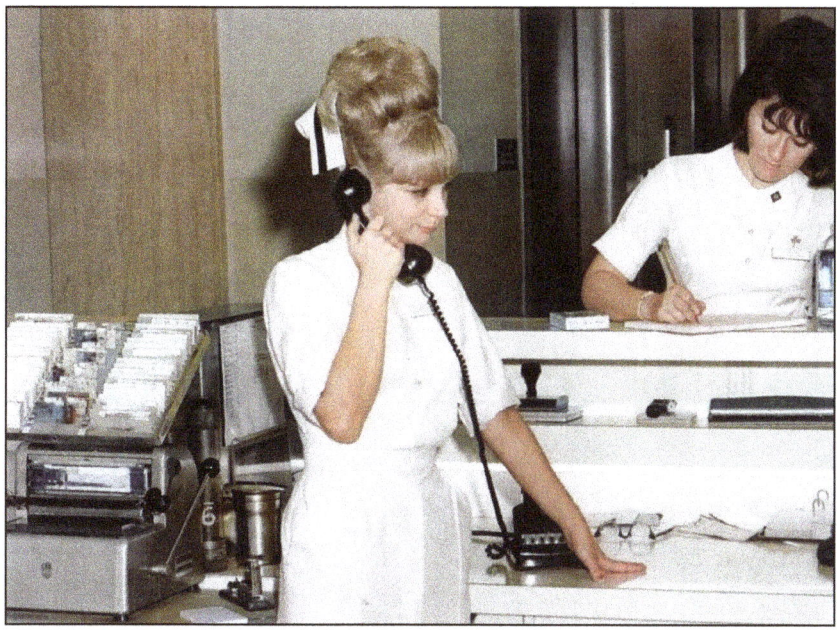

Figure 08.61. A nurse on the phone and a nurse writing, 1970s. C. Note the Addressograph on the left with patients' cards above it. Every patient had a card (first metal, then plastic) containing their name, medical record number, and other important information. Nurses inserted the card into the Addressograph and stamped every page in a patient's chart.

Figure 08.62. Nurse Erma Gallenburg on the phone and writing. Gallenburg was the night nursing supervisor at Mt. Sinai Hospital, 1964. C. (Images Courtesy of Cedars-Sinai Medical Center)

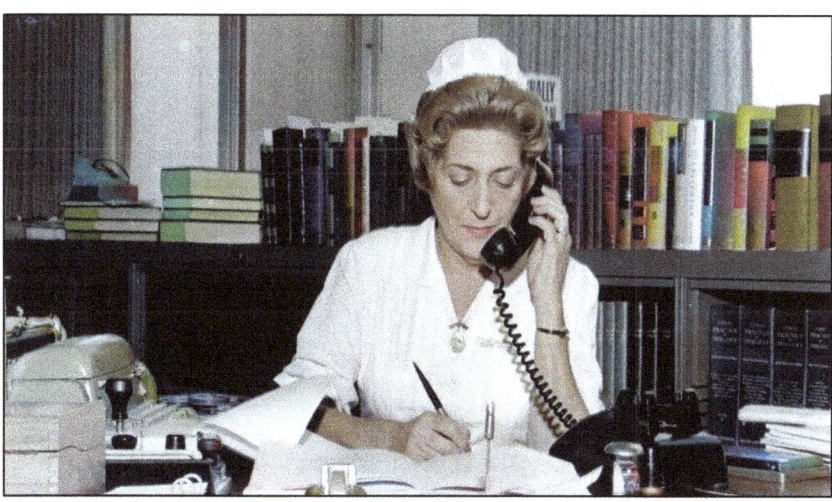

Chapter Eight

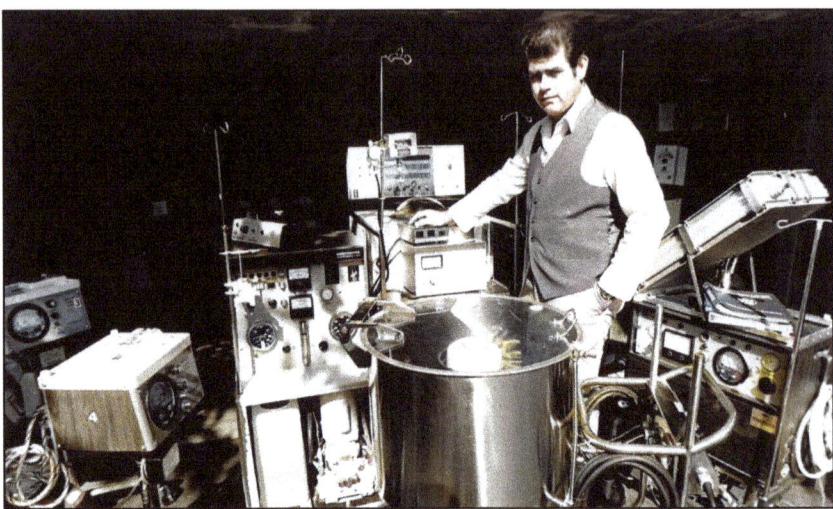

Figure 08.63. Ray Duarte with his Museum of Hope machines, n.d. He preserved seventeen pieces of equipment as a testimonial to the patients who used them. C. (Courtesy of Ray Duarte)

Ray Duarte collected outdated dialysis machines over many years for his Museum of Hope. The 1950–1971 machines were from earlier stages of kidney dialysis treatments. Hospitals donated machines for his collection; Duarte and his corps of volunteers rescued others before sanitation trucks picked them up. He displayed his dialysis museum at regional and national kidney conferences and at rayduarte.com. His collection included a 100-liter pump tank, one of the first machines marketed on a large scale.

After his 1971 graduation from RN school, Duarte worked in Los Angeles County General's Renal Ward 4000. Renal nurses became proficient in the care of patients undergoing kidney transplants, peritoneal dialysis, and hemodialysis. They were trained in self-care, home care, inpatient care, and acute care hemodialysis—a training style that no longer exists.

While in training, Duarte's instructors warned him there was a twenty-five percent probability he would contract hepatitis and a one percent probability of mortality. Later, he learned the risk was a forty percent chance. The nurses pulled patients' names out of a hat to determine which lucky patient would receive the difficult-to-obtain renal care. Nurses primed the artificial kidney filters with formaldehyde. With blood flows of 300 cubic centimeters to 500 cubic centimeters per minute, nurses and patients were extremely fearful of air entering the lines. Many patients died. [57]

Duarte published technical articles in *Dialysis and Transplantation* magazine and creative short stories in various anthologies.

Everything but the Utility Sink

Sharon Rogone became an LVN in 1976. After receiving her Associate Degree in Nursing from San Bernardino Valley College in 1980 she worked as a neonatal nurse in the Los Angeles area. She soon realized the need for basic, well-designed equipment.

During the 1980s, neonatal intensive care nurses had to improvise the many devices they needed to care for premature infants. Manufacturers made few tools to fit the size of a tiny preemie. In 1990, Rogone started her own company, "Small Beginnings," to develop her ideas.

Her product inventions included the Bili Bonnet (a shield to protect the baby's eyes during phototherapy), specialized diapers, pacifiers, positioning devices, and suction tools. She sold her products to major hospitals in Los Angeles, Chicago, and New York, and international sites.

The Smithsonian, in Washington D.C., placed her patented products in their archives. They listed her in three categories: a woman entrepreneur, a woman inventor, and the medical category for neonatal intensive care products.

Rogone said everyone is an inventor. "Every time you wish you had something that would do this and that, you are an inventor. If you pursue it, it is an invention. However, people simply do not pursue. The pursuit, and the perseverance to follow up on your ideas, is what makes the difference." [58]

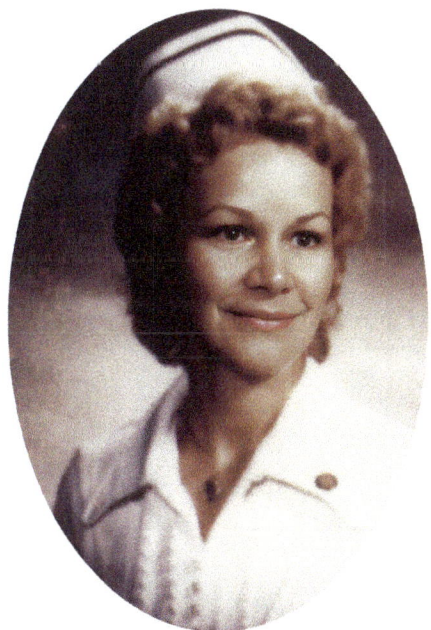

Figure 08.64. Sharon Rogone's nursing school photo, 1980. (Sharon Rogone)

Chapter Eight

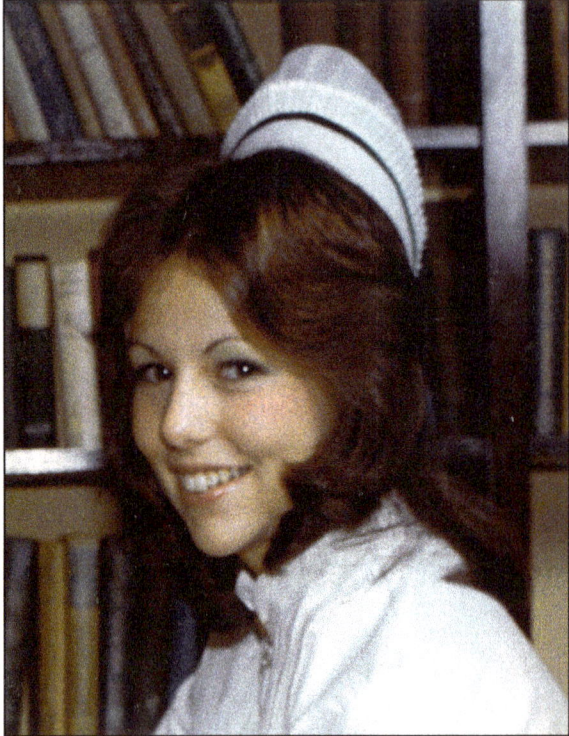

Figure 08.65. Lynn Campanaro on the day she received her diploma from Westchester Hospital School of Nursing, 1974. (Lynn Campanaro)

Lynn Campanaro said she wanted to become a hairdresser; however, her father insisted all his daughters obtain a college education: he wanted her to become a nurse. Campanaro soon realized nursing suited her. One of her five sisters also became a nurse.

When Campanaro graduated in 1974, patients who required long-term care at Westchester Hospital were wards of the state. They never left. They lived in the hospital their entire lives; nursing students who graduated from training programs thirty years apart could discuss common patients they had cared for during training. Rules were different in the 1970s: nurses were allowed to smoke at the nurses station even though patients with oxygen were lying in beds nearby the desk.

Campanaro advanced her diploma degree and obtained a Bachelor of Science and then a dual Master of Science in Nursing and Informatics. After twenty-eight years in pediatrics and research, she moved to Los Angeles to work as a supervisor in laser surgery. Campanaro never regretted changing career paths, but she still liked to cut and style her friends' hair.[59]

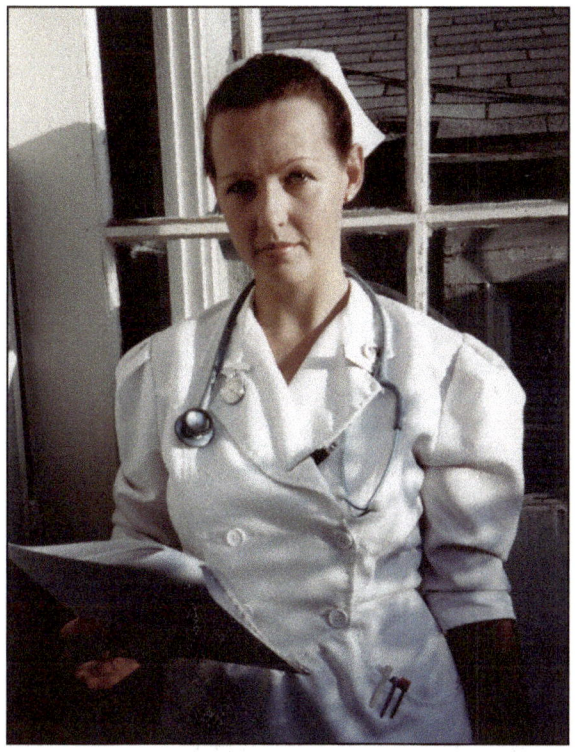

Figure 08.66. Fey Reichman starred in her former husband's film school movie, *All in a Day's Work,* 1993. Although she wore a nurse's cap for the movie, she never wore a cap for work. He derived the title from a phrase written on an old Nurse Mate shoebox. The movie plot involved a nurse who murdered her husband. (Courtesy of Fey Reichman)

Reichman graduated from *krankenpflegeschule* (nursing school) in Munich, Germany, in 1985. Nursing students in Germany could study either midwifery or nursing. Reichman put her name on the school's waiting list. She wanted to become a midwife, but nursing school was available first. Their academic pathways were further divided: nurses studied either adult or pediatrics.

At mealtimes in the hospital, the kitchen wheeled in carts with huge steaming pots of food. The nurses ladled out patients' food from the large pots—individualized food trays did not exist. Nurses reused bandages. The laundry washed them, and the nurses re-rolled them every day.

Reichman took additional pediatric classes when she moved to California to conform to U.S. requirements. She passed the nursing board exam in 1994 and began working with HIV patients. After her first position, Reichman worked in several nursing specialties and as a certified massage therapist. [60]

Chapter Eight

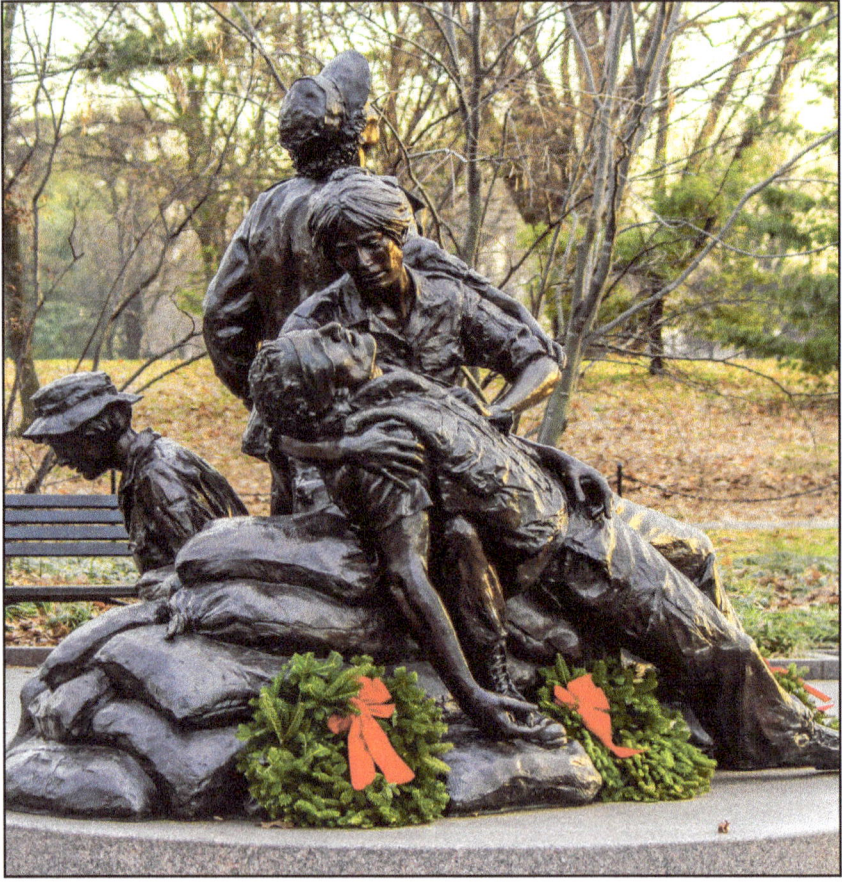

Figure 08.67. Vietnam Women's Memorial at the Vietnam War Memorial, Constitution Gardens, Washington D.C., Dec 21, 2013. (By James DeMers)

The Army Nurse Corps and Vietnam Veteran, Diane Carlson Evans, first conceived the idea of creating the Vietnam Women's Memorial in 1983. Not everyone agreed with her idea. Evans and the other founders experienced controversy and rejection.[61]

They faced challenges for many years: fundraising, resolutions to get passed, Senate and House amendments, Fine Arts Commission rejections and approvals, and presidential legislation. After ten years the sculpture was constructed at the Vietnam War Memorial site in Washington, D.C., and dedicated on November 10-12, 1993.

The sculptor, Glenna Goodacre, arranged the four figures-in-the-round, creating an interesting composition from all angles. Sandbags support the nurses as in Vietnam. She modeled it, in part, after Michelangelo's "Pietà."[62]

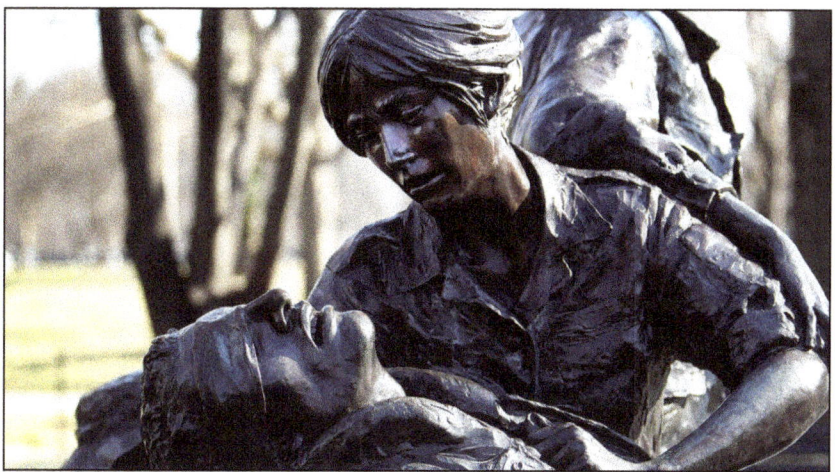

Figure 08.68. Close-ups of a nurse comforting a wounded soldier on her lap, another kneels, staring at the soldier's empty helmet with an expression of frustration and despair, a third looks up in search of a medevac helicopter, March 1, 2022, Photos courtesy of Marvin Lynchard, DOD.[63]

The Vietnam War lasted from 1954 to 1975. The U.S. engaged in the conflict from 1961 to 1975: 6,250 U.S. nurses served during the war. Eight died.[64]

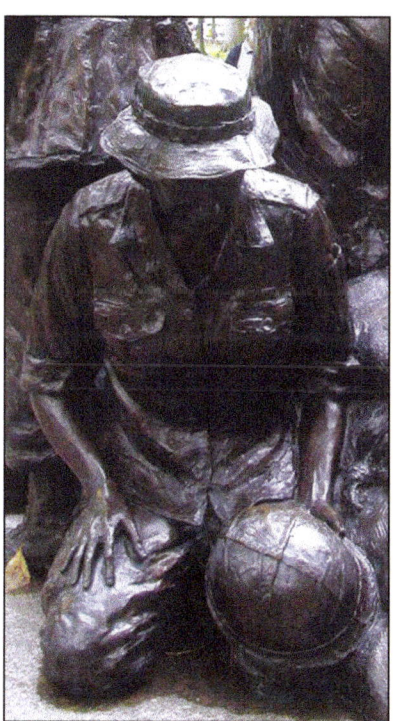
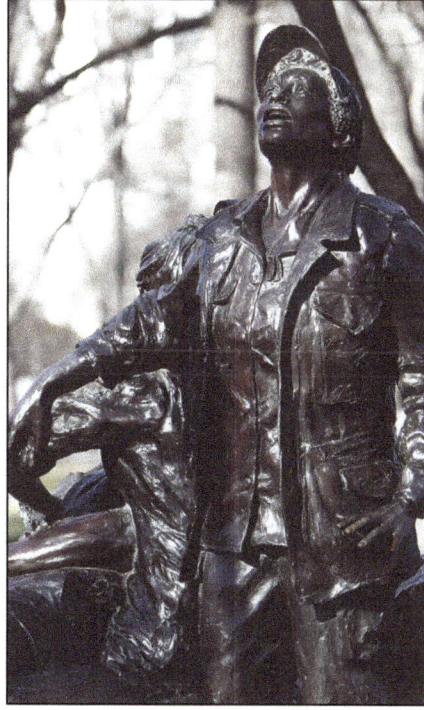

Chapter Eight

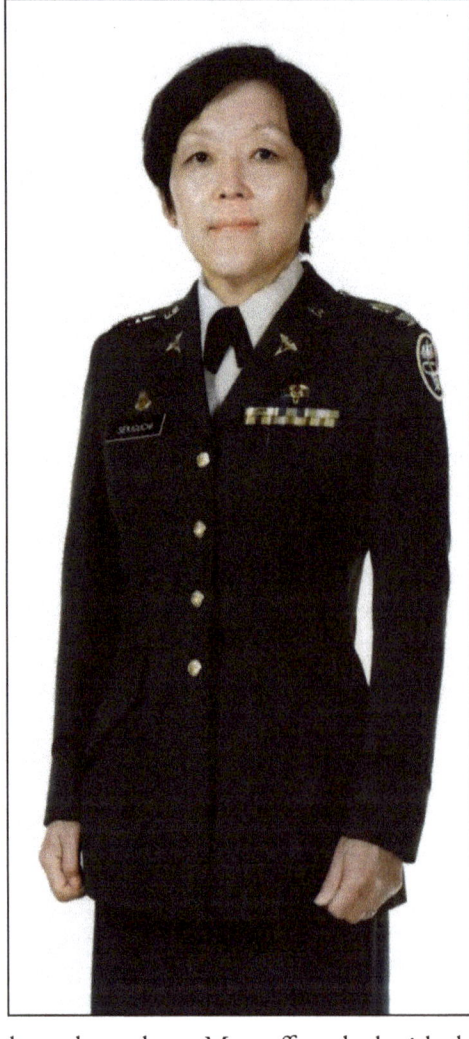

Figure 08.69. June Sekiguch, n.d. C. (Courtesy of Military Women's Memorial)

Born in Los Angeles, June Sekiguchi was a chief nurse in the Army when she received orders that her staff would assist the Navy with the infamous Operation Babylift.[65]

At the end of the Vietnam War, on 3 April 1975, Saigon City was attacked. The United States Government decided to evacuate Vietnamese orphans in a plan called Operation Babylift. Over three weeks, they evacuated approximately 2,000 children out of Vietnam and flew them to Canada, Europe, and Australia.

Sekiguchi said, "Deep within the furrows of my heart, I remember some of the innocent victims of disengagement from birth families and re-engagement with their new American families. To this day, I wonder about each of the children and hope to be able to hear about them. My staff worked with the Navy as long as we were needed to process these innocent victims of war."

One of the casualties of war and its aftermath was inadequate documentation; not all the children were true orphans. Some birth parents and relatives, who later immigrated to the United States from Vietnam, requested custody of children already placed into families.[66]

Sekiguch obtained a Master of Nursing and Master of Business. She received a Meritorious Service Medal, with two Oak Leaf Clusters; an Army Commendation Medal; a National Defense Service Medal; an Army Service Ribbon; and an Overseas Service Ribbon. Sekiguchi retired with the rank of colonel.[67]

Figure 08.70. Patricia Shields n.d. C. (Military Women's Memorial)

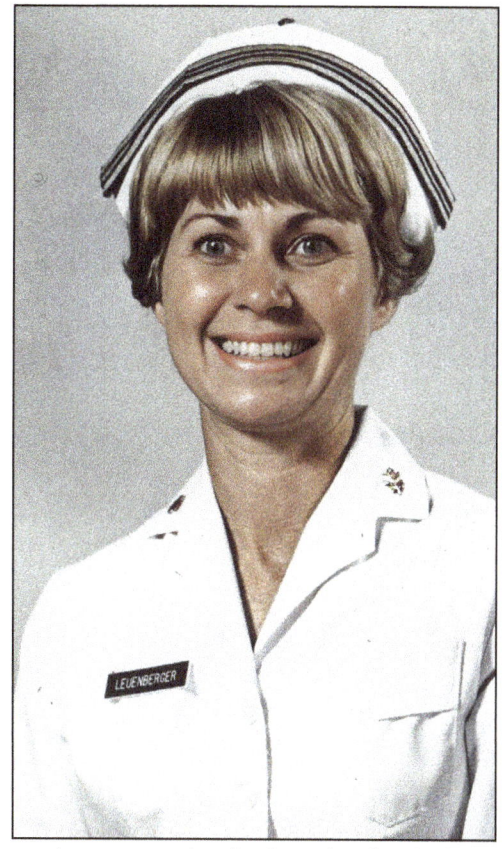

In 1954, Los Angeles native Patricia Leuenberger Shields joined the military branch called Women Accepted for Volunteer Emergency Services (WAVES).

The WAVES, a female non-nursing branch of the Navy, was established during World War II. WAVES held rank and received military pay. [68]

Most WAVES performed clerical work. Shields received additional hospital training and became part of the WAVES Hospital Corps.

They assigned her to the Naval Hospital in Corona, California. Shields hoped she could save enough money to attend nursing school when she finished her active duty.

In March of 1955, Congress passed "The Career Incentive Act." It included a nursing education program that selected a few Hospital Corps WAVES to attend four-year collegiate nursing programs—completely paid by the Navy.

The program was called the Navy Enlisted Nursing Education Program (NENEP). Shields was one of the first ten nurses to participate. The Navy sent her to the University of Colorado at Boulder. NENEP students wore the WAVE uniforms with a new arm patch.

When the other private nursing students went home in the summer, the NENEP students stayed at the Naval Hospital in the Great Lakes. Shields received a Bachelor of Science in Nursing and served in the Navy Nurse Corps in Vietnam until 1976.

She retired with the rank of Commander and received the National Defense Service Medal and the Vietnam Service Medal. [69]

Chapter Eight

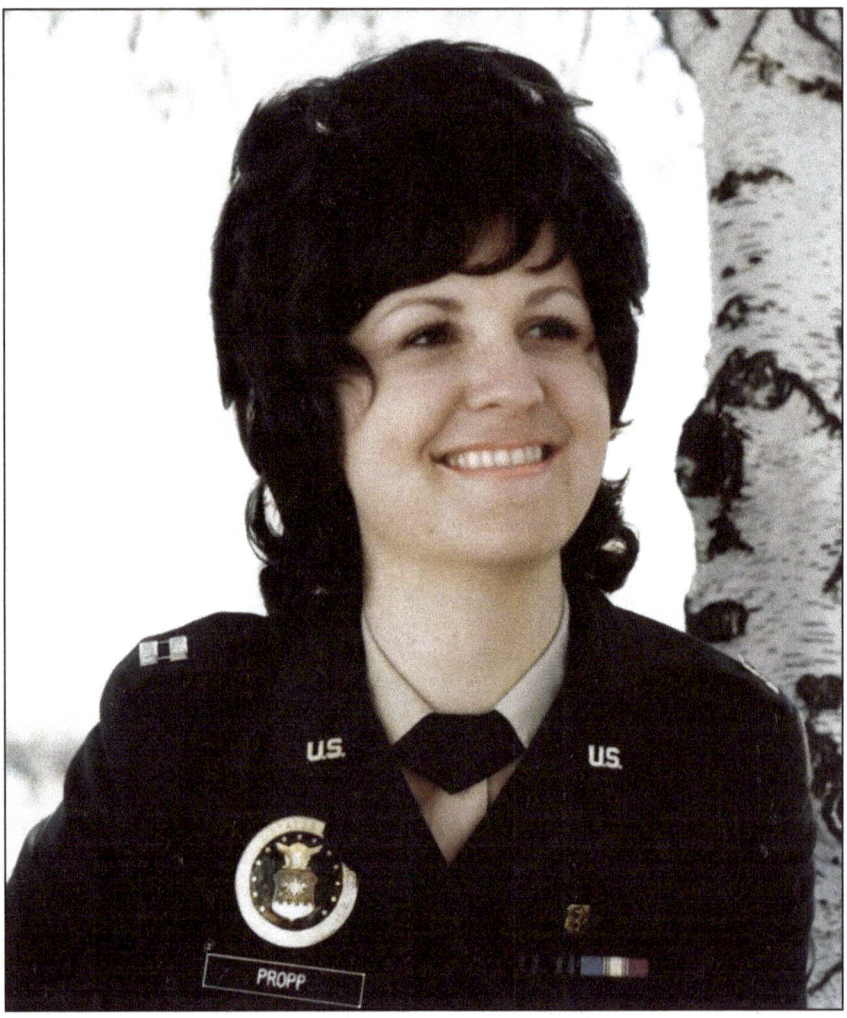

Figure 08.71. Los Angeles native, Lieutenant Colonel Janet Propp Weaver, n.d. C. She served on active duty in the Air Force Nurse Corps from 1968 to 1976 and in the reserves until 1994. (Military Women's Memorial)

Janet Propp Weaver became part of an unexpected five-month recall to active duty when Desert Shield/Desert Storm began in Iraq. Weaver said, "I remember that Friday night phone call on November 9, 1990, 'By orders of the President of the United States, you are hereby called to active duty in support of Desert Shield.'" With that order, she returned to a primary care nursing role that she had not practiced for seventeen years. She was amazed, however, that she could function as a nurse again after all those years away from bedside nursing. She said her confidence grew each day despite the stress of the acute care setting. [70]

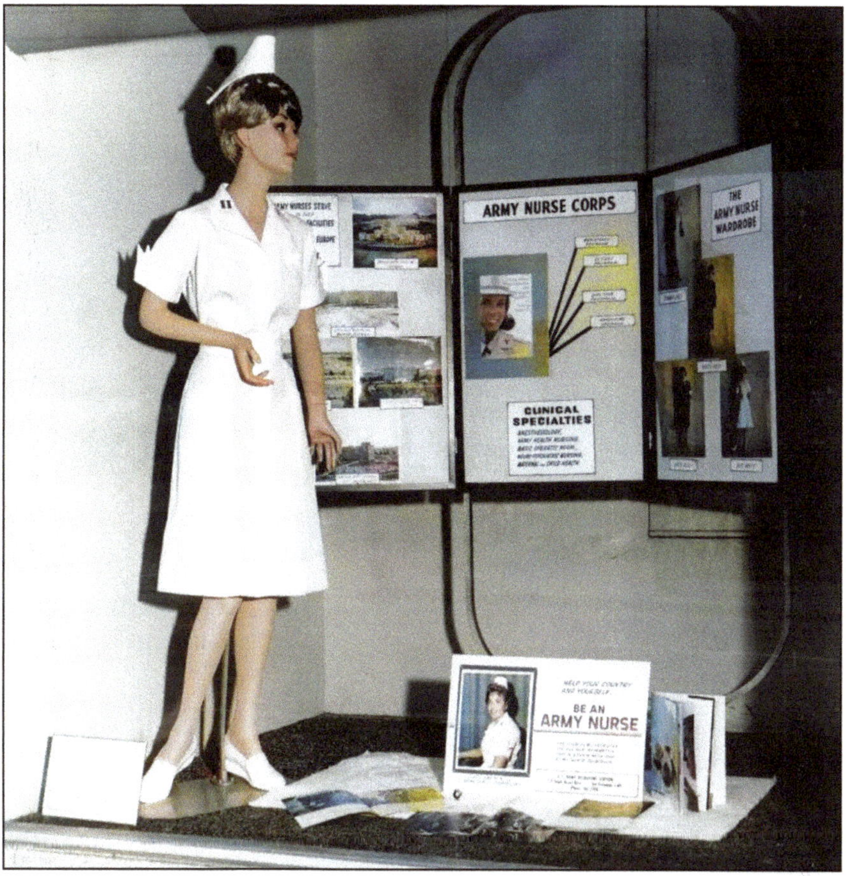

Figure 08.72. Colonel Judith Illi Petrello's Army recruiting windows in a Los Angeles JC Penney store, c. 1966. C. (Military Women's Memorial)

Figure 08.73. Colonel Judith Illi Petrello's Army hospital uniform.

She served in the Army Nurse Corps from 1961 to 1982 and as a recruiter for the Army Recruiting 6th Base in Los Angeles, from 1965 to 1966.

Petrello received an Overseas Service Ribbon, Meritorious Service Medal, Army Commendation Medal, Army Meritorious Unit Commendation, National Defense Service Medal, and an Army Service Ribbon.[71]

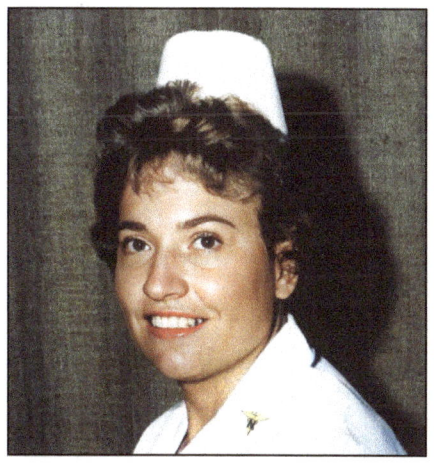

Chapter Eight

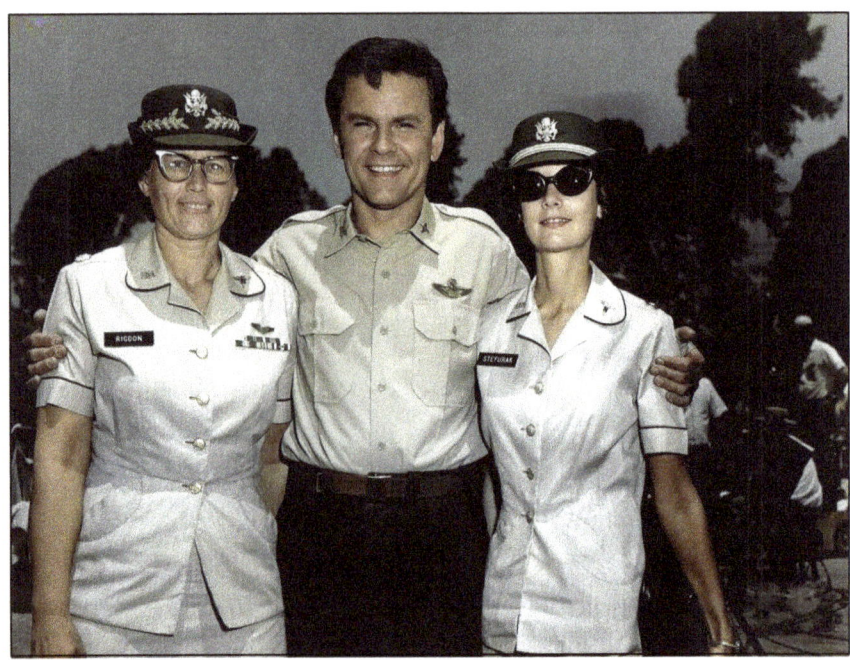

Figure 08.74. Army nurses pose on the set of the television series "Hogan's Heroes" in Hollywood. Major Rigdon, left, Robert Crane, and Captain Stefurak, 1967. C. (Military Women's Memorial)

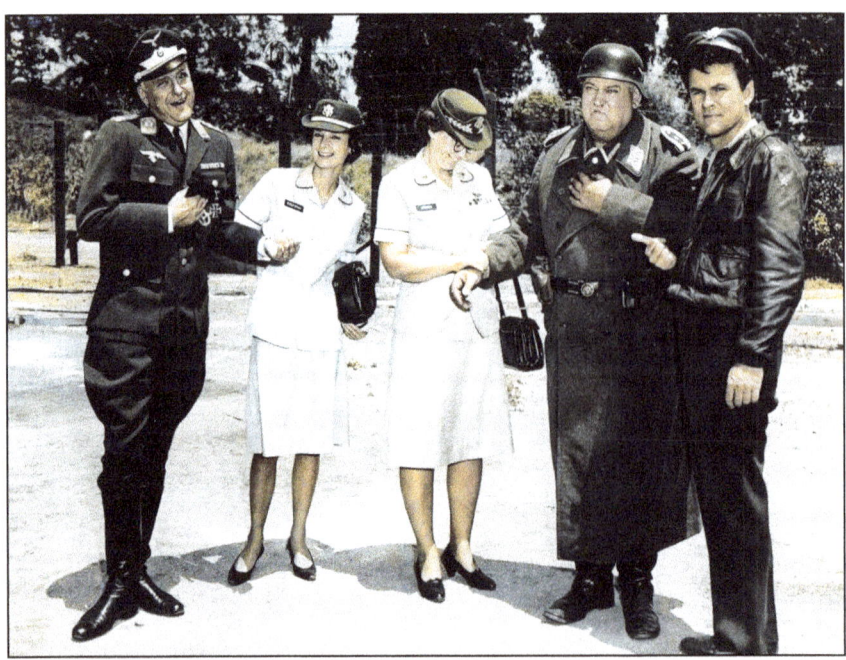

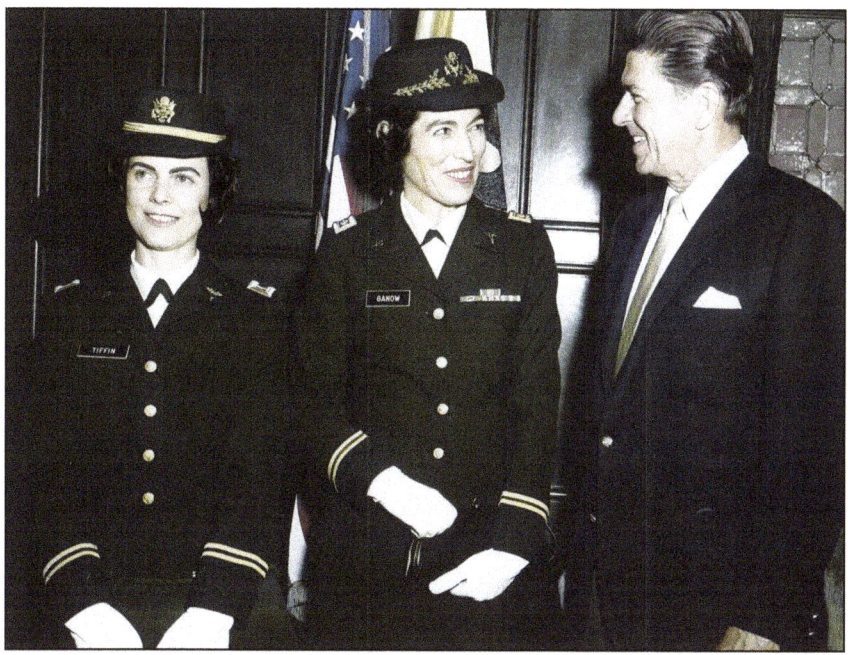

Figure 08.75. Army nurses Captain Tiffin, left, and Major Ganow greet Governor Ronald Reagan in Los Angeles, 1967. C. (Courtesy of Military Women's Memorial) [72]

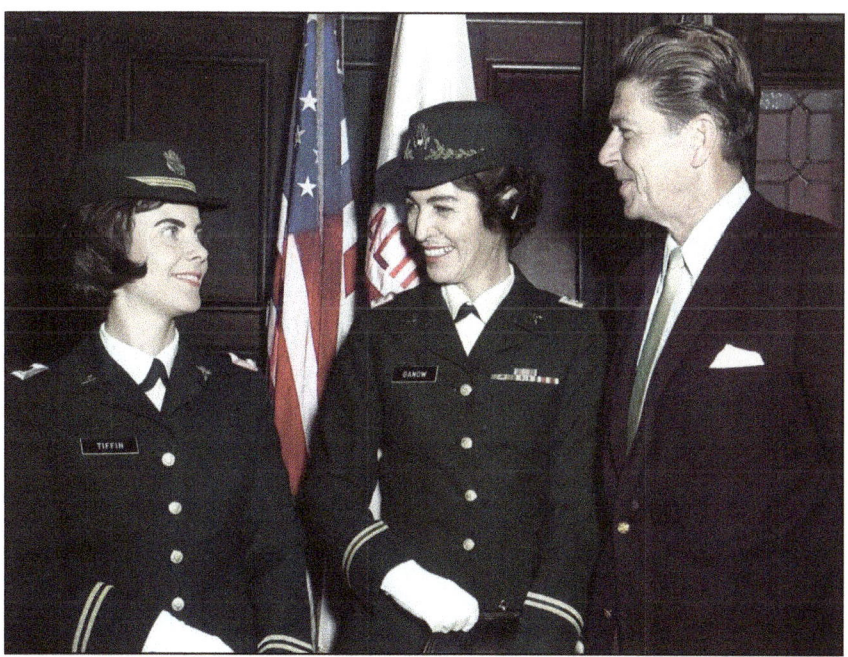

Baccalaureates, Associates, Theorists: 1946-1987

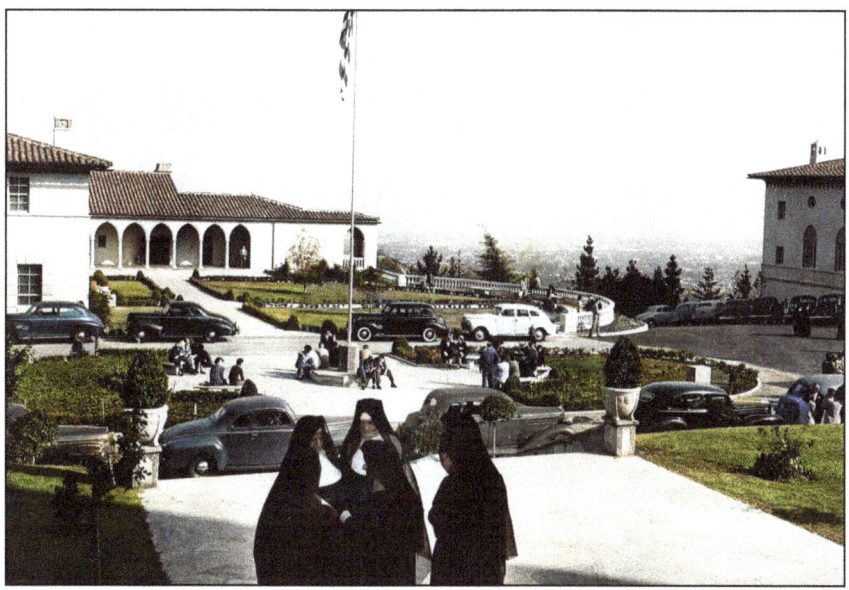

Figure 09.01. Mount St. Mary's College campus in the 1940s. (Courtesy of Mount St. Mary's University)

In 1948, two nursing leaders from two different institutions on the Westside advanced nurses education in Los Angeles. No evidence exists that the two leaders discussed it, but both had similar ideas: hospitals should not own nursing students, and nursing students should be treated the same as other college students. Both women worked to move Los Angeles nursing students from hospital-based apprentice models to college-based classes and degrees.

The Sisters of St. Joseph of Carondelet assigned Sister Rebecca Doan to start a nursing program at Mount St. Mary's College; the Provost at the University of California in Los Angeles (UCLA) recruited Lulu Wolfe Hassenplug to start their program. Mount St. Mary's never owned a hospital, and UCLA's hospital did not open until 1955, so both deans needed to locate sites that would allow their students to obtain clinical hours.

They found willing hospitals: the new baccalaureate students practiced alongside the diploma nursing students and returned to their respective colleges to study the sciences. Despite this accomplishment, hospital-based diploma programs continued for three additional decades. Both colleges organized about the same time. Mount St. Mary's first five students graduated in 1952 and UCLA graduated their first eight in 1954.

Chapter Nine

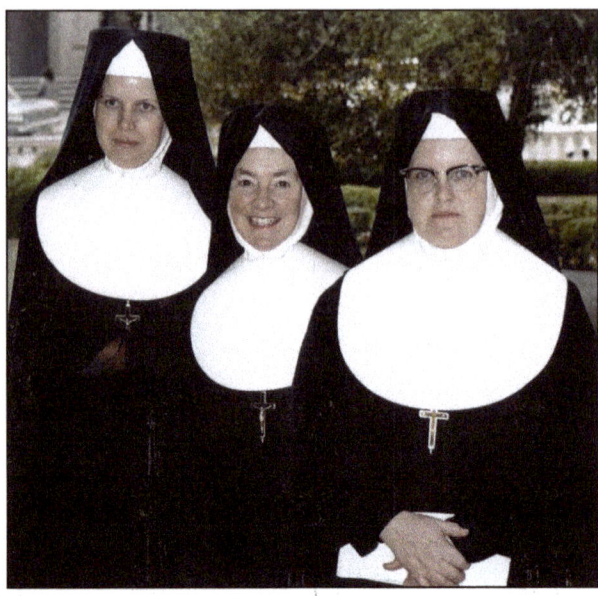

Figure 09.02. Sister Cecilia Louise Moore, Sister Mary Patricia Sexton, and Sister Genevieve Marie Gaughan, 1962. (Mount St. Mary's University)

Sister Rebecca Doan and Sister Genevieve Marie Gaughan started the nursing program in 1946. The order sent both Sisters to the Catholic University in Washington, D.C., to obtain a Master in Education. Sister Doan became the director, and Sister Gaughan the clinical instructor.[1]

Sister Doan was soft-spoken on the outside but dynamic on the inside. Although small of stature, school graduates often said, "She seemed a lot bigger when I was a student." Born as Mildred Rebecca Doan, she wanted to be a teacher but could not afford tuition. Nursing school diplomas cost less. She entered the Sisters of St. Joseph of Carondelet order in 1932.

The Board of Nurse Examiners accredited the program in 1950.[2] The first five students spent two years and two summers in clinical rotations at St. Francis, St. Vincent's Hospital, Queen of Angels, Brentwood Veterans Hospital, and Childrens Hospitals. They had studied two prior years in the classroom. Sister Doan didn't believe students should learn by working for a hospital—she thought a college education was the better method.

The National League of Nursing (NLN) required the chairperson to have a PhD, so Sister Doan obtained a doctorate from UCLA in 1957.[3] The college received retroactive NLN accreditation that same year.[4] Sister Doan served as president of the Mount from 1961 to 1967, and she worked in the nursing department until 1971.[5]

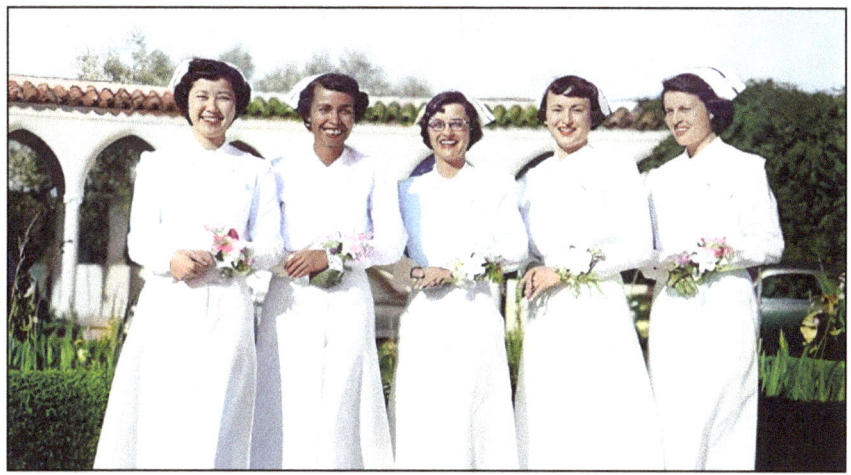

Figure 09.03. The first five graduates from Mount St. Mary's College SON: Mary Ishida Yoshimoto, Vivian Burgess, Ruby Mae Bunyard, Maureen Boylan Scherzberg, and Marie Astier Devine, in June 1952. Among the first graduates were a Japanese American, an African American, an Irish American, and a French American nurse. (Mount St. Mary's University)

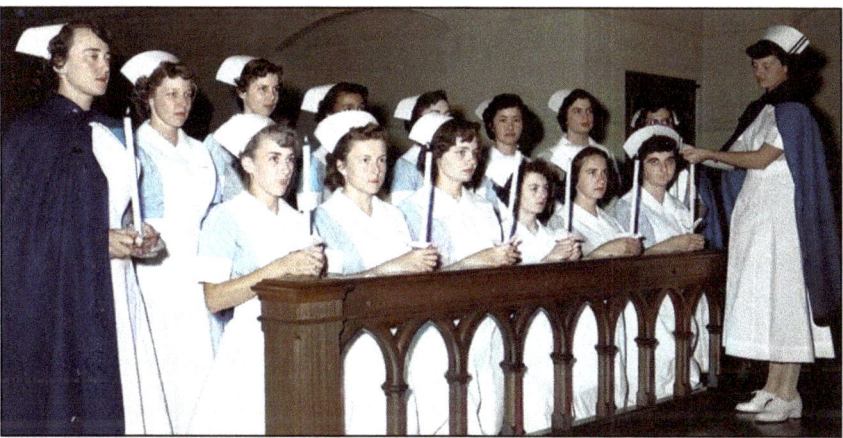

Figure 09.04. A capping ceremony for the class in 1951. Maureen Boylan Scherzberg is placing the cap. (Courtesy of Maureen Boylan Scherzberg)

Maureen Scherzberg became a Flying Tiger nurse in 1956. The Flying Tigers developed the first commercial transcontinental air-cargo route. During the Korean War they transported troops; after the war they transported supplies and military families between Asian and Burbank airports. They used nurses on board the planes because prop planes made long flights and passengers became ill. In 1976, Scherzberg graduated from the University of California, Davis, in the first graduate degree nurse practitioner program.[6]

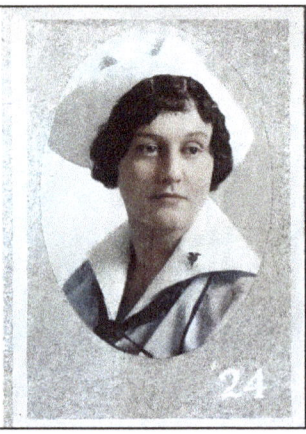

Figure 09.05. Lulu Hassenplug (then Lulu Wolf) in her 1924 graduation yearbook, Army School of Nursing.

Hassenplug first entered a hospital for a tonsillectomy at age twelve. She witnessed the nurses care of the children and believed she could improve it. Nine years later, in 1924, she graduated from the Army School of Nursing. She taught at Piedmont Hospital in Georgia and then received a Bachelor of Science from Columbia University Teachers College in 1927.

Hassenplug questioned the traditional methods used by schools to teach nurses—she did not see the value of students as service tools. She said that folding linens and other menial tasks did not teach them to become professional nurses. Hassenplug used her new concepts in 1948 when she was appointed dean of the first School of Nursing at the University of California, Los Angeles.

She produced a university-based program: nursing students were integrated into university life the same way as other students; they were not housed in special dorms. They could marry. She motivated her students toward graduate education. She set a goal for the School of Nursing to have its own dedicated building.[7-8]

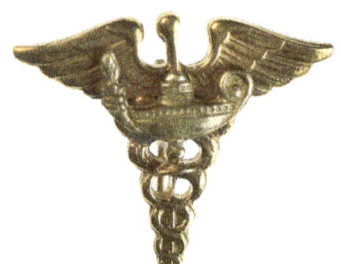

Figure 09.06. Army School of Nursing graduate pin from 1924. Author's collection.

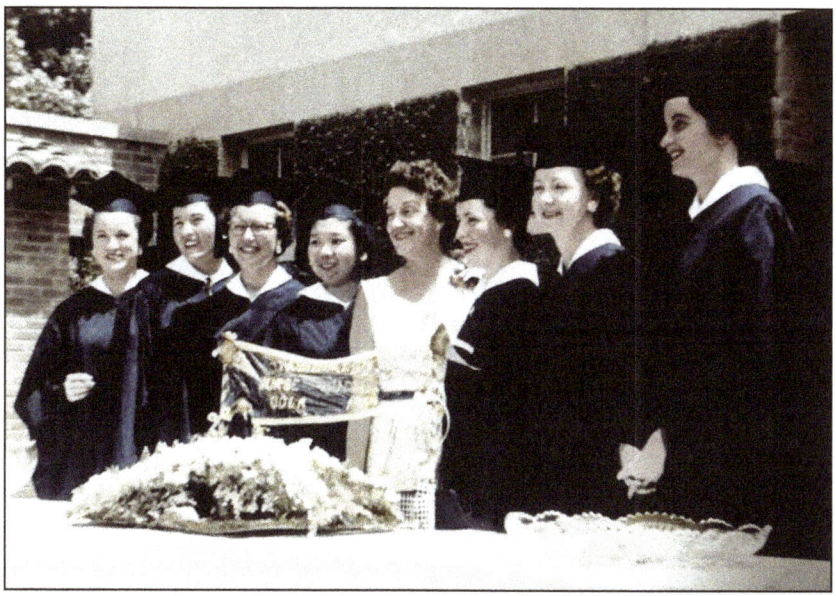

Figure 09.07. The first UCLA School of Nursing graduating class, 1954: Marie Forman, Sheila Garrett, Doreen Hawcroft, Akiki Tiara, Dean Lulu Hassenplug, Roberts Langton, Mary Bell, and Betty Howard, left to right.

Figure 09.08. UCLA School of Nursing faculty at the 1954 graduation: Harriet Coston, Madge Sledge, Maura Carroll, Charity Kerby, and Jo Elliot, left to right. C. (Courtesy of UCLA School of Nursing)

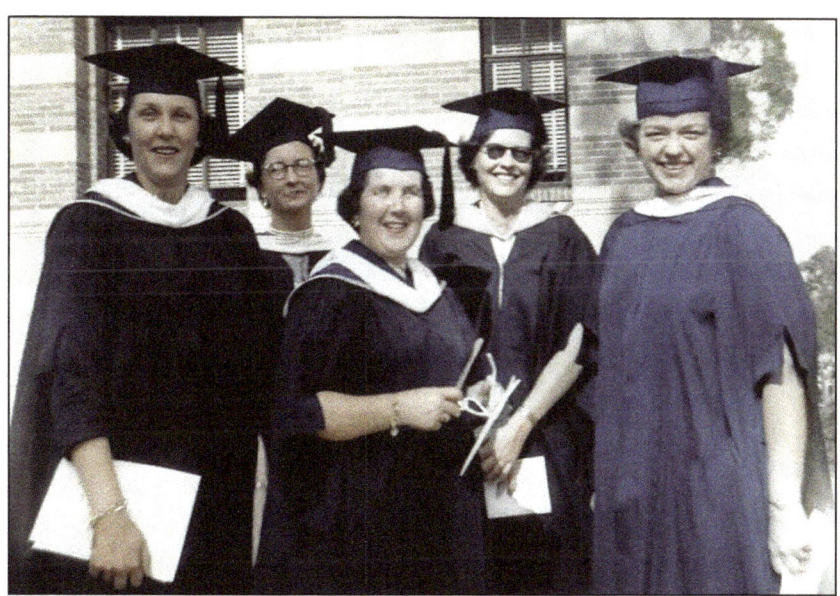

Chapter Nine

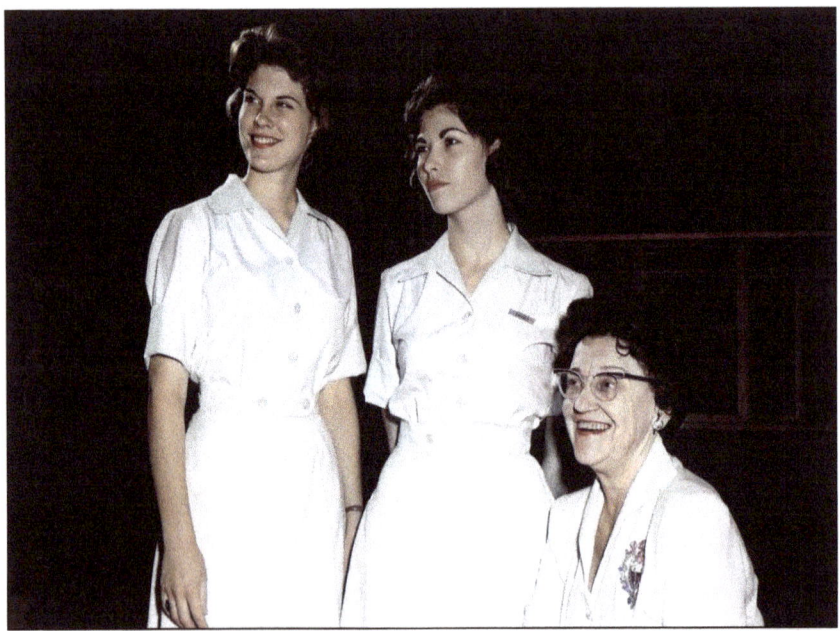

Figure 09.09. UCLA nursing students Lindsay King, left, and Andrea Kaplan, center, with Lulu Hassenplug, 1958. C. (Photos courtesy of the History & Special Collections, Louise M. Darling Biomedical Library, UCLA).

Hassenplug said, "A nurse should be recognized by the expert care she gives, not by what she wears." She had to wear a cap and white uniform in school, but she never made UCLA nursing students wear a cap—even in 1950.[9]

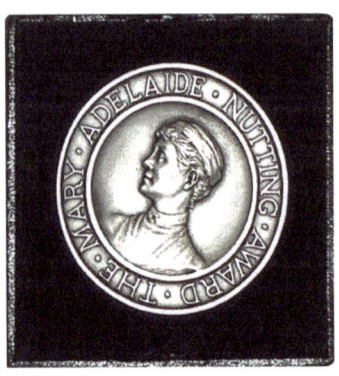

Figure 09.10. Hassenplug's 1965 Mary Adelaide Nutting Medal in its Case.

Hassenplug received many awards, including two honorary doctorates, the Alpha Tau Delta Gold Key, the Jessie M. Scott Award, the *Los Angeles Times* "Woman of the Year" in 1958, and the Mary Adelaide Nutting Award in 1965. In 1944, the National League for Nursing Education created the Mary Adelaide Nutting Medal in her honor and awarded Hassenplug the first medal.

Nutting helped to establish the Army Nurse Corps. She was the first woman to hold a professorship at Columbia University and the first university professor of nursing in the world. In 1934 Nutting was named honorary president of the Florence Nightingale International Foundation.[10]

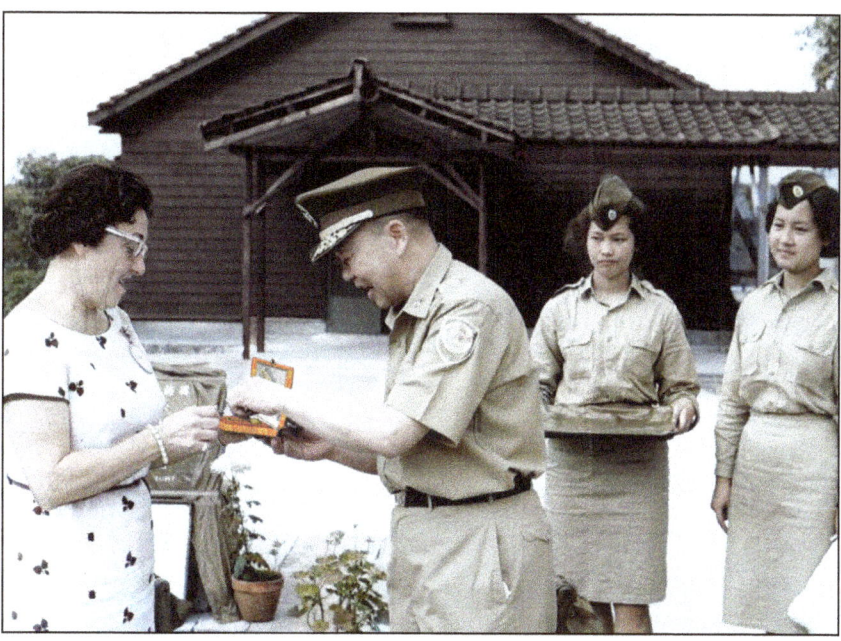

Figure 09.11. Lulu Hassenplug at the groundbreaking ceremony for the new dorm as Dr. Chi-Tsh Loo and two student nurses present her with a commemorative golden shovel, 1964. C. In 1962, the National Student Nurses Association raised money to replace the overcrowded student nurse dormitory at the National Defense Medical Center in Taipei, Taiwan.[11]

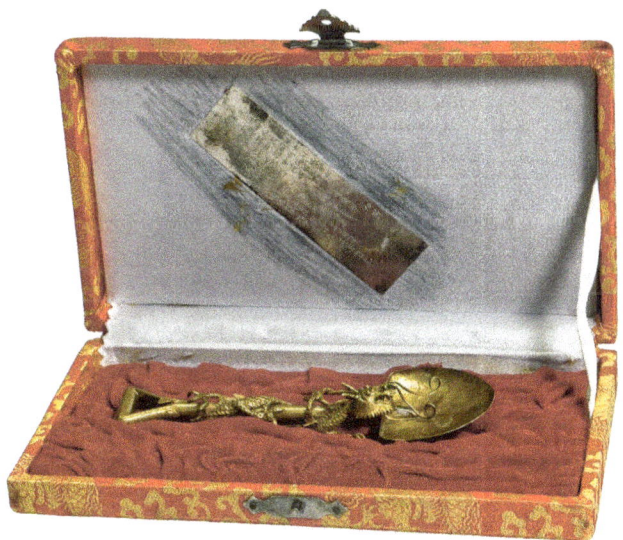

Figure 09.12. The golden shovel. (Photos courtesy of the History & Special Collections, Louise M. Darling Biomedical Library, UCLA)

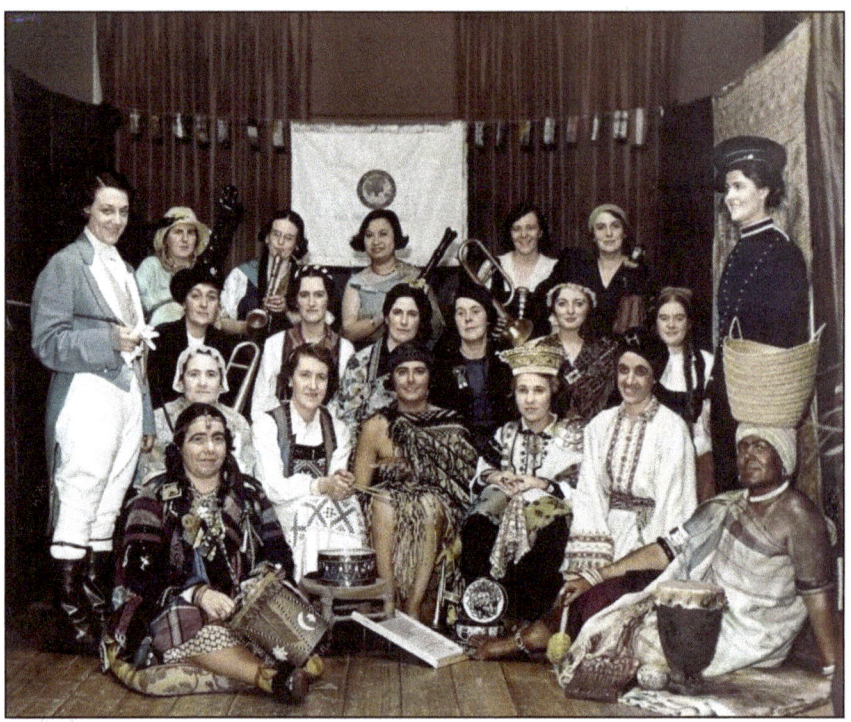

Figure 09.13. Nurse musicians performed a concert for the Florence Nightingale International Foundation meeting in England. Ringmaster Lulu Hassenplug, standing at left, represented the U.S. Nurses attended from fifteen countries. Other countries represented in the photograph are Austria, Denmark, Latvia, Czechoslovakia, Bulgaria, Norway, Sweden, Finland, Ireland, Canada, New Zealand, and England, 1937. C. (History & Special Collections, Louise M. Darling Biomedical Library, UCLA)

The concept of the Florence Nightingale International Foundation began at the International Council of Nurses meeting in Cologne, Germany, in 1912. Ethel Bedford Fenwick wanted to create an educational foundation, not a museum, as a living memorial to Florence Nightingale. World War I delayed the progress; the foundation finally opened in 1934.

Initial membership included the fourteen counties that had an International Council of Nurses chapter. The Foundation awarded a certified postgraduate course (in nursing specialties and public health) to nurses who made an international contribution to nursing. The Foundation remained linked to the International Council of Nurses.

Hassenplug received the Florence Nightingale Foundation International Fellowship in 1936—the second American granted that honor.[12]

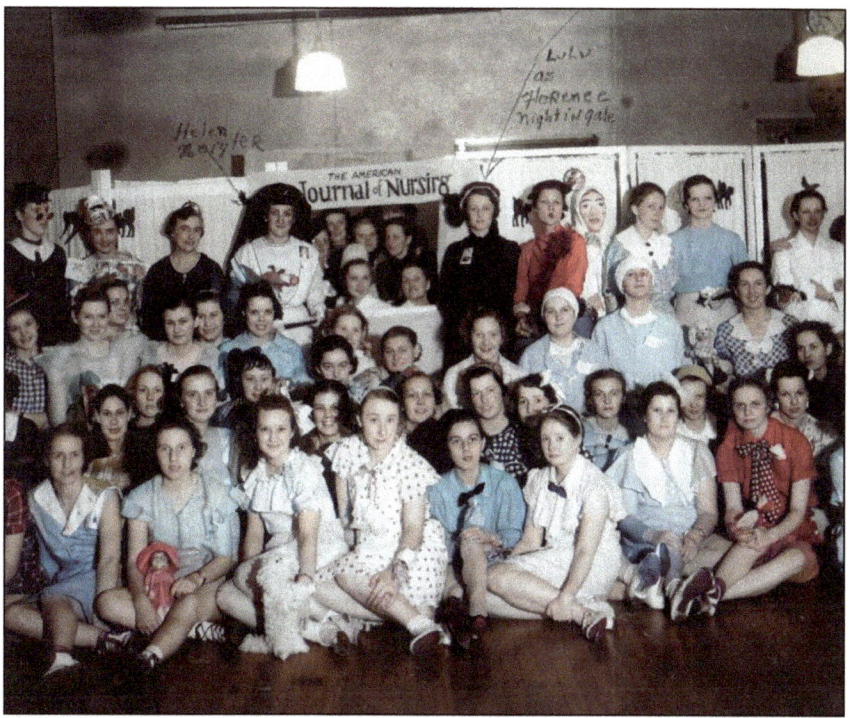

Figure 09.14. A 1935 Halloween party to celebrate the 35th anniversary of the *American Journal of Nursing*, taken in Cabaniss Hall at Virginia Commonwealth University. The arrow at the top on the right side points to Lulu Hassenplug, dressed as Florence Nightingale; the arrow on the left points to Helen Zeigler, 1935. C. (Courtesy of History & Special Collections, Louise M. Darling Biomedical Library, UCLA)

Both Zeigler and Hassenplug taught at Virginia Commonwealth University Medical College. In 1938 Hassenplug became an associate professor at Vanderbilt University School of Nursing—she later advanced to a full professor. In the same year, Zeigler was appointed dean and professor at Vanderbilt. She must have been Hassenplug's good friend, as she is the only other person whose name Hassenplug wrote on the photo.

In 1924, the Rockefeller Foundation sponsored a conference focused on the issue of public health nursing education in the U.S. The meeting resulted in the formation of the Committee for the Study of Public Health Nursing, which later expanded to include hospital nursing. The Foundation sought to raise the prestige and standards of the entire nursing profession by upgrading nurses education, through the establishment of university affiliations and national accreditation procedures. Vanderbilt was one of the first five schools to receive the Rockefeller Foundation funding. [13]

President Lyndon Johnson signed HR 11241 on 4 September 1964. This amendment to the Public Service Act increased opportunities for training professional nurses. It provided loans, diploma school subsidies, traineeships, and established a National Advisory Council on Nurse Training. Hassenplug became a member of the National Advisory Committee. [14]

Figure 09.15. The pen Johnson used to sign HR 11241, September 4, 1964.

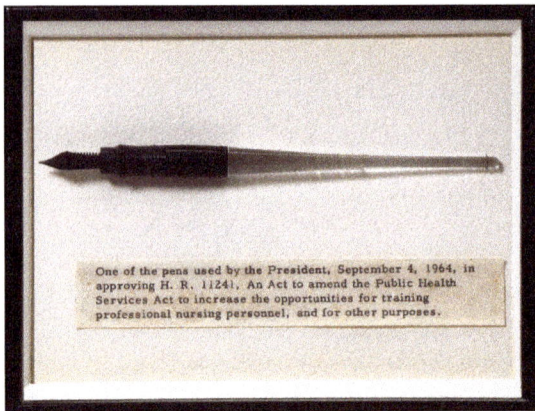

Johnson signed HR 5894 on 8 November 1967. The amendment removed restrictions on the careers of female officers. The Act allowed the promotion of line officers to the grades of Captain and Commander, allowed for the possibility of a Rear Admiral for the Nurse Corps, removed age restrictions, allowed active duty enlisted time to be counted for retirement purposes, and increased Nurse Corps membership in Selection Boards. Hassenplug received both the fountain pen and the ballpoint pen the president used to sign the acts. (Special Collections, Louise M. Darling Biomedical Library)

Figure 09.16. The pen Johnson used to sign HR 5894, November 8, 1967.

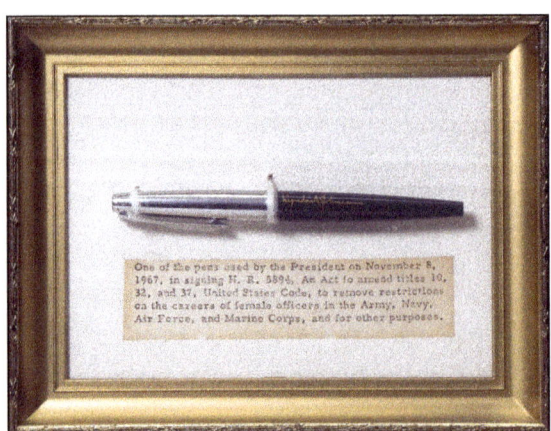

In 1974, the Council of Continuing Education for Health Occupations mandated nurses earn three continuing education units for re-licensure by 1977. However, many nurses had sought continuing education even before the requirements existed. [15]

Marjorie Squaires headed the UCLA Extension (UNEX) program that began in the mid-sixties. In 1966, she directed the pilot for a public television series on KCET. The shows included educational units about patient stress when hospitalized, post-hospital needs of medical-surgical patients, special techniques at the bedside, and methods to help patients face death. Seventy hospitals enrolled 6,120 nurses.

Governor Reagan appointed Squaires to the California Board of Nursing. She served as the administrator of all nursing programs in continuing education from 1967 to 1972. She wrote many grants, including the National Institute of Mental Health grant "Dynamic of Prejudice—Implications in Nursing," an idea that developed after the Los Angeles riots of 1965. She formed a committee and held planning meetings in Watts. Black and White nursing leaders organized three conferences to improve relationships and address the needs of nurses in minority groups.

Squaires received her nursing diploma from Seaside School of Nursing in Long Beach. She earned a bachelor's and master's from the University of California, Los Angeles. She was an avid reader and a member of the Long Beach Soroptimist organization. In 1972 she left UCLA and joined the University of Wisconsin–Milwaukee College of Nursing as an associate professor and assistant to the dean. [16]

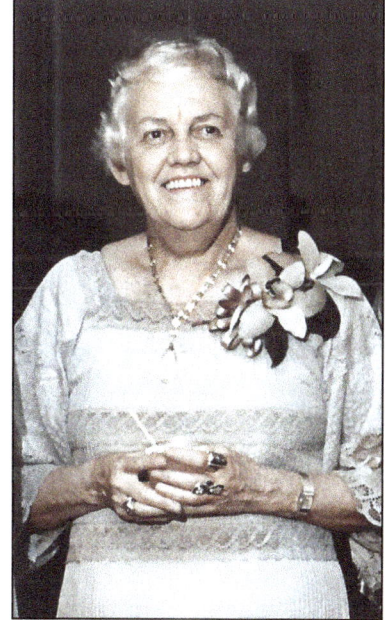

Figure 09.17. Marjorie Squaires, 67, at her professor emerita retirement party in 1979. C. (University of Wisconsin–Milwaukee College of Nursing)

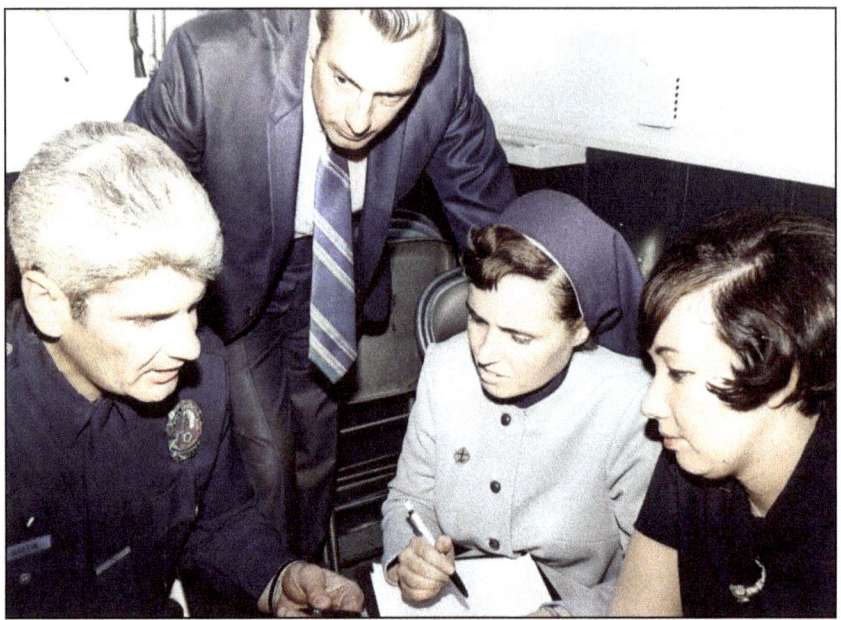

Figure 09.18. Sister Callista Roy teaching Los Angeles police recruits how the Roy Model could be adapted for use in their work, 1970s. C. (Courtesy of Mount St. Mary's University)

Sister Callista Roy was born at Los Angeles County General Hospital. Roy entered the Sisters of Saint Joseph of Carondelet and graduated with a BSN from Mount St. Mary's College in 1963. She is best known for her 1976 nursing theory, the Roy Adaptation Model for Nursing Practice.

She received a Master in Nursing, a Master in Sociology, a Doctor of Sociology, and a post-doctorate fellowship in neuroscience-nursing, administration, and ethics at UCLA. She had faculty appointments at many universities. Her list of research projects is as lengthy as her list of honors, awards, federal appointments, and publications.

At UCLA Roy attended a pediatric seminar by Dorothy Johnson that required a term paper. Roy asked Johnson if she should use Johnson's Behavioral System Model; Johnson encouraged Roy to pursue her own ideas. Many schools have since used Roy's theory for research at the masters and doctoral levels—it was translated into twelve languages. Her theory states that health and illness represent one inevitable dimension of a person's life, and to respond positively to environmental changes, that person must adapt.

Roy was bedridden for twelve years, erroneously diagnosed with the disease encephalomyelitis, until she had a curative surgery for an acoustic neuroma.[17]

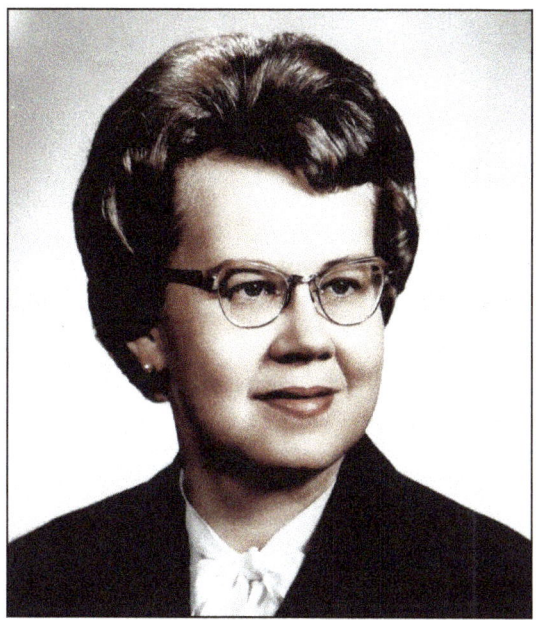

Figure 09.19. Dorothy Johnson, n.d. C. (Vanderbilt Univ. Special Collection)

Dorothy E. Johnson graduated at the top of her class from Vanderbilt University School of Nursing's baccalaureate program, in 1942. They awarded her their prestigious Vanderbilt Founder's Medal. She then obtained her Master of Public Health from Harvard in 1948. She worked in public health and as a pediatric nursing instructor.

She joined UCLA as faculty in 1949 and helped Lulu Hassenplug develop their baccalaureate nursing program. In 1955 she went to Vellore, India, to assist with the development of a baccalaureate nursing program. When she returned to UCLA, she taught exclusively in the master's program, maternal-child health specialty (the first two students graduated in 1953). She led a formal doctoral planning committee in 1968—four students graduated with the first Doctor of Nursing Science in Los Angeles in 1991.

Johnson was best known as a nursing theorist, detailed in her publication "Behavioral Systems Model for Nursing." Her theory stated that individuals strive to maintain stability and homeostasis by adapting their behaviors to the perceived changes or stressors within and without their environment. The ability of a person to adjust to their internal or external environment predicates their success or failure. [18]

Johnson retired at the height of her theorist career after open-heart surgery in 1978. She moved to Key Largo, Florida, to pursue a study of seashells. [19]

Chapter Nine

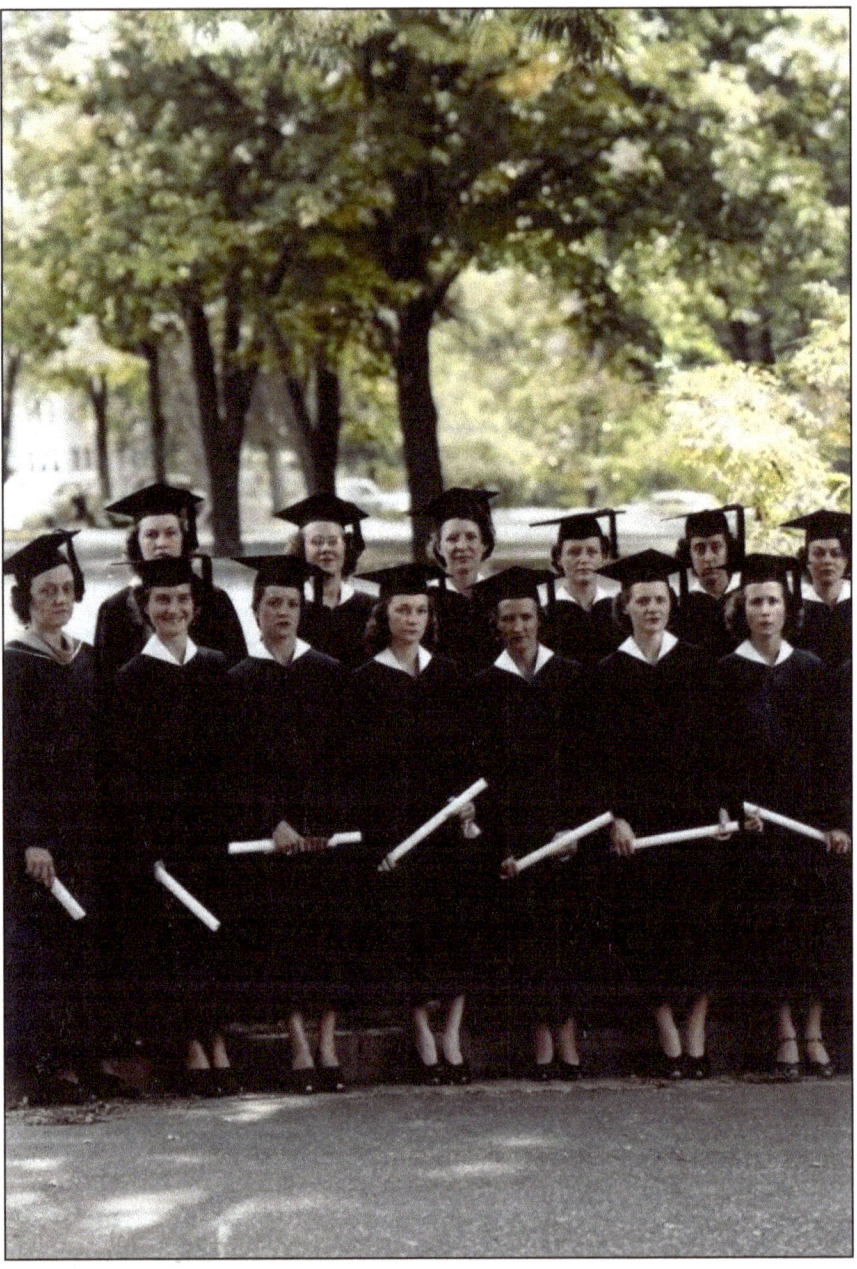

Figure 09.20. The Vanderbilt University School of Nursing, graduate class of 1942. Assistant Professor of Nursing, Lulu Wolf Hassenplug, is in the front row, far left. C. (Vanderbilt University Medical Center Special Collections)

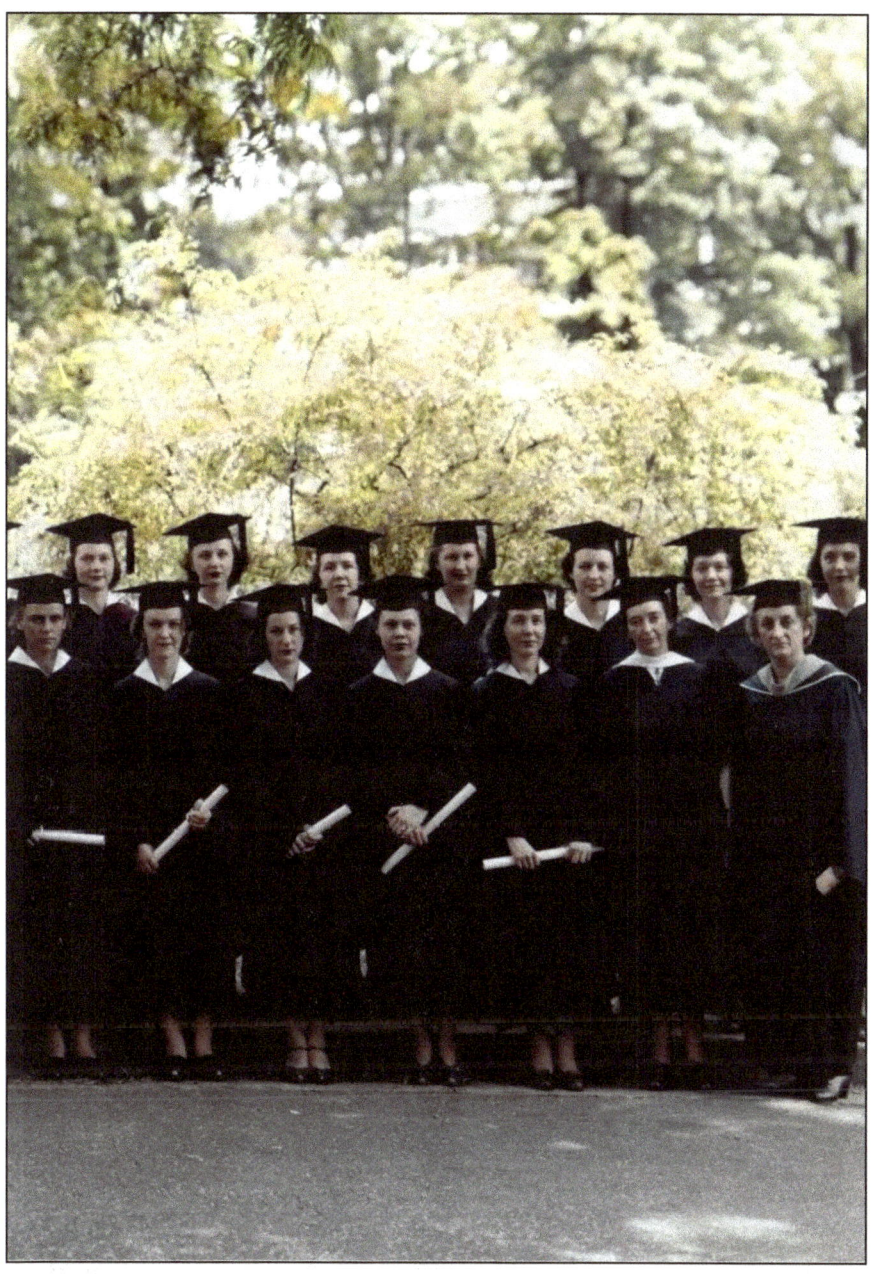

Dorothy Johnson, a new graduate nurse, is standing in the back row, second from the left. Seven years after her graduation, Dorothy Johnson joined Lulu Hassenplug as a faculty member at UCLA.

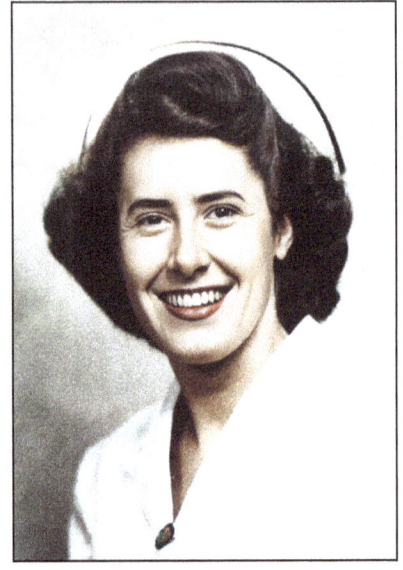

09.21. Betty Neuman at her People's Hospital Nursing School graduation, in Akron, Ohio, 1947. C. She later worked as a staff nurse, industrial nurse, and school nurse in Los Angeles. She received a Bachelor of Science in Nursing, a Master of Mental Health, a Master of Public Health from UCLA, a Doctor of Clinical Psychology, and two honorary doctorates.

In 1967, Neuman developed the Community Mental Health Program for UCLA. Prior to this, nurses had never worked in community outpatient settings. The program included the first course in mental health consultation. Neuman could not find tested literature to help her develop the course, so her students validated the teaching.

However, she is best known for her holistic nursing theory, the Neuman Systems Model, published in 1972. The components of the model were based on four concepts: Client/Person, Environment, Health, and Nursing. Neuman traveled the world and taught her theory to students in many different countries. [20]

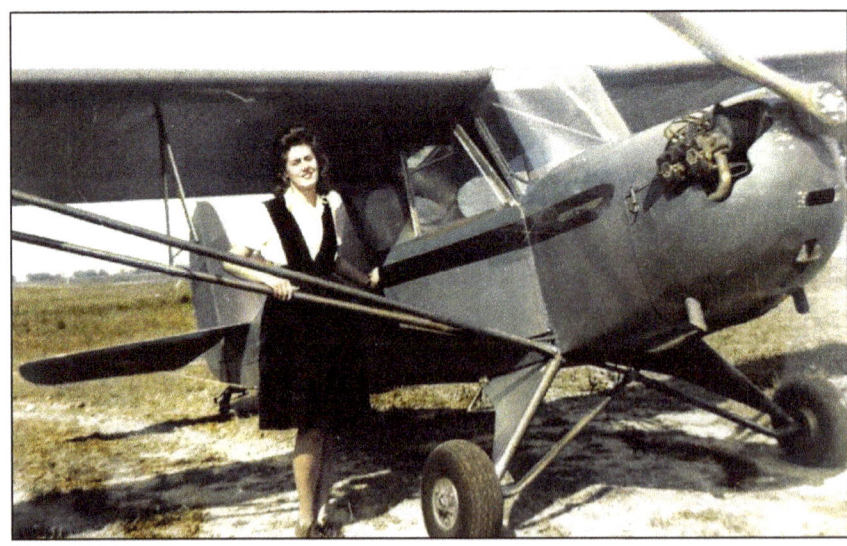

Figure 09.22. Neuman beside her Cessna at Santa Monica Airport, 1951. C. She learned to fly in her twenties. (Courtesy of Neumann College Library)

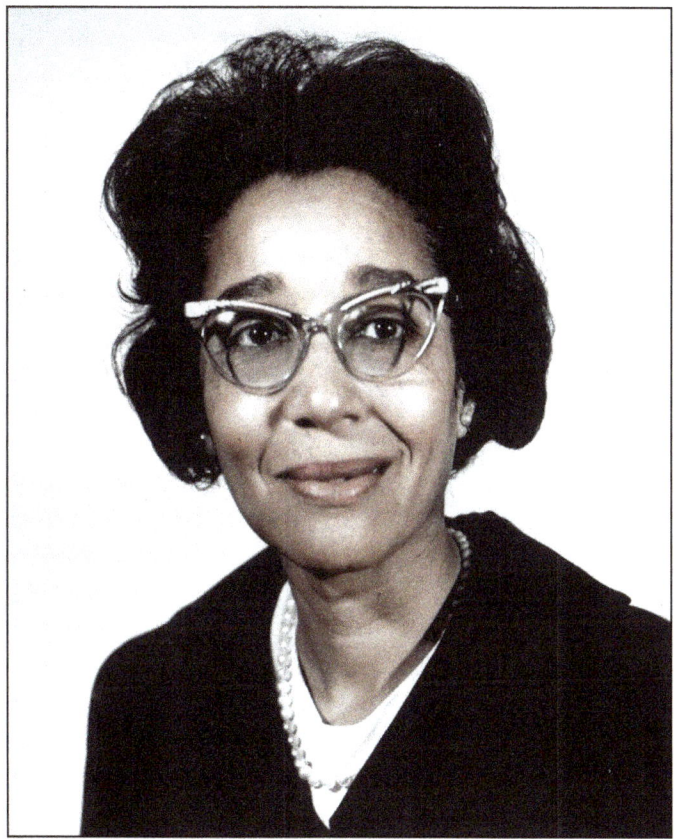

Figure 09.23. Laurie Gunter, first geriatric nurse specialist, n.d. C. (Courtesy IUPUI University Library Special Collections and Archives)

Laurie Gunter graduated from Meharry College of Nursing in 1943. After obtaining her PhD in Human Development, she began to specialize in geriatric nursing. She taught at UCLA from 1961 to 1971. She wrote the first geriatric curriculum nursing text, *Education for Geronic Nursing*, in 1979, with Carmen Estes.[21] Gunter organized the first International Conference on Geriatric Nursing in Los Angeles in 1981 and helped develop the first Geriatric Certificate Program for the American Nurses Association. [22-23]

When she began her studies, a scant amount of literature concerning normal aging was available. Gunter changed that—she published more than one hundred papers, journal articles, chapters, and books on geronics. Gunter and Estes coined the term geronic to eliminate the constant need for clarification between the study of geriatrics and gerontological (later called gerontology). Penn State bestowed her an honorary alumna, and Sigma Theta Tau awarded her outstanding contributions to nursing research. [24]

Chapter Nine

Bonnie Bullough became a nurse through the Cadet Nurse Corps program in 1944. She met her husband, Vern, at a hospital in California where he served in the Army. She worked in surgery, pediatrics, and as a public health nurse. She earned a Master of Science in Nursing at UCLA, a PhD in Sociology, and completed a family nurse practitioner certificate. In 1968 she became assistant professor of nursing and associate professor and chair of the primary care section at UCLA.

In 1972 she developed the nurse practitioner certificate program at UCLA, which later became the NP master's program. In 1975 she joined California State University, Long Beach (CSULB), as a professor of nursing—she established their first master's program for NPs. [25-26] Bonnie reported the beginning of the physician backlash against NPs at the American Nurses Association conference in 1984. She published articles about NPs, including the "Professionalization of Nurse Practitioners" in the *Annual Review of Nursing Research*, 1995. [27]

From 1979-1989 she was dean of the School of Nursing at SUNY Buffalo. In 1993 she joined the nursing faculty at the University of Southern California.

She wrote individually and co-wrote with her husband books and articles about nursing and human sexuality. She edited thirty books and fifty articles; she refereed 160 articles, plus over twenty book chapters. She gave hundreds of lectures, including some as a Fulbright Professor, at the University of Cairo.

Vern Bullough became an eminent sexologist, medical historian, active humanist, and a pioneer in the study of alternative sexual behaviors. Vern and Bonnie assembled the finest collection of materials based on sex and gender. He helped found the American Association for the History of Nursing and became the president of the Society for the Scientific Study of Sexuality. He completed a Bachelor of Science in Nursing at CSULB at fifty-three. [28]

Vern received the Distinguished Humanist Service Award from the International Humanist and Ethical Union. He was the author, co-author, or editor of fifty books; he contributed chapters in another seventy-five, one hundred refereed articles, and hundreds of popular articles. [29]

He lectured in fifty states and more than twenty countries. Vern and Bonnie shared the Alfred Kinsey Award for distinguished sex researcher in 1995. [30] He championed the separation of church and state.

In the sixties, Bullough and Bullough traveled around the world to observe hospital and nursing activities, practices, and policies. Vern began donating his research library to the CSUN library in 1973 and assisted the acquisition of several archival collections from his friends and colleagues. [31]

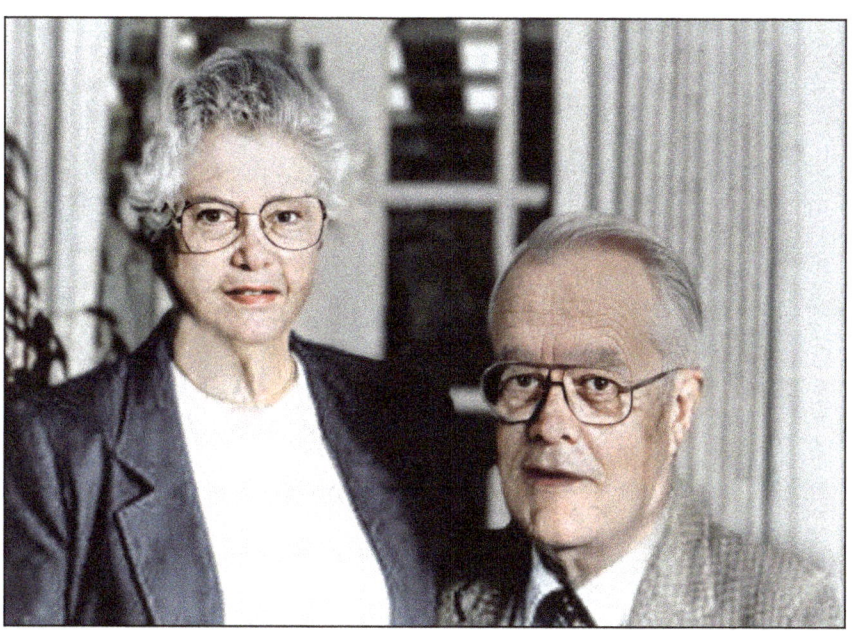

09.24. Bonnie & Vern Bullough. C. (California State University, Northridge)

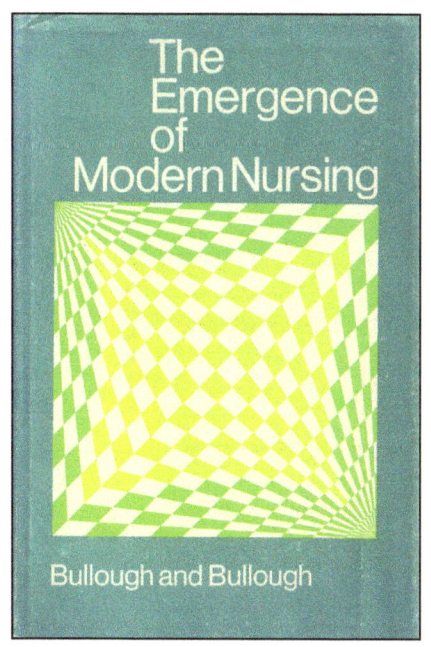
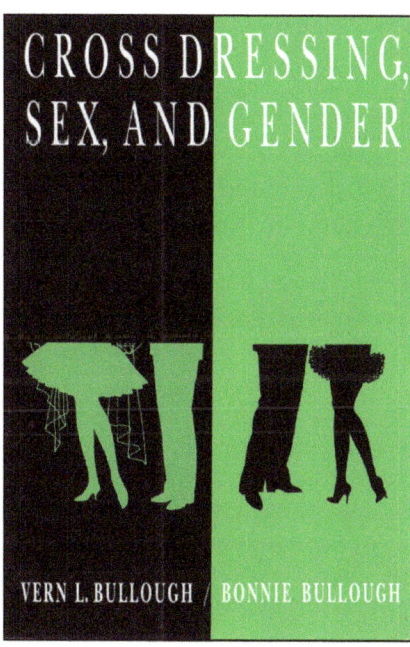

09.25. The Bulloughs' first book, *Emergence of Modern Nursing*, 1964, and their book *Cross Dressing, Sex, and Gender*, 1993. (Macmillan Company)

Chapter Nine

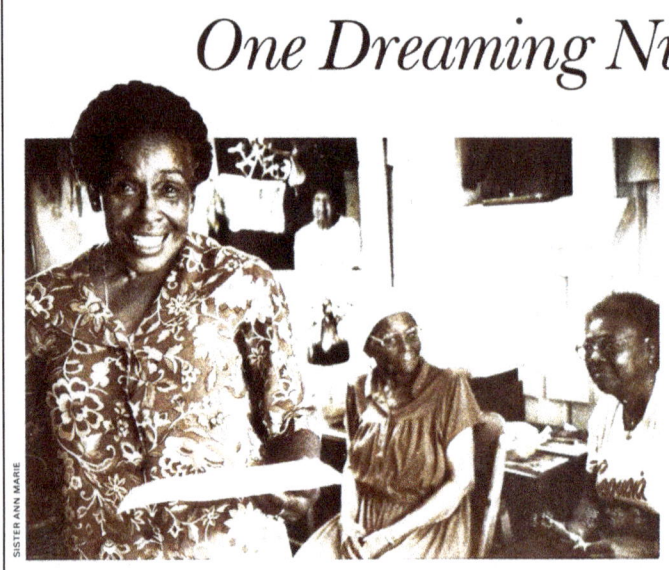

One Dreaming Nurse

With Vivian Burgess inside her Phillip's Manor are three of the residents. Presenting Vivian for her award was fellow alumna Joella Hardeman Gipson '50, attending from Wayne State University.
The Sunday festivities began with a record attendance at Mass, followed by a champagne luncheon outside on the chapel terrace. White umbrella-tables were festooned in balloons and flowers and set with linens in shades of pink to purple.

Figure 09.26. Vivian Burgess at Phillip's Manor for Creative Living, 1987. C. (Courtesy of Mount St. Mary's University)

Vivian Burgess made history as one of the first nursing graduates at Mount St. Mary's College. She was also the first Black woman at the college. Burgess said, "When Sister Rebecca Doan approached a local hospital about allowing us to do our clinical work there, they rejected our group because I am African-American. So Sister Rebecca said, 'I will just take this program elsewhere,' and she did."

Burgess worked at Queen of Angels and then 25 years at the University of Southern California School of Medicine. When she retired, in 1979, USC gave her a ticket to Paris, Rome, and London, and $500.00 spending money.

In 1985, she opened an independent senior home in the Crenshaw area called Phillip's Manor for Creative Living. She modeled the home after a Scandinavian cooperative living project. As an experiment, she moved a 90-year-old man into the house she owned in Watts. She realized companionship and meal planning were absent from her project, so she refined her ideas. In 1984 she purchased a home in Crenshaw and opened Phillip's Manor with two residents; it quickly filled to its capacity of seven.

In 2006, Pope Benedict XVI conferred to Burgess the honor of Dame Commander in the Order of the Knights of St. Gregory—the highest honor a layperson may receive in the Catholic Church.[32]

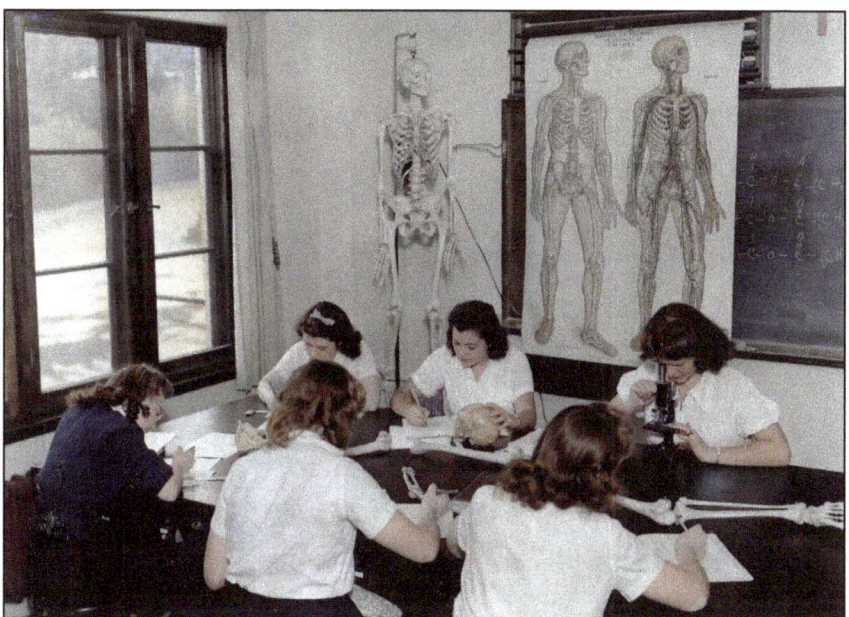

Figure 09.27. Students studying anatomy and physiology at the Mount, n.d. C. (Courtesy of Mount St. Mary's University)

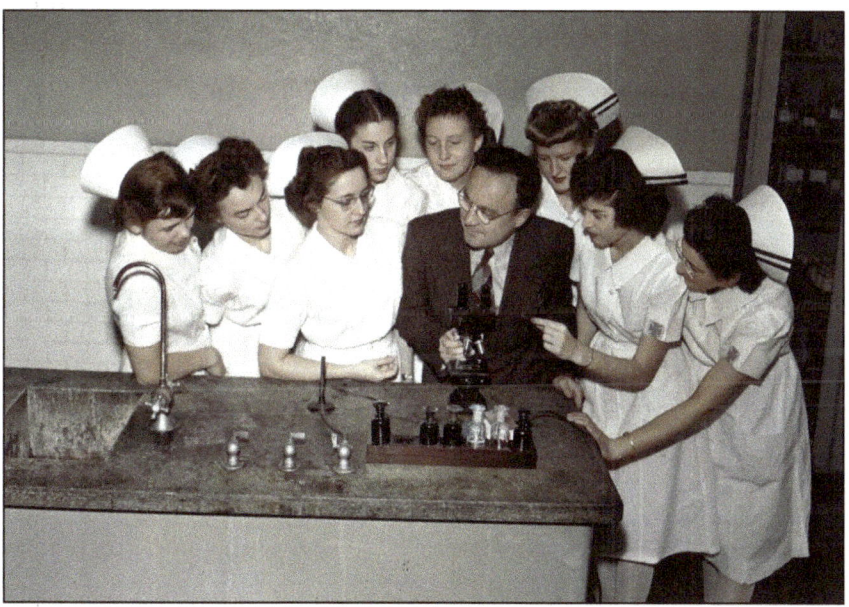

Figure 09.28. Students learn about the microscope at Los Angeles County Hospital, 1947. C. (Courtesy of Special Collections, Charles E. Young Research Library, UCLA)

Chapter Nine

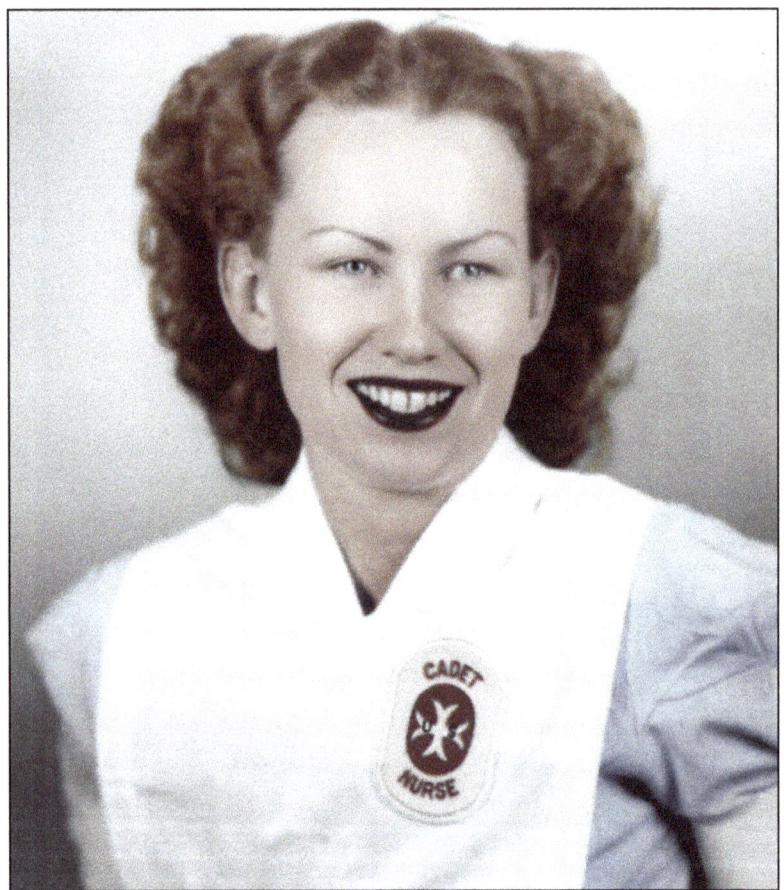

Figure 09.29. Joyce Kelly wearing the Cadet Nurse patch on her senior year uniform, 1947. C. She attended nursing school in Texas, the final year the government offered the Cadet Nurse program.

In 1959, Kaiser Permanente Hospital in Los Angeles hired Joyce Kelly as one of their first five nurse anesthetists. Kaiser needed more anesthetists and asked Kelly how they could attract more to the hospital. She told them to advertise nationally, pay more than anyone else, and start a nurse anesthetists school. They did all three and asked Kelly to become the first director of Kaiser Permanente School of Anesthesia. She accepted but wanted more. She wanted the program to become the first nurse anesthetist graduate degree program in the United States. She sought out a university—California State University, Long Beach, accepted her proposal.

The first Kaiser nurse anesthetist class graduated in 1974. Kelly completed her nurse anesthesia program at Baylor Hospital in 1956 and a graduate degree in Healthcare Management. She obtained a PhD at the age of sixty. [33]

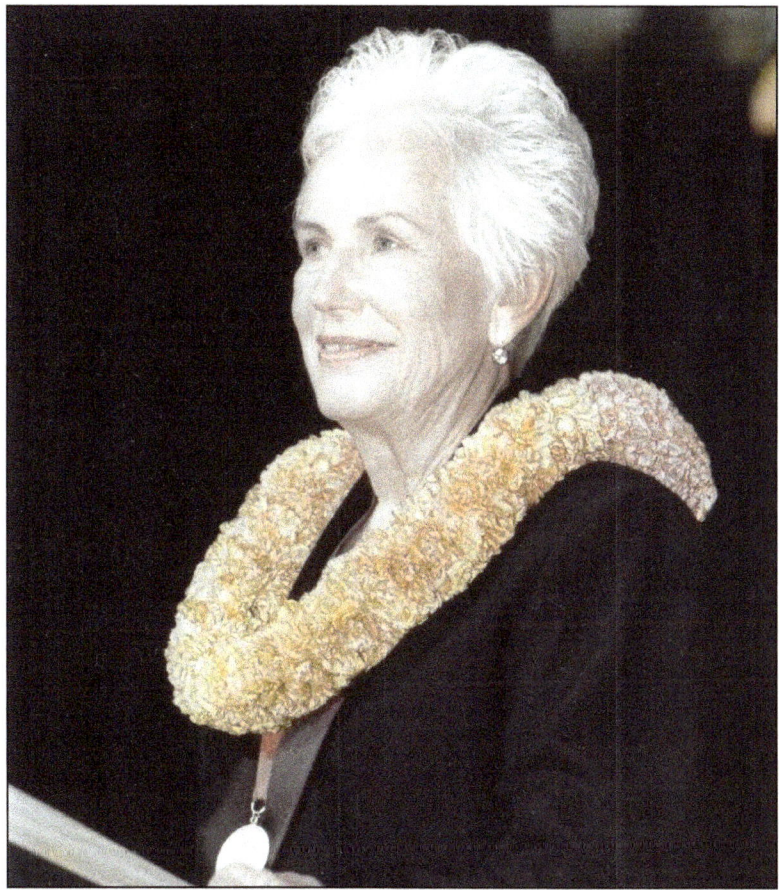

Figure 09.30. Joyce Kelly in 2002 receiving the Agatha Hodgins Award for Outstanding Service from the American Association of Nurse Anesthetists, the organization's highest award. [34] C. (Photos courtesy of Joyce Kelly)

Physicians used to say nurse anesthetists were created in the United States and did not exist in other countries. Kelly traveled the world, witnessed the proliferation of nurse anesthetists worldwide, and wrote the paper "An International Study of Fundamental Programs for Nurses Providing Anesthesia." She presented this paper at the Fourth International Symposium on the History of Anesthesia at the University of Hamburg, Germany, in 1997. Kelly taught at nurse anesthetist programs in China, Russia, Japan, Korea, Nigeria, Denmark, Thailand, and Vietnam.

Kelly became the first recipient of the Helen Lamb Award in 1980. Lamb personally selected Kelly to be the first recipient of the award named in her honor. [35] Lamb founded the School of Anesthesia at Barnes Hospital in 1929 and helped create the "Flying Fortress, Barnes Model" anesthesia machine.

Chapter Nine

Patricia Snyder was driving to visit her parents in January of 1957 when she saw a plane crash in the Pacoima Junior High School athletic yard. She rushed to help. A four-engine plane had collided at 20,000 feet with a jet fighter. That started her lifelong service with the Red Cross of Los Angeles.

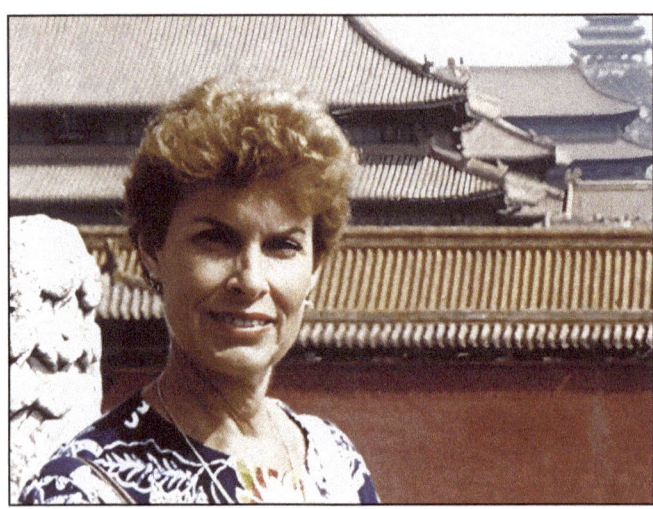

Figure 09.31. Patricia Snyder, in 1988, during a trip to the Forbidden City in China, with the Red Cross of Los Angeles. (Courtesy of Pat Snyder)

She helped during the 1983 Coalinga earthquake and when the Sylmar Veterans Hospital collapsed in 1971. Her first time away from home, in 1977, she flew to the Appalachian floods to assist people in the decimated areas of Kentucky, Tennessee, Virginia, and West Virginia.

Later in her Red Cross career, she travelled to Guam, Saipan, Samoa, and other countries. She lived in Mexico City for five months after the 1985 earthquake. After the 1986 Aero México plane crash in Cerritos, she went door-to-door looking for casualties. Snyder said she could never have dreamed of having a life filled with these experiences, traveling to many countries.

Snyder wrote four Red Cross books: *Disaster Preparedness, Emergency Survival, Safety and Survival in an Earthquake,* and *Assisting the Disabled and Elderly.* In 1984 the Red Cross gave her the highest award: the Harriman Award for Distinguished Volunteer Service—the first nurse to receive the award.

Snyder belonged to a family of nurses: her grandmother, Lena Gates, was a nurse in the early 1900s; her mother, Beatrice Young Macpherson, graduated in 1926; and her daughter, Kathy Klepic, graduated in 1974.

Snyder graduated from Hollywood Presbyterian Hospital School of Nursing in 1952. She lived in the dorm. She said the housemother constantly checked the nursing students. They had to wash their shoelaces every night and be in by eleven; late arrivals had their privileges revoked.[36]

Gertrude Hutchinson is descended from a family of nurses: her mother, her aunt, and her cousin all graduated from the diploma program at United Hospital School of Nursing, New Brighton, Pennsylvania (called Beaver Valley Hospital during her mother's training). She graduated in 1971.

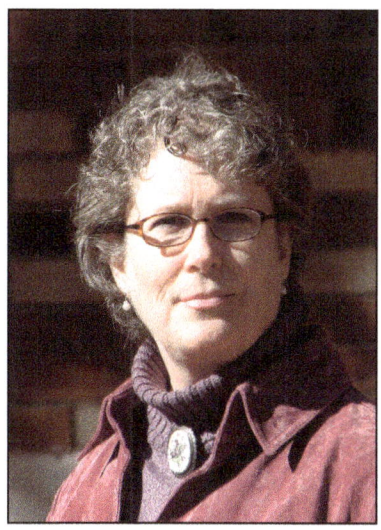

Figure 09.32. Gertrude Hutchinson at the Bellevue Alumni Center in 2008. (Courtesy of Gertrude Hutchinson)

She worked in the emergency room for nineteen years, critical care for nine years, and a level II nursery for eight years. Hutchinson moved to Los Angeles in 1994. She worked at several hospitals and as a critical care transport (CCT) nurse for Schaffer Air Ambulance in Los Angeles and flew in fixed-wing airplanes for out-of-state transport.

However, Hutchinson loved history her entire life so she decided to make a change. She obtained a Master in Information Systems from the University of Albany, and a Master in Public History. One day she found her dream job—the archivist at the Bellevue Alumni Center for Nursing History in Guilderland, New York. The Center has preserved the history of nursing for the entire state of New York; they made their archival records and manuscript collections available to the public.

Hutchinson researched nurse histories from the fifty-five collections and maintained the Center's large holdings of archival records from schools of nursing, visiting nurses associations, hospitals, other employers of nurses, collections of individual nurses personal papers, oral histories, and rare manuscripts. She presented programs to groups on history, created displays, and conducted oral interviews for the Nursing History Oral History Program.[37] In 2016 she completed her Doctor of Nursing Science in Leadership and Education from The Sage Colleges, New York.

She added to her impressive credentials by becoming the director of history and education and the archivist at the Bellevue Alumnae Center for Nursing History, in the Center for Nursing at the Foundation of New York State Nurses; archivist at the American Association for the History of Nursing; adjunct professor at SUNY Empire State College; and assistant professor at Russel Sage College. In 2018, the Professional Organization of Women of Excellence Recognized (POWER) honored her on the famous Reuters Billboard in New York City's Times Square.[38]

Chapter Nine

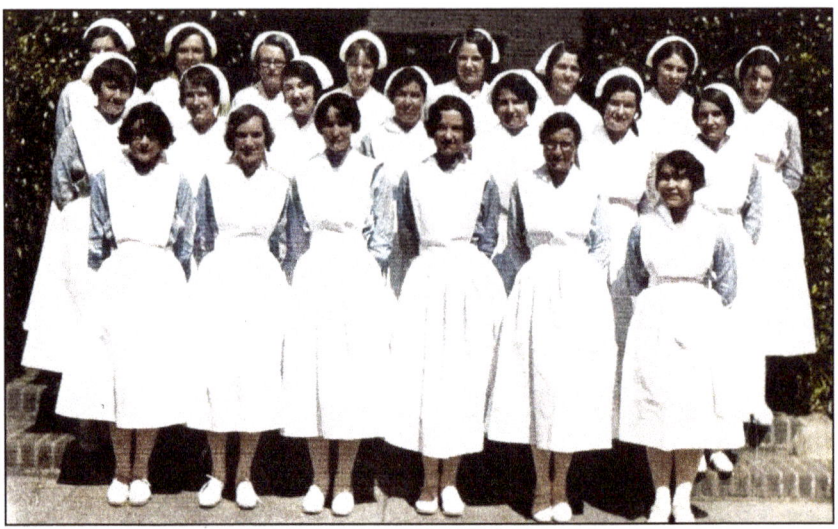

Figure 09.33. The 1932 graduating class from the Pasadena Hospital School of Nursing, the first group of nurses to complete a dual program: diploma nurse and a junior college certificate, 1932. C.

Since the middle of the 1920s, junior colleges had offered basic science classes to students in hospital schools of nursing. They were classes for nurses only; credits, however, did not transfer to colleges.[39] Pasadena Hospital School of Nursing adopted a unique program in 1930: the nursing school became part of Pasadena Junior College (PCC). The students earned twenty-eight college credits and received a junior college certificate and a hospital diploma. Four faculty members at PCC were employees of the hospital.[40]

In 1951 Mildred Montag, at Teachers College, Columbia University, received funding for an experimental program to find a "shortened and better method of preparing registered nurses." Montag also wanted nurses to continue their education if they desired. Traditional hospital diploma programs did not offer this choice because hospital training did not earn transferable college credits. After a rigorous selection process, she chose six junior colleges for the pilot program, including Pasadena City College.[41]

All colleges in the experiment offered a two-year program, except PCC. It differed from the other five programs because the California legislature required nurses to study for a minimum of three years.[42] The college solved this issue by requiring student nurses to practice a one-year internship following the two years of study. After three years they received an Associate in Nursing (ADN). The pilot program began in September 1953 and remained through four years of funding. After the pilot program ended, PCC continued their ADN program.[43]

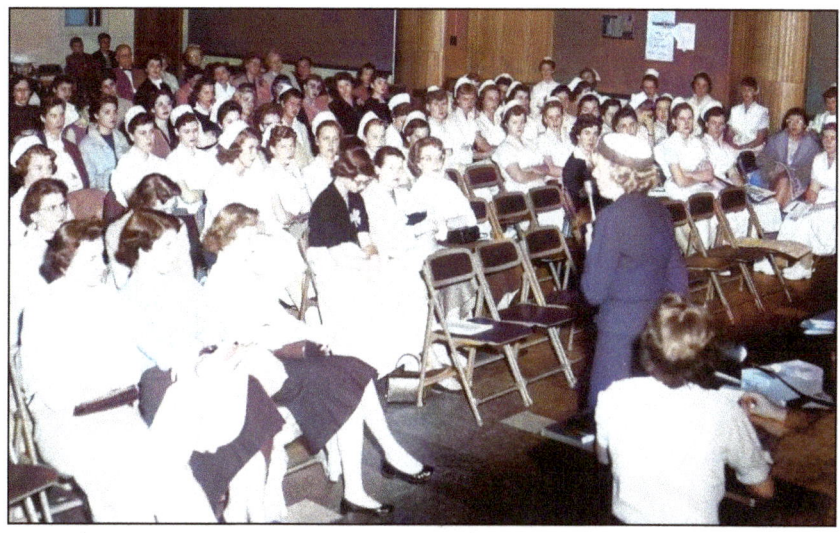

Figure 09.34. Dr. Mildred Montag meeting with nursing students in Harbeson Hall at Pasadena City College, c. 1960. C. (Photos courtesy of Pasadena City College Shatford Library/Pasadena Digital History)

In 1957, the California legislature addressed the concern that the state needed more nurses. They modified the existing law, requiring nurses to study for three years, and allowed junior colleges to offer a twenty-four-month course of two academic years and two summer terms, or the equivalent time. [44]

Figure 09.35. First graduating class of the Pasadena City College Nursing program, 1956—the first ADN program in Los Angeles County. C. [45]

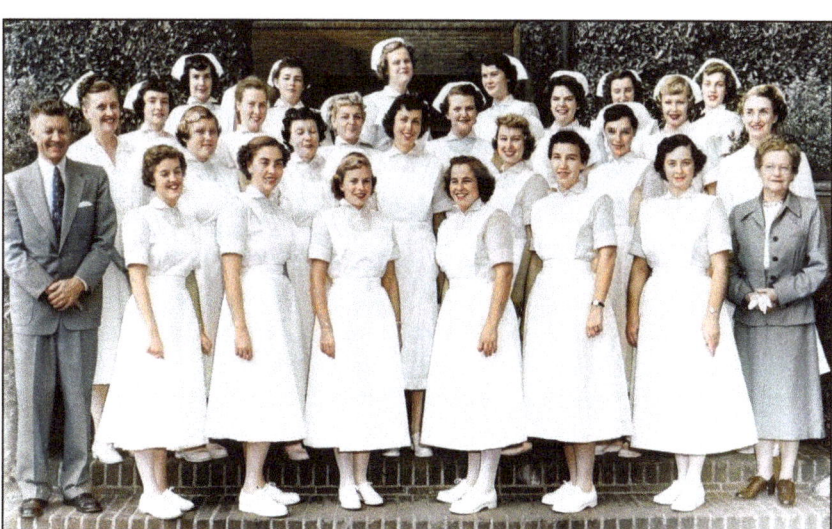

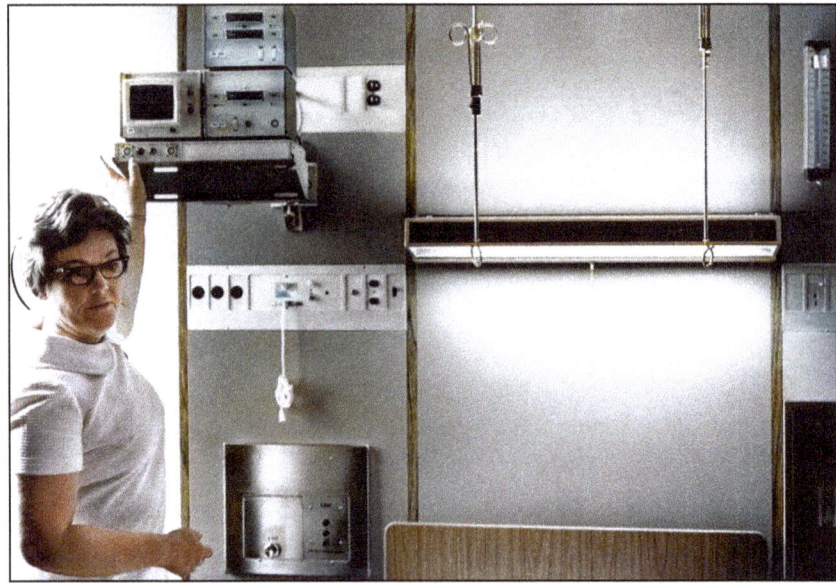

Figure 09.36. Barbara Jury in the newly opened telemetry unit, on the fifth floor ICU, at California Hospital, c. 1970. C. (Courtesy of California School of Nursing Alumni Association)

When Barbara Jury graduated from California Hospital's diploma program in 1950, she also received a Bachelor of Sciences (BS) from the University of Southern California (USC). She attended one graduation in a white uniform and another in a black cap and gown. Since 1941, California had tried to offer nurses a bachelor's degree through this method. All students entering in 1941–1942 were BS students with an entrance requirement of sixty-four college credits. The nursing shortage during WWII forced the hospitals to alter their college prerequisites requirement.

Jury first worked as a staff nurse, and then after she obtained a Master of Nursing from UCLA in 1961, California Hospital promoted her to the director of the School of Nursing. One of her goals at that time was to achieve National League of Nursing (NLN) approval for the school. After years of preparation, the school received accreditation in 1966.

She was director of nurses in the hospital from 1966 to 1978 and then moved to her favorite position in risk management. She valued her involvement in monitoring the quality of healthcare delivery. Jury remained active in the California Hospital School of Nursing Alumni Association long after retirement; she worked hard during the sixties to keep the organization going. She always appreciated the history of nurses—the California Hospital School of Nursing 1949 yearbook, *The Summary*, listed her as historian. [46]

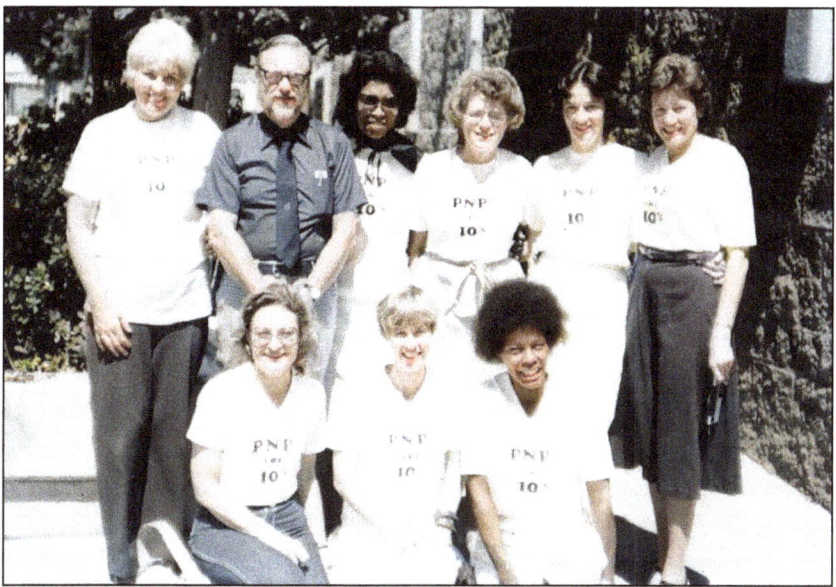

Figure 09.37. The University of Southern California's pediatric nurse practitioner students with physician instructor: Willis Wingert, Sandra Clauss, Barbara Ellis, Zeleen Franklin, Bell Harding, Heidi Haugh, Wilhelmina In'T Hout, and Joyce Jacob in the first row, far left. C. (Courtesy of Joyce Jacob)

Joyce Jacob's speech therapist told her she would make a good nurse. That made sense: her mother and stepmother were nurses. Her father was an orthopedic surgeon at California Hospital, and she was born there. She graduated from California Hospital School of Nursing in 1960. She first worked as a school nurse at McDonald Elementary School (for the disabled) until the 1975 law passed that said special education must be taught in regular schools.

In 1980 she heard about a new pediatric nurse practitioner (PNP) certificate program at the University of Southern California (USC). They accepted eight nurses. She trained at the USC Pediatric Pavilion Clinics. The PNP students were not well accepted, but they continued to practice anyway. They graduated in July 1981 after completing 1,634 clinical and 394 theory hours.

She later obtained a Master of Education from California State University, Los Angeles. Jacob worked as a PNP in the Child Health Disability Program (CHDP) for eleven years and then as a coordinator.[47] Jacob served as president of the National Association of Pediatric Nurse Practitioners (NAPNAP) in the 1980s and was the former president of the California School of Nursing Alumni Association.[47]

Chapter Nine

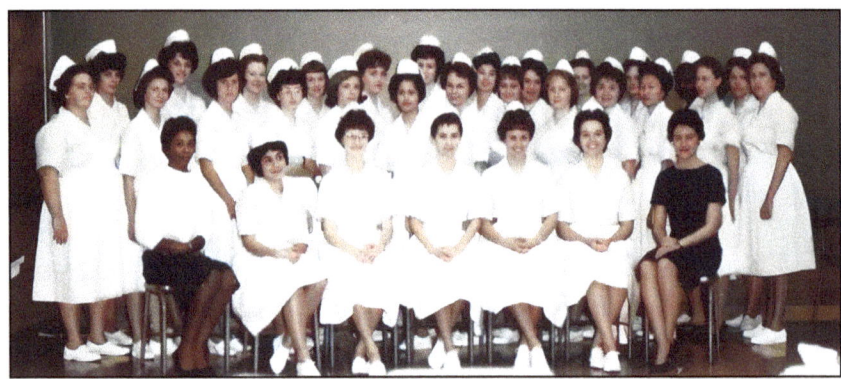

Figure 09.38. Los Angeles State College Nursing Class, c. 1960. C. (CSULA)

Los Angeles State College opened on Vermont Street in 1947 at the current campus of Los Angeles City College. Initially, both schools shared the same campus. In 1955, Los Angeles State College moved to its current location near the 10 Freeway. In 1964, it joined the State College System and changed its name to California State College at Los Angeles. Their first BSN program began in 1956, and the students graduated in 1960. [48] The college obtained university status in 1972 and became California State Univ., Los Angeles.

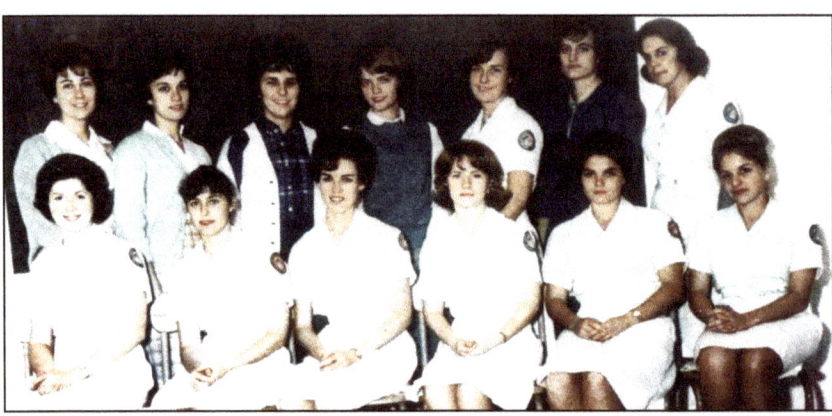

Figure 09.39. The first BSN graduating class at California State University, Long Beach, School of Nursing, June 1965. C. Jo Ann Breece, Patricia Burbeck, Velda Kuykendall, Judith Long, Kathy Schwabl, Janice Storker, Nancy Sonntag, Karen Lindgren, Pennie Jorgensen, Judith Johnson, Sally Schilling, Janice Paine, Geraldine Hingsbergen. C. (CSULB SON)

That same year CSULB hosted the first International Sculpture Symposium ever held in the U.S. and the first at a college or university. Six sculptors from around the world and two from the U.S. have created many of the monumental sculptures seen today on campus. [49]

286

Baccalaureates, Theorists, Associates

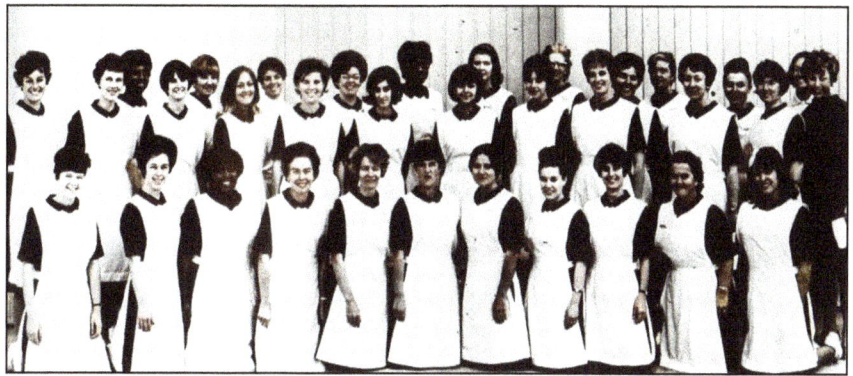

Figure 09.40. The first nursing class in their first year at Santa Monica City College, 1968. C. Santa Monica City College received 120 applicants the first year they offered a program for registered nurses. They accepted only thirty-four. [50-51] (Courtesy of Santa Monica Community College)

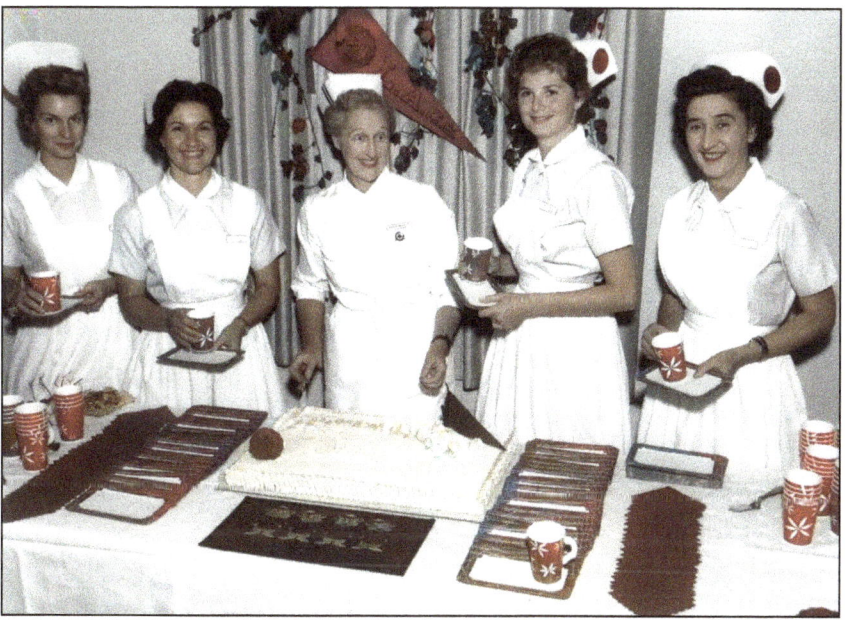

Figure 09.41. The cake says, "Congratulations Graduates," and the banner flag behind them says L.A.C.C. for Los Angeles City College, n.d. C. (Courtesy of Cedar-Sinai Medical Center).

Community colleges were usually not aligned with one hospital; the colleges needed to contract with city hospitals so their nursing students could gain clinical experience. Most would contract for a specific area in one hospital (medical, surgical, pediatrics, etc.). Students moved from hospital to hospital.

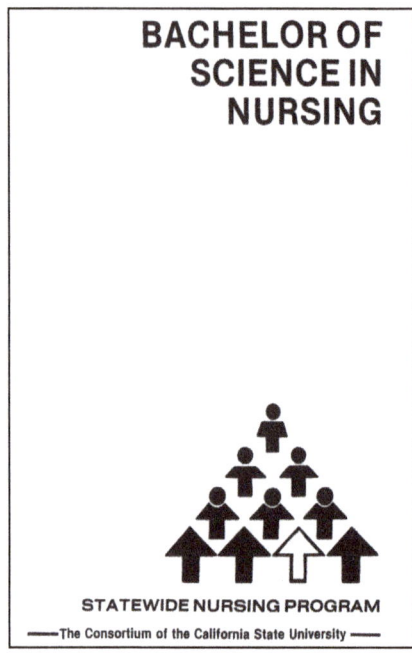
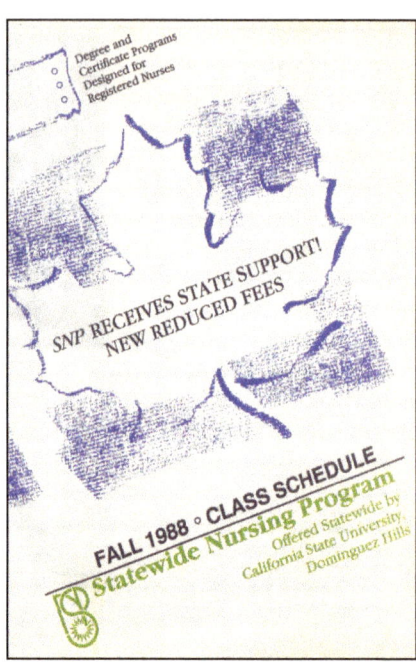

Figure 09.42. A schedule for the Statewide Nursing Program, Consortium.
Figure 09.43. A schedule for the Statewide Nursing Program, CSUDH.

The California State University Consortium/Statewide Nursing Program/ California State University, Dominguez Hills, School of Nursing created one of the most unique and complex nursing programs the state had ever offered.

In 1973, the California State University system began an external degree program called the Consortium. They advertised it as the "1,000 Mile Campus." This allowed working adult students to obtain distance learning degrees; college classes were held in a variety of locations near students' homes. Students could study at a pace that suited their work and family lives. Although the Chancellor's office of the CSU, in Long Beach, administered the program, the State did not fund it. The Consortium developed and functioned as 100% self-supported by student fees. [52]

By the mid-1980s, the Hospital Research and Education Trust study and the California Association of Hospitals and Health Systems recommended public and private institutions develop a master plan for nursing education to combat the acute nursing shortage of "professional nurses" and "technical nurses." The 1965 concept and nomenclature of the professional Bachelor of Science vs. the technical ADN/diploma nurse continued to permeate educational development ideas. [53] Still, in the 1980s 55% of RNs held only a diploma, 22% a BSN, and 18% an ADN. [54]

Baccalaureates, Theorists, Associates

Although California programs existed for a generic BSN, an RN to BSN path did not. In 1978, the CSU Chancellor's Office invited chairs from CSU nursing programs and other professional nursing groups to form a committee to discuss the needs of RNs who wished to obtain a BSN. A path to increase masters-prepared nurses would also be required to fill increasing faculty shortages. The group determined few spaces existed in current programs, and working RNs had difficulty attending traditional programs. The team reviewed external degree programs and adult learning principles.[55]

Based on the group's findings, the State began a program in 1981-82, within the Consortium called the Statewide Nursing Program (SNP), which offered two degree paths: an RN to BSN and a Master of Science in Nursing (MSN). The team developed a unique curriculum—working RNs could study on weekends and evenings, at their own pace, at 170 local hospitals and community college facilities statewide. They submitted a grant application to the W.K. Kellogg Foundation to create the learning materials: workbooks, syllabi, audio and visual media, and curricula. While waiting for the grant, several health care agencies contributed start-up funds in the spring of 1981.[56]

In January 1982, CSU received 2.3 million from the Kellogg Foundation to fund the SNP's course development and program dissemination. The courses were divided into one and two-unit modules, equal to one traditional credit hour.[57] The first courses were offered in the Long Beach area.[58]

Like traditional programs, an academic year consisted of two semesters and one summer session but with rolling admissions, which allowed a student to enter at any point. The students enrolled in one module at a time. They could utilize all USC, UC, community colleges, and medical libraries, plus collaborative hospital learning resource centers. The regular and adjunct SNP faculty taught these courses. Registered nurses with preceptor expertise facilitated student performance courses/field work at instructional sites.

In 1983, the National League for Nursing granted the SNP undergraduate program an eight-year accreditation. In the spring of 1983, twenty RNs completed the BSN; the first 16 MSN students graduated in March 1985.[59] By 1986-87, the SNP accounted for nearly 80 percent of the Consortium's enrollment.[60] More than 1,000 nurses had earned a BSN with an enrollment of 3,000 students.[61] The SNP successfully initiated the first RN to BSN program in Los Angeles County—probably the first in California.

In 1973 the fees were $85 per credit unit (601 inflation dollars in 2024) and various other fees.[62] By 1986, fees had increased to $150 per unit and a $250 mentoring fee. Enrollment greatly decreased because of the fee hikes. They lowered fees to $138 per unit; still, the high costs slowed the students progression. Many gave up due to family responsibilities and work schedules.

Chapter Nine

Officials determined the Consortium could not maintain financial stability through self-supporting mechanisms. They decided to close the Consortium in 1987 yet hoped to maintain the SNP. The California Postsecondary Education Committee endorsed a plan for CSU to seek support from the state. The Chancellor was determined to transfer the program intact and maintain its statewide mission.

The CSU administration began soliciting several CSU campuses for their interest in assuming the SNP. Other CSU campuses already offered nursing degree programs; California State University, Dominguez Hills (CSUDH), did not. CSUDH could thereby eliminate the potential conflict between operating the two styles of programs. Dominguez Hills considered this offer. Following a "freewheeling discussion," the president appointed a task group to outline the conditions for CSUDH to assume responsibility. On 2 July 1987, the Chancellor and CSUDH's President Bronwell signed the SNP transfer document. Dominguez Hills became the first public campus in California to operate a statewide instructional program. [63]

Effective 1 July 1987, Dominguez Hills assumed the responsibility to operate the existing Consortium's MSN and BSN Statewide Programs, manage the Nursing Department staff, and maintain the non-traditional dimensions of the programs. [64]

The transfer process to Dominguez Hills consisted of three phases:

1. Physical relocation of the SNP Consortium's employee and accounting records and the establishment of suitable campus facilities (they bought temporary trailers to function as the Department of Nursing)
2. Budget creation for the state's support
3. A transition year (the 1987-88 academic year) to convert the Consortium self-supported status to a campus-operated, state-supported status [65]

The university calculated they would incur higher expenses for travel to off-campus teaching sites and for communication (mail, telephone, and data) to 3,000 statewide students—especially in the transition years. The transfer required decision, training, and organization of multiple details. The State agreed on a higher faculty-to-student ratio of support for two years: they would calculate the 1990-91 cost of operating the SNP at the normal campus-wide full-time equivalent student (FTES) ratio. [66]

The University reduced student fees in 1988 to those of all campus-based CSU students: $226 per semester for 6 or fewer units (600 inflation dollars in 2024) and $358 for 6.1 or greater units. Substantial savings over the 1987 Consortium fees of $414 for 3 units. The ten statewide geographic instruction areas, A to J, continued. The program articulated with the community college nursing programs to serve as an advertisement for the CSUDH/SNP and as insight for ADN students to see a path forward to a BSN. [67]

By 1991, some classes were videotaped and shown at off-campus classes—students interacted with the instructor by phone. In 1994, the program began offering web-based/internet courses in addition to the classroom. Eventually, they phased out classroom instruction; by 2000, all classes were internet-based. They added other advanced degrees and certificates—all conducted online except for the required clinical portions. [68]

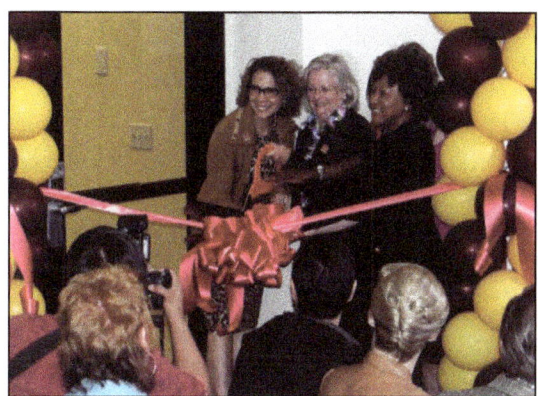

Figure 09.44. Cutting the ribbon on the new state-of-the-art nursing skills lab. L to R are President Mildred García; Carole Shea, the former SON director; and Patricia Hinchberger, lecturer and the director of the MEPN program, Nov. 8, 2010.

In 2010, the school dedicated its first Clinical Skills Lab. The Chancellor's Office allocated 1.6 million dollars for CSU nursing facility improvements system-wide. [69] In 2022, the House Appropriations Committee funded $700,000 for additional upgrades. [70]

Figure 09.45. Three MEPN (Masters Entry Program into Nursing) students: Scott Dcragisich, Joseph de Veyra, and Poppy Purcell in the skills lab, November 8, 2010.

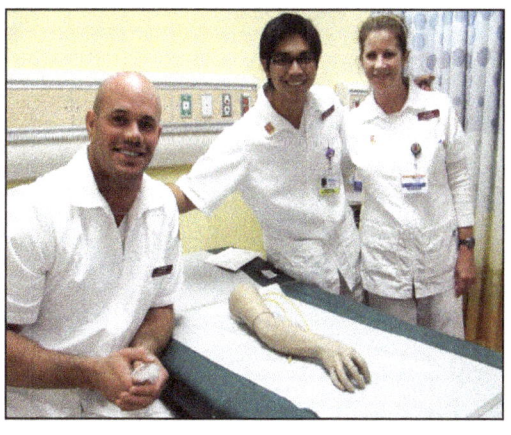

In 2008, the SON initiated their only classroom-based program—an MEPN—but it ended due to declining NCLEX scores. The last cohort graduated in 2015. [71]

While the school no longer formally uses the Statewide Nursing Program moniker, it is still utilized for state financial reasons. [72] In 2024 it is simply California State University, Dominguez Hills, School of Nursing.

Books to Protest and Collect

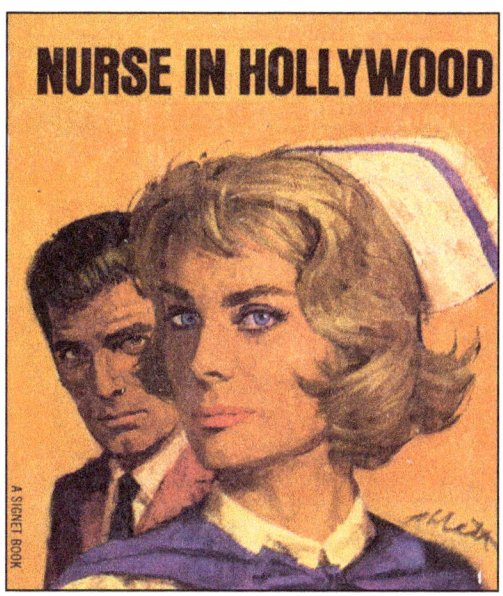

Figure 10.01. Cover of the nurse novel, *Nurse in Hollywood*, 1965. Hollywood producer discovers nursing student Kitty Walters and asks her to choose: her dream of becoming an RN or every girl's dream of becoming a star.

In the 1940s, nurses became a popular subject in the media. Incorrect portrayals occurred throughout history, and occasionally nurses protested; however, during this period the focus on nurses increased. Comic books, romance novels, and movies portrayed nurses in unrealistic roles. Products also used nurses in advertisements to boost sales because nurses were trusted.

Nurses were often viewed as sexual objects. The drama was heightened. Their work was mainly clerical as they toted charts and followed doctors around the hospital halls. The opposite also persisted: images of nurses as purely altruistic women or as rescuing angels. Scientific interests, intelligence, or plain hard work were less intriguing. Men were rarely shown in nurse roles either; if men were shown, it was not as a lead character.

Women within the feminist movement felt particularly appalled by the proliferation of nurse romance novels because the plots frequently revolved around a nurse's solitary goal of marrying a doctor. Some nurses rallied against these images; some did not see them as a threat. As culture progressed, the advertisements and romance novels were perceived as quaint, and nurses started to display personal collections of the novels as memorabilia.

Chapter Ten

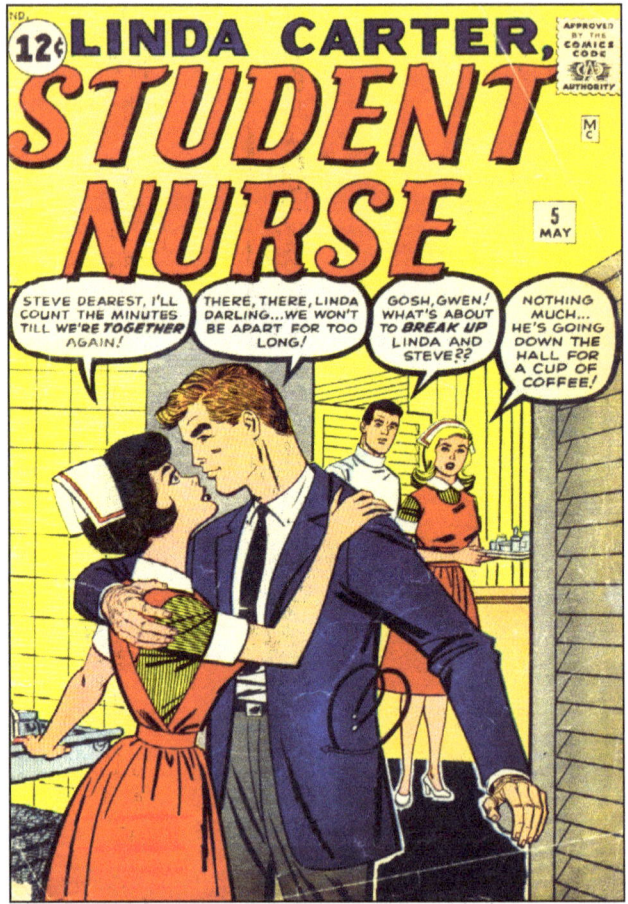

Figure 10.02. *Linda Carter, Student Nurse* comic book cover, May 1962, No. 5, Issue 9. Linda is distraught over a separation from her boyfriend, Steve. The doctor wonders what traumatic event will break up Linda and Steve. Gwen reveals that the couple will only be separated because Steve is leaving to buy a cup of coffee. (© Marvel Characters, Inc. Used with permission)

In September 1961, Marvel Comics announced *Linda Carter, Student Nurse,* destined to become your most beloved friend. Carter passed food trays, dated, and gossiped. The supervising nurse, Nurse Barker, closely watched her fledgling student nurses.

Two handsome young doctors competed for Carter's affections—much to the disgust of her beautiful, scheming classmate Gwen Glitter. Naïve Carter considered Glitter her true best friend and confided in her. Glitter's wicked plots against Carter, however, always backfired and ironically helped Carter to succeed.

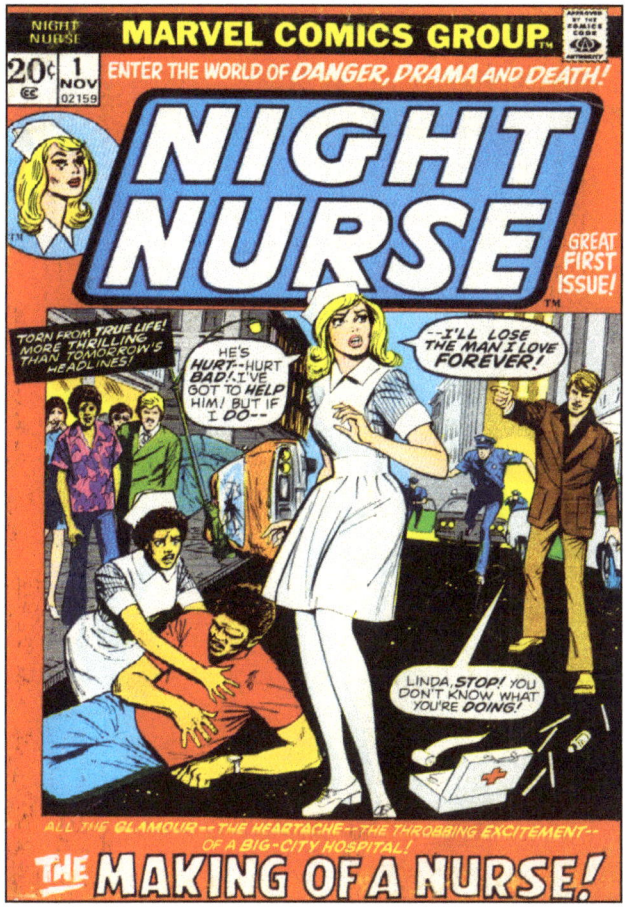

Figure 10.03. The premier issue of *Night Nurse*, November 1972. (© Marvel Characters, Inc. Used with permission)

Marvel published the first issue in their last series of nurse comic books, *Night Nurse*. They created only four issues. Again, they used the name Linda Carter but made no mention of her student nurse days, and her hair color had changed to blonde. Linda and her roommates experienced adventures on the night shift at Metro General, including bomb threats and serial killers.

Carter fell in love with a wealthy businessman. He forced her to choose: marry him or work. She chose work and watched him walk away. Georgia Jenkins, from the inner city a few blocks from Metro General Hospital, provided free medical care to the people from her old block on her days off. Christine Palmer intended to make a life without her father's money. Her father threatened if she didn't come home by Thanksgiving, "Don't come home at all." She stayed at Metro General and became a surgical nurse.

Chapter Ten

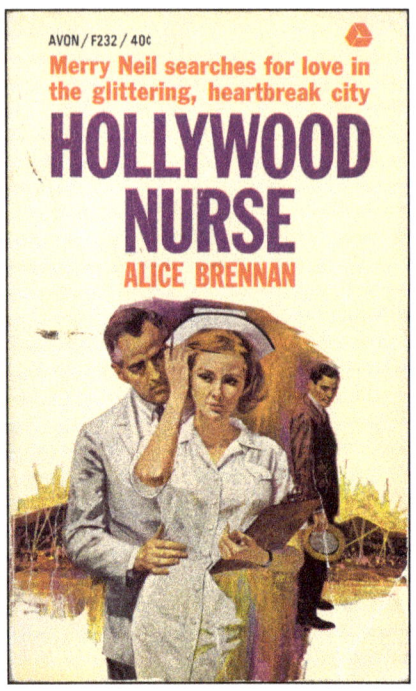 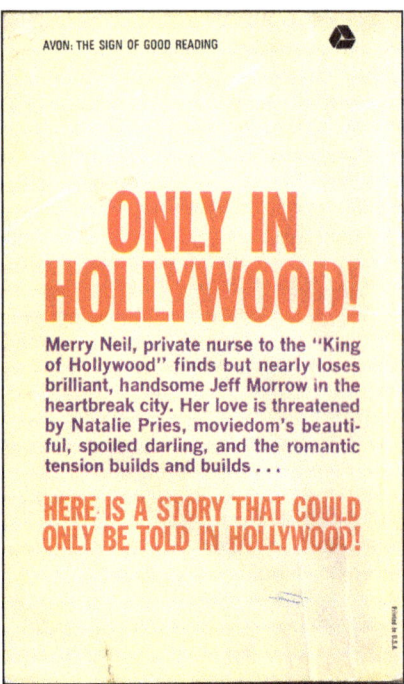

Figure 10.04. *Hollywood Nurse*, 1966. Los Angeles nurse images sold romance.

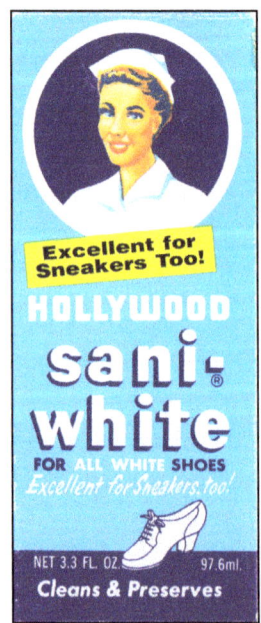

Figure 10.05. Sani-white, 1950. Los Angeles nurse images sold shoe polish.

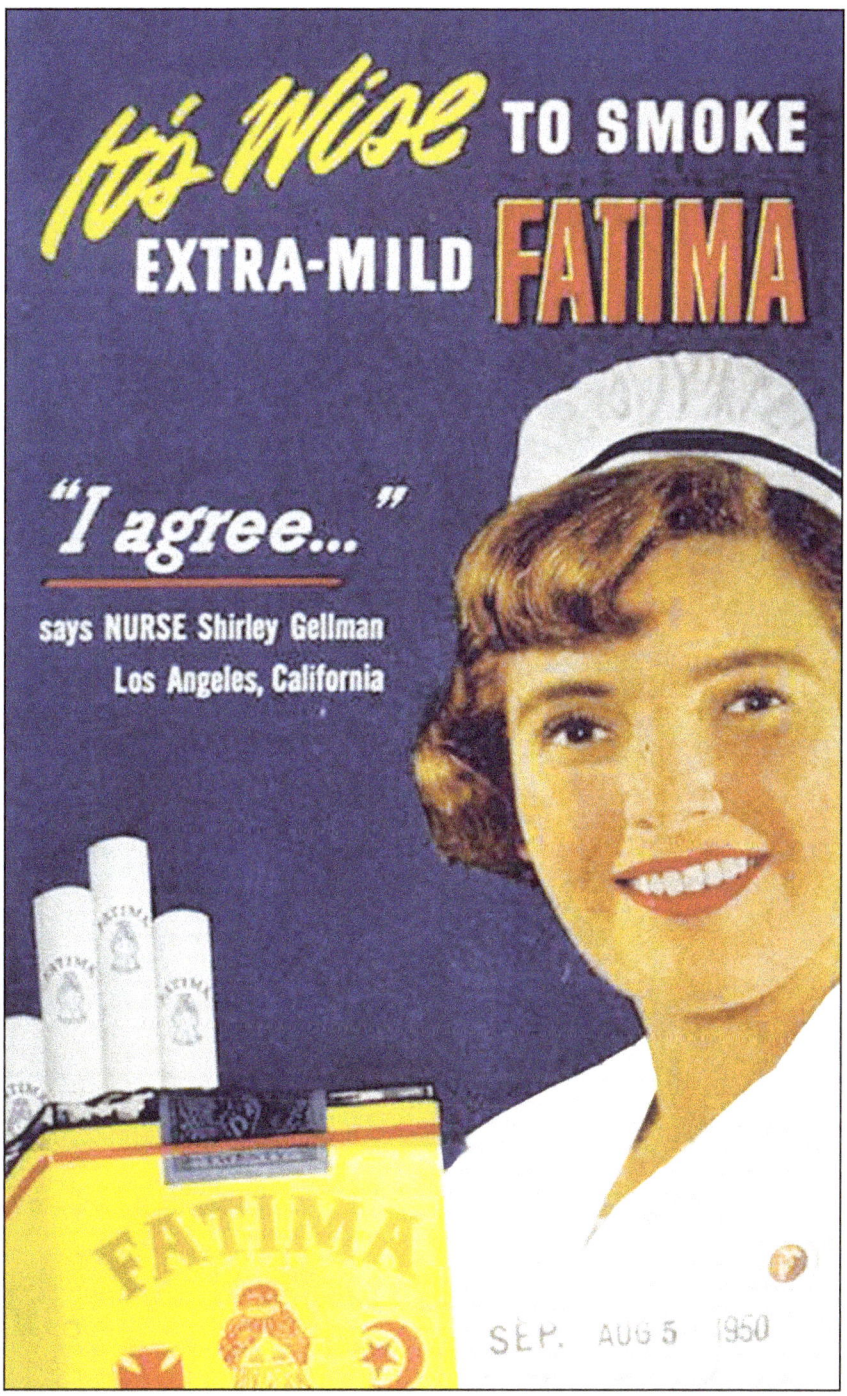

Figure 10.06. Fatima ad, 1950. Los Angeles nurse images even sold cigarettes.

Practitioners, Scientists, Organizations: 1970-1996

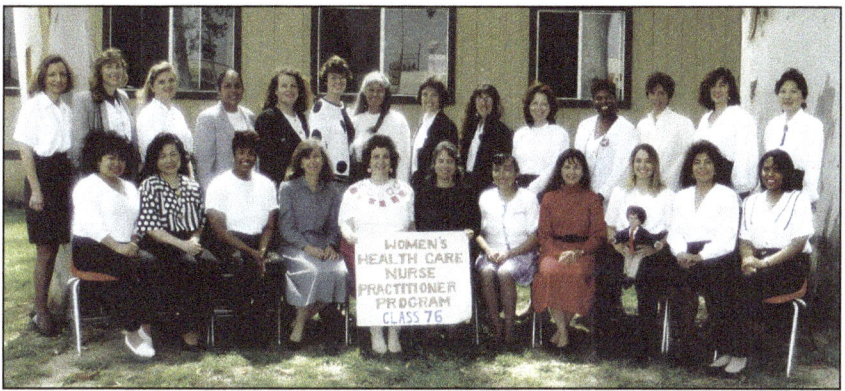

Figure 11.01. The 76th graduating class of the Women's Health Nurse Practitioner Program (WHCNPP), Harbor-UCLA, 1992. Instructors Linda Goldman, left, and Sharon Schnare, right, hold the class sign. The author is in the front row, third from the right, holding a talking mascot doll. He spoke gentle, supportive phrases the busy NP students wanted to hear, such as, "Let me rub your feet."

In 1965, Professors Loretta Ford, RN, and Henry Silver, MD, initiated the first NP program in the United States at the University of Colorado—a pediatric NP specialty. Not everyone agreed with their idea. Ford said, "I think if you care deeply, you're willing to stick your neck out." [1-2]

On 30 June 1971, the WHCNPP at Harbor-UCLA graduated the first nurse practitioner class in California. WHCNPP also trained the first NPs for Guam, Samoa, and the Navajo Nation.[3] Physicians Robert Bragonier and Don Ostergard trained the initial instructors Mary Lindsay, Martha Jones, and Mary Gramlich. Bragonier was a tireless champion for women's healthcare, reproductive rights, and the nurse practitioner role.[4]

At its inception, the program began to supply NPs for Title X clinics. Title X was a federal grant program for family planning and sexual health services. Later, the school became affiliated with CSU Long Beach and other universities. Qualified NP students could simultaneously obtain a Master of Science in Nursing from a university and an NP certificate. WHCNPP expanded to offer a family nurse practitioner supplement for graduate NPs.

Regulations eventually required all NP programs to award a master's degree, and more universities began NP programs. The WHCNPP graduated 1,874 NPs over thirty-seven years. The final class graduated in 2007.[5]

Chapter Eleven

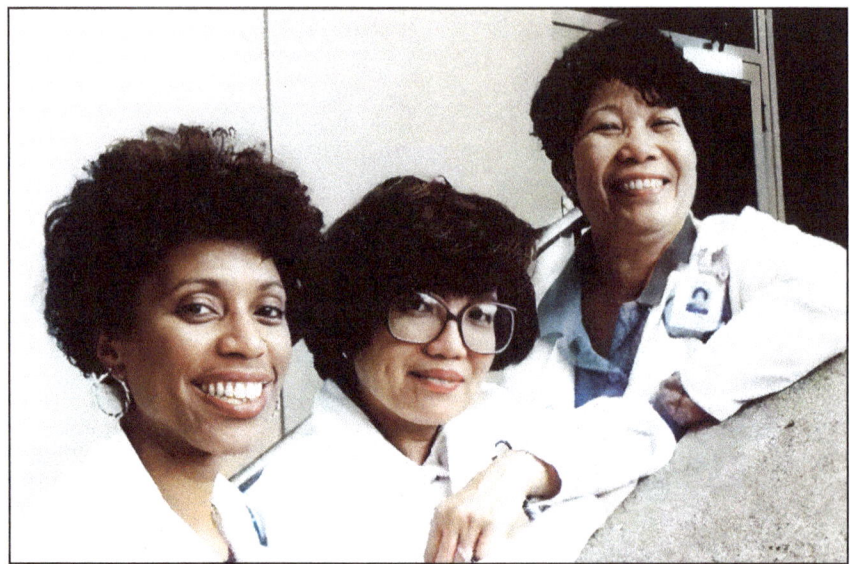

Figure 11.02. Nurse epidemiologists pose for their Employee Team of the Month award. Sandra Bible, Elsie Fontanilla, and Romea Fama, left to right, April 1991. C. (Courtesy of Cedars-Sinai Medical Center)

Elsie Fontanilla never found an infection control problem she could not solve. When the Department of Health had a question, they called her for a solution. Fontanilla obtained a Bachelor of Science in Nursing in the first class at St. Luke's College of Nursing, Philippines, in 1970. The hospital's original school of nursing began in 1907 as the predecessor of the college.

Fontanilla immigrated to Los Angeles in 1971 because her mother liked the area. In 1974 she joined Cedars of Lebanon Hospital. The Joint Commission on Accreditation of Hospitals (JCAHO) began to require infection control standards for accreditation in 1977. Fontanilla became an infection control nurse to write new policies. She realized infection control nurses must monitor all aspects of the hospital: construction projects, sterilization processes, monitoring of hand hygiene, cleaning products, surveillance of infectious outbreaks, and teaching employees about infection control. She had the power—and responsibility—to immediately halt any practice that did not comply with infection control standards.

When the hospital became Cedars-Sinai Medical Center, the job became more complex: Fontanilla changed the title of infection control (IC) nurse to nurse epidemiologist and the IC Department to the Department of Epidemiology. In the 1970s, Los Angeles began a chapter of the Association for Professionals in Infection Control and Epidemiology; Fontanilla became involved at its inception and remained a leader in the field.[6]

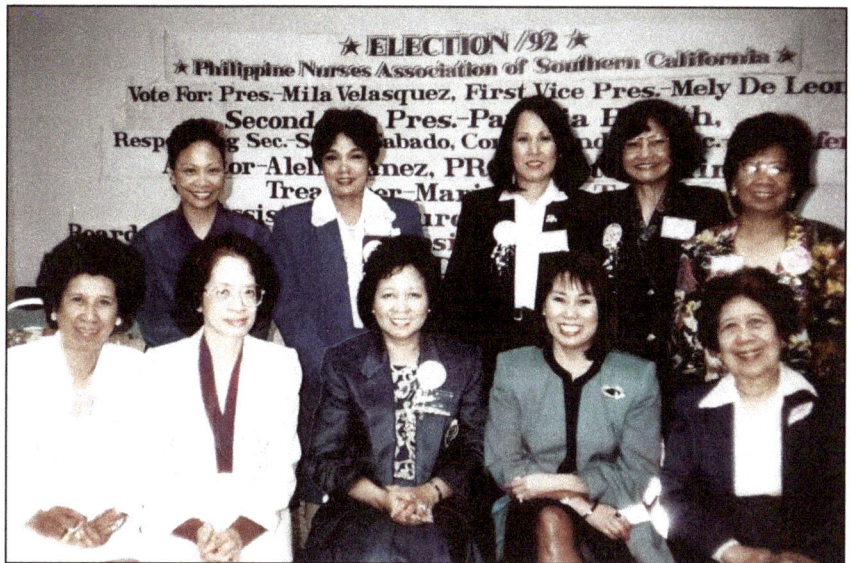

Figure 11.03. The Philippine Nurses Association of Southern California (PNASC) members and board candidates at their 1992 board elections: Mely de Leon, Clarita Miraflor, Mila Velasquez, Patricia Hoerth, Angelina Torres. Standing are Ely Alferos, Aleli Ibanez, Imelda Trinadad, Josie De Jesus, and Leto Ordinario, left to right. C. (Courtesy of Mila Velasquez)

The PNASC started in Los Angeles in October 1960 (as the Filipino Nurses Club) in the home of Blas and Angelina Torres—years before the national organization began. educator and public health supervisor, Juanita Virgilio Inocencio, was the founding president.

The Exchange Visitors Program sought to ease the nursing shortage during the Vietnam War by allowing foreign nurse graduates (FNGs) to immigrate. Initially, only ten percent of FNGs passed the licensing exam. The law required immediate deportation upon failure. Leticia Jue, Mierfe Calica, Elsie Fontanilla, and Delia Goggins led a campaign to extend the unrealistic six-month FNG Interim Permit. Jue became the first Filipina to serve on the State Board Review Panel. They found sixty percent of test items were flawed. They revamped the questions and extended FNG permits to twelve months.

Mila Velasquez, sitting at the center, received a Master of Nursing from the University of the Philippines in 1975. She moved to Los Angeles, helped revive the PNASC, and served as its president for many years. At first she worked as a clinical specialist at the Veterans Administration (VA), then in the 1990s the Department of Veterans Affairs chose her to attend a post-masters NP program at Uniform Services University of the Health Sciences in Maryland. She then worked at the VA as an NP for ten years.[7-8]

Chapter Eleven

Betty Smith Williams conducted the first meeting for the Council of Black Nurses, Los Angeles, in her living room. Williams was the first African-American nurse to wear the cap of the Frances Payne Bolton School of Nursing, Case Western Reserve University. She had obtained a Bachelor of Science in zoology at Howard University, so she qualified for a program that allowed students with a bachelor's degree to study for a Master of Nursing, which she received in 1954.

The following year, she moved to Los Angeles. Nurses with a master's degree were rare in 1955, but they were highly sought after because the recently developed bachelor degree programs needed professors. Although they had never hired a Black professor before, Mount St. Mary's needed her. She became the first Black nursing professor in California. Williams taught Sister Callista Roy and later helped the Mount implement Roy's theory in the nursing department.

Williams received a Doctor of Public Health from UCLA. She held faculty positions in nursing at UCLA and California State University, Long Beach. She was the first Black assistant dean in the School of Nursing at UCLA, and the first Black dean at the School of Nursing at the University of Colorado Health Sciences Center in Denver.

Williams met Barbara Johnson, a graduate of the Mount's third nursing class, at the Los Angeles City Health Department. They were concerned that Black nurses did not have a forum to advance their cause. In 1967, they invited several nurses to meet at William's home. This was the beginning of the Council of Black Nurses. This nucleus developed a citywide meeting in which they established the organization's goals. Within three years they met nurses from San Francisco's newly established Black nurses group.[9]

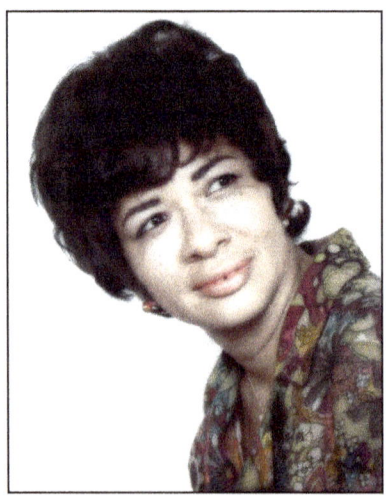

Figure 11.04. Betty Smith Williams, 1968. (Photographs courtesy of Betty Smith Williams)

Williams received her Master of Nursing from the Frances Payne Bolton School of Nursing, Case Western Reserve University. Bolton was a congresswoman who supported nurses, public health issues, and championed nursing education bills—including the passage of the 1943 Bolton Act (the Cadet Nurse Corps). In 1923, Bolton endowed the School of Nursing at Case Western Reserve University.[10]

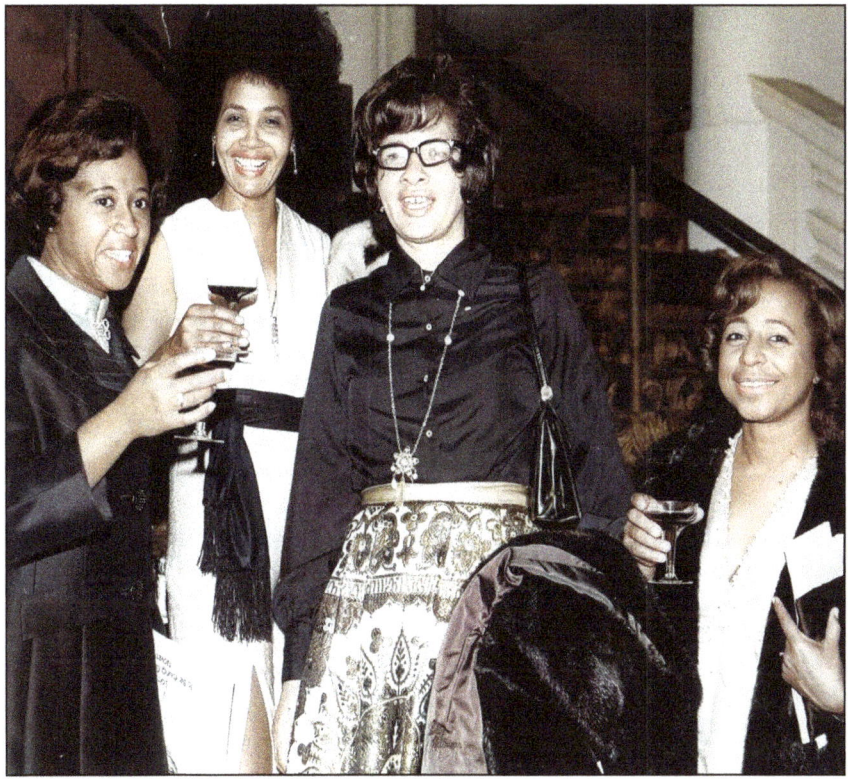

Figure 11.05. The Council of Black Nurses organization leaders at the Scholarship Theatre Party Reception. Barbara Johnson, co-founder; Rosalie Jackson, vice president; Betty Smith Williams, co-founder & first president; and Omeria Butts, member, left to right, c. 1970. C. (Betty Smith Williams)

In 1969, Williams obtained a grant for a California Statewide Conference. Black nurses from different states attended. In 1971 she cast the motion that founded the National Black Nurses Association (NBNA).

In 1995, Williams was elected as the seventh national president of the NBNA. In 1998, the NBNA became the founding organization of the National Coalition of Ethnic Minority Nurse Associations (NCEMNA). Williams was a co-founder and the first president of NCEMNA.

Williams believed minority nurses should belong to both general nurse associations and ethnic minority associations. General nursing organizations focused on the welfare of the profession. The ethnic minority groups, however, focused on improving the health status of their communities. "We provide and promote for our community of concern," Williams said. "We have an inside track and experiential knowledge of the culture." [11]

Chapter Eleven

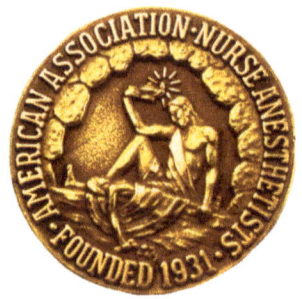

Figure 11.06. American Association of Nurse Anesthetists pin. The figure is of Hypnos, the God of Sleep, retiring to the Cave of Night to seek rest. He holds a bunch of poppies to foster sleep and pleasant dreams. He sits atop the lamp of learning to maintain vigil. Morpheus, the God of Dreams, watches and protects Hypnos as he sleeps. The pin is colloquially referred to as the Morpheus. [12]

The idea of organizing nurse anesthetists into an acting body began at the 1930 biennial convention of the American Nurses Association when Agatha Hodgins presented a paper concerning this idea. The organization became official in 1931. In 1935, the California Association affiliated with the National Association of Nurse Anesthetists (the predecessor of the American Association of Nurse Anesthetists).[13]

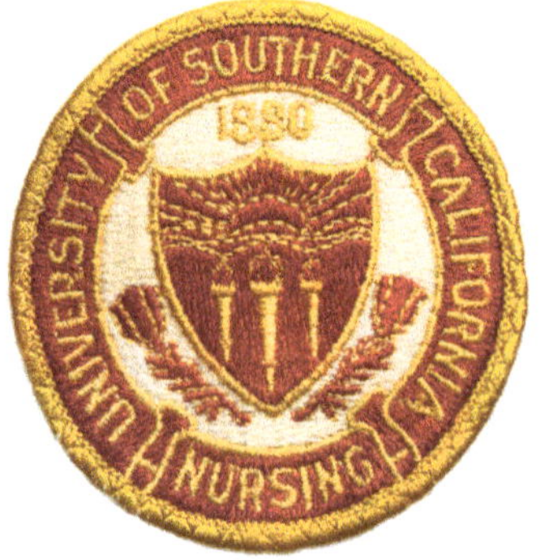

Figure 11.07. The USC Nursing School patch, 1980s.

The University of Southern California (USC) opened in 1880, yet the Department of Nursing didn't begin until 1981—one hundred years later.[14] The department offered a bachelor's degree and several graduate programs: family nurse practitioner, geriatric nurse practitioner, enterostomal therapy, nurse-midwifery, nurse anesthesia, and nursing administration.

On 2 November 1991, during a project to meet a service course requirement, five USC nursing students aboard a Flying Doctors of Mercy airplane helped save the lives of colleagues. Four planes were flying side by side when one plane hit electrical wires and crashed in Sinaloa, Mexico. Nursing students Houston, Greene, Schmuecker, Romero, and Hahn cut their stethoscope tubing for tourniquets and clothing for bandages. The *Los Angeles Times* story appeared on the front page; a made-for-TV movie detailed their experience.[15]

Despite media attention and the program's successes, the Nursing Department closed in 2004.[16] According to Assistant Professor Janet Schneidermanne, one of the reasons cited for the demise was that the nursing department had "a different vision and mission than the parent institution."[17]

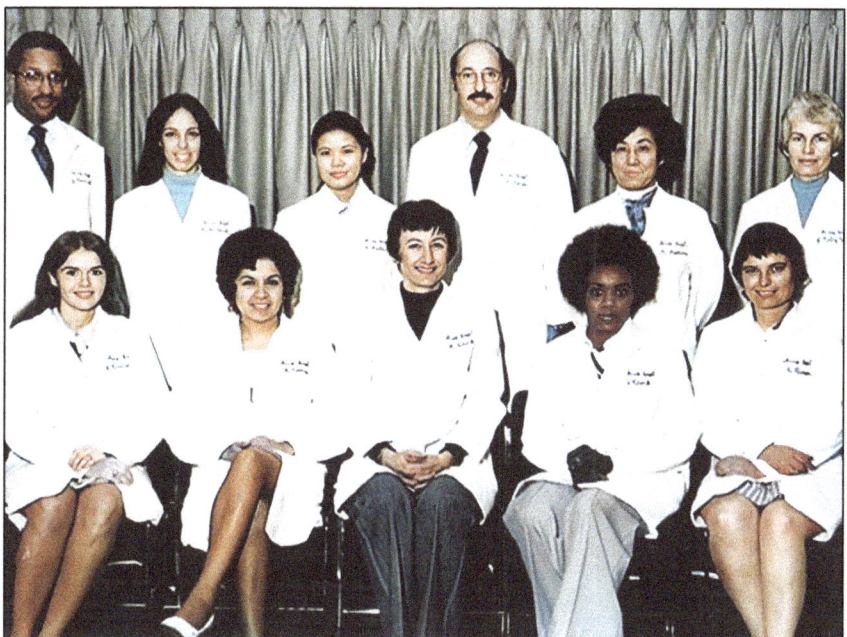

Figure 11.08. The first graduating class of Kaiser Permanente School of Anesthesia, 1974. C.

In 1978 they affiliated with California State University, Long Beach, and became the first program in the United States to award a Master of Science in Nursing with a clinical specialty of nurse anesthesiology.[18] (Courtesy of Kaiser Permanente School of Anesthesia.)

Figure 11.09. On the right is Ida Rodgers, the first member of the first chapter of ATD (Alpha Tau Delta), with Barbetta Jackson Tulley in the middle and Beebe, 1971 C. The UCLA chapter hosted the first ATD Convention to celebrate the fraternity's 50-year anniversary.

ATD, the first professional nursing fraternity, began at the University of California at Berkeley in 1921.[19] Alpha Chapter was also called the Lady of the Lamp. (History & Special Collections, Louise Darling Biomedical Library, UCLA)

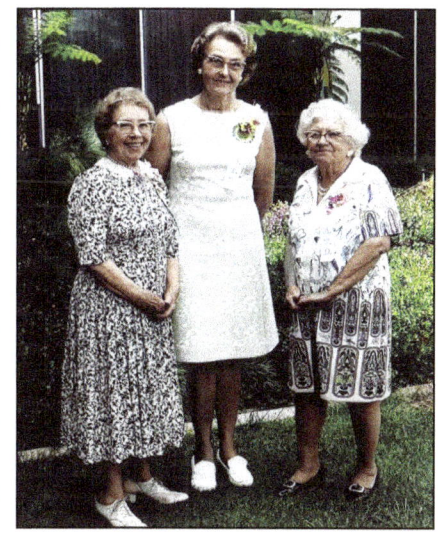

Chapter Eleven

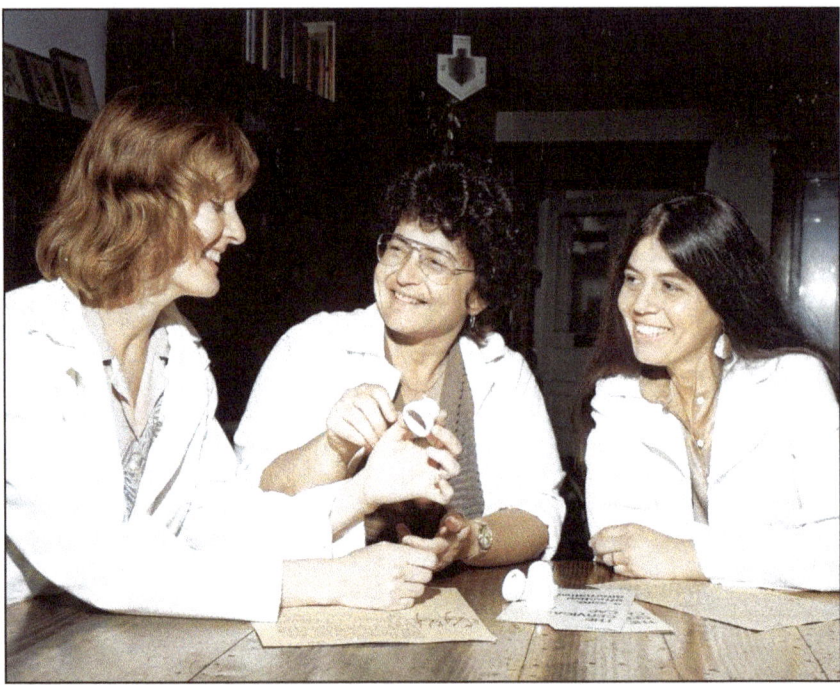

Figure 11.10. Nurse Practitioner Renee Potik, center, in her Venice home with Nurse Practitioner Mary Ann Forgette, left, and Physician Assistant Alexandra Voines, 1980. C. (Special Collections, Charles E. Young Research)

Renee Potik brought the contraceptive cervical cap to the West Coast. She had read about the cap in a feminist magazine in 1979, but it was not yet FDA-approved. Potik flew to New Hampshire to learn from a clinic that imported the cap from Great Britain. When word circulated about the new contraception device, women clamored to try it. She started a cervical cap research project with Gerald Bernstein, MD. [20] The FDA finally approved the Prentif cap in 1988. [21]

Potik became the first private practice nurse practitioner in Los Angeles; she joined a group of doctors and paid her share of the office bills. When her patients required a surgical procedure, she accompanied the patient into surgery and performed positive visualization techniques—no extra charge. She became a colposcopist (a medical practitioner who uses an instrument that magnifies the cells of the cervix and vagina to permit direct observation and study of cervical tissue).

Potik also practiced at a clinic for the homeless on Skid Row and later at a clinic for farm workers. She graduated from the Women's Health Care Nurse Practitioner Program at Harbor-UCLA in 1978. [22]

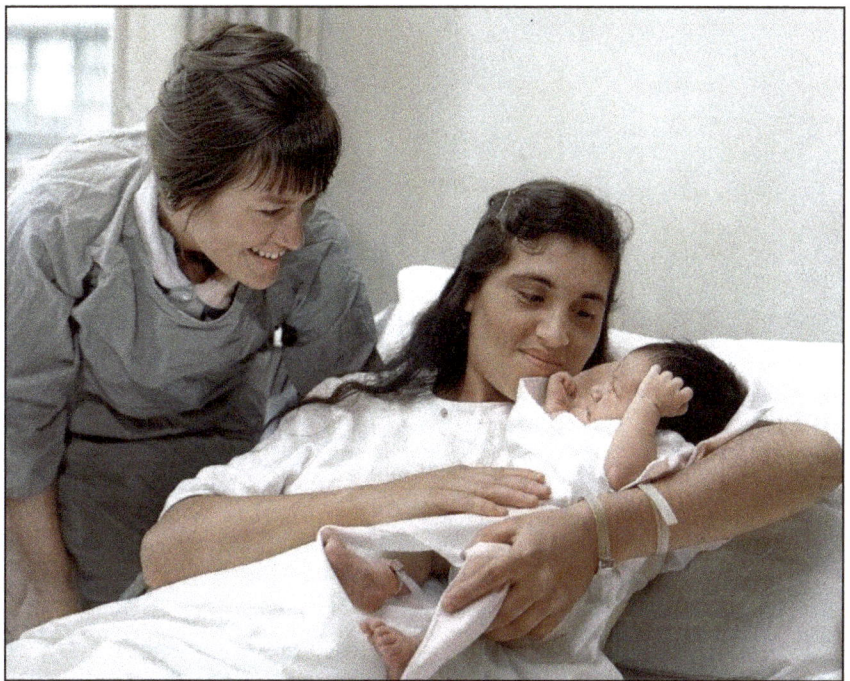

Figure 11.11. Nurse Midwife Wanda Mueller, left, after she delivered her twenty-fifth baby. The mother was Nicando Guitterez, March 26, 1974. C. (History & Special Collections, Louise M. Darling Biomed Library, UCLA)

California stopped licensing lay midwives in the 1930s. In 1973, California law continued to specify nurse-midwives could provide only prenatal care. No professional programs trained midwives until a new state law permitted the Department of Health to authorize select paramedical programs.

Los Angeles County Hospital initiated the state's first pilot program for nurse-midwives. In 1974, three nurse-midwives began delivering babies at Women's Hospital, County-USC: Irene Matousek, Sister Ann Keating, and Wanda Mueller. [23-24] The first U.S. school of midwifery opened at Bellevue Hospital, New York, in 1911. Ten midwife pupils from seven nationalities lived in the rear house of a twelve-bed hospital at 223 East 26th St. [25]

In 1925, Mary Breckenridge developed the Frontier Nursing Service of Kentucky. The service used public health registered nurses, educated in England, to staff nursing centers in the Appalachian Mountains. They often traveled to deliveries on horseback. [26]

The American College of Nurse-Midwifery was incorporated on 7 November 1955 as the professional organization for Certified Nurse-Midwives. [27]

Chapter Eleven

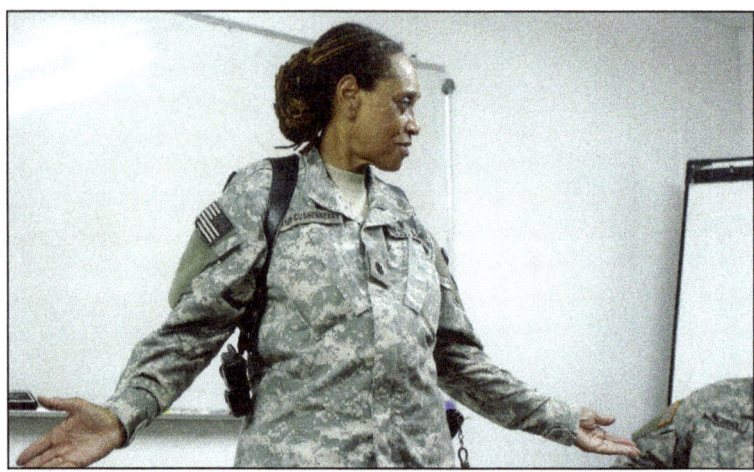

Figure 11.12. H. Frances Hayes-Cushenberry teaching a stress reduction class at Camp Liberty, 2007. (H. Frances Hayes-Cushenberry)

H. Frances Hayes-Cushenberry graduated from Compton College in 1976. At first she thought an associate in nursing was sufficient schooling. She worked in obstetrics at King Drew Medical Center, and later she applied to the King Drew Nurse Anesthetist program—they told her she was not academic material. They were wrong. Between 1984 and 2006, she obtained a Bachelor of Science in Nursing; Midwifery Certification; Master of Mental Health, Nurse Practitioner; Juris Doctor; Doctor of Education; and Master of Forensic Science. She viewed school as a stress reliever.

She enlisted in the Army in 1989, completed her active duty in 1993, and was placed in the reserves. In 2004, the Army called her to active duty at Camp Liberty in Iraq. She used her mental health training for the Combat Stress Team. Many soldiers suffered from anxiety and depression. She helped prepare them to return to the field. Some soldiers wanted to go home, but they couldn't. She emphasized the importance of a positive outlook in stressful situations.

After fourteen months, she returned to Los Angeles and joined the faculty at Compton College. Ironically, in 1973 she had failed her initial attempt in that nursing program. When her students worried because they failed a class, she told them, "Don't worry. Just try again."

The Army called her back to Iraq in 2006—she neither expected nor desired a second tour. Soldiers were worn out. Nurses had developed compassion fatigue and needed counseling. After her second fifteen-month tour, she returned to Compton College.[28] Later, she taught nurse-midwifery at Charles R. Drew University,[29] and nursing at El Camino College.[30]

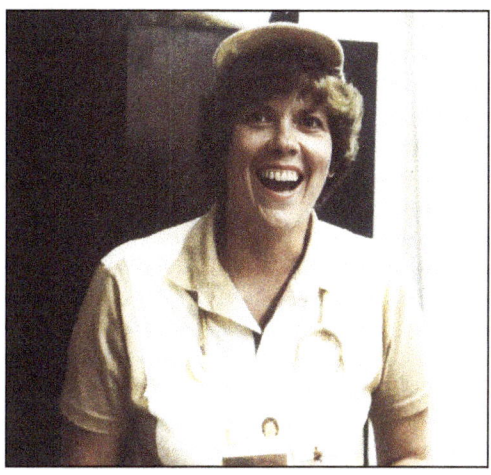

Figure 11.13. Deborah Parkman Henderson, in charge of critical care, during the games at the Pasadena Rose Bowl at the 1984 Los Angeles Olympics. (Courtesy of Deborah Henderson)

In 1984, Deborah Parkman Henderson became the administrator of the California Emergency Medical Services for Children project at Harbor-UCLA Medical Center. The project standardized the quality of care for children. She helped implement an Emergency Department Approved Pediatric program; she developed protocols for rural and urban settings and supervised nurses in rural California.

She standardized the pediatric code cart at Harbor-UCLA amid many disagreements regarding which supplies should be included. She developed a training program for airway management—2,800 paramedics in Los Angeles and Orange counties used her program.

Henderson realized emergency department nurses, especially those in rural areas, might not have access to Pediatric Advanced Life Support (PALS) courses; the Emergency Nurses Association funded her idea to write a manual. She co-edited the *Pediatric Emergency Nursing Manual* published by Springer Publishing in 1994. Staff from twelve states participated in the development of the case base, self-learning manual. Nurses as far away as Australia used the book. In 1998, she branched off into injury prevention, asthma education, and disaster issues.

Henderson's father was a diplomat; she was educated in France, Germany, and Switzerland in her early years. She obtained an ADN at Pasadena City College in 1978, and a PhD in Medical Education at USC in 1997. Additionally, she holds a Bachelor of Arts in Human Relations and a Master of Arts in Human Development.[31]

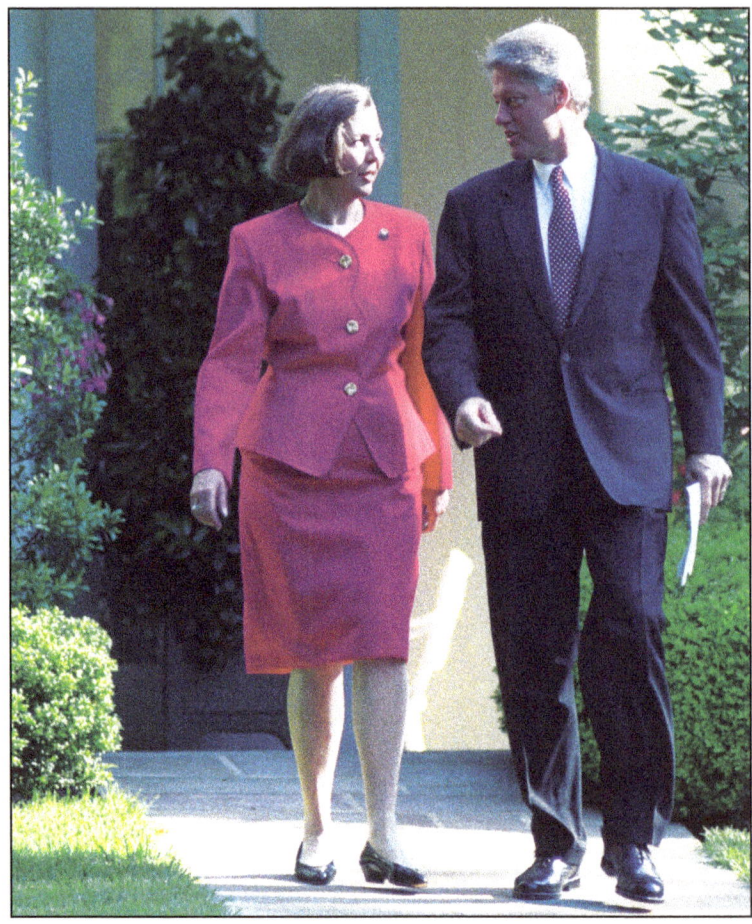

Figure 11.14. Kristine Gebbie with President William Clinton at the White House on the day of her appointment, June 25, 1993. (Courtesy of William J. Clinton Presidential Library)

President Bill Clinton appointed Nurse Kristine Gebbie as the first national AIDS policy coordinator (AIDS Czar) in 1993. She resigned her post after one year.[32] Gebbie had championed issues concerning AIDS since the early 1980s. She formed an advisory commission that set standards for AIDS testing, created anti-discrimination measures, and fought to protect patient confidentiality. She became the first nurse appointed as the state health director in Oregon and as the secretary of health in Washington State.

Gebbie obtained a Bachelor of Science in Nursing at St. Olaf College in 1965; a Master in Community, Mental Health Nursing at UCLA; and a Doctor of Public Health. She taught at UCLA from 1968 to 1971.[33-34] Virginia Clinton Kelly, Clinton's mother, was a nurse-anesthetist in Arkansas.[35]

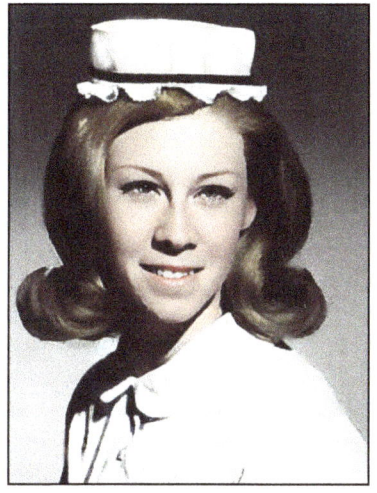 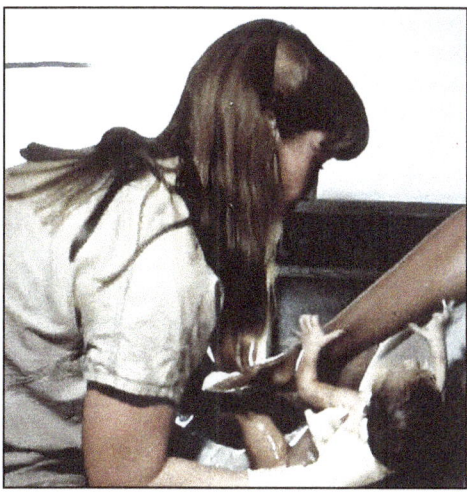

Figure 11.15. Dianne Susan Moore's BSN graduate picture and Moore delivering a baby at a Los Angeles birthing center. (Courtesy of Diane Moore)

When Dianne Moore was eleven, her grandfather fractured his neck. He lay in bed in a hospital ward, unable to sit up because doctors had immobilized his vertebrae. He was thirsty, and they did not have bendable straws; she didn't know how to give him a drink. She called the nurse. The nurse came in, plopped a whole ice cube into his mouth, and said, "There." He started choking, and Moore was horrified. She knew she could do better. In fact, she thought she could be a top nurse. She had good grades, enjoyed science, and realized nurses could have long careers.

Moore graduated from Hunter College with a BSN in 1968, obtained a Master of Nursing at UCLA, a Master of Public Health at Columbia, a Nurse Midwife Certification (CNM) from SUNY Brooklyn Downstate Medical Center, and a PhD at New York University.[36] As a CNM, she became the founder and chief midwife of Westchester County's first freestanding birth center. She worked in a private CNM birth center in Culver City, CA.

She obtained many appointments: director of nursing, Fresno City College; director of midwifery, the Birth Center at the Beth; assistant professor, Columbia Presbyterian Medical Center, UCLA & H.H. Lehman College; preceptor for midwifery students in the Community Nurse-Midwifery Program, Kentucky Frontier Nursing Service, and at Case Western Reserve University. *Who's Who in American Nursing* featured her in their book.

Moore became founding dean of nursing at West Coast University, College of Nursing, in L.A. She designed test scores, not prerequisites, for entry into the school. She championed innovative educational methods at WCU.[37]

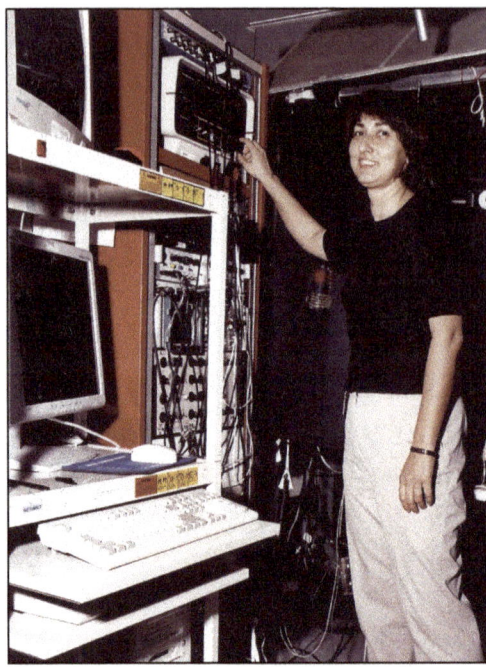

Figure 11.16. Mina Attin at UCLA, 2005. (Photo by Yvette Roman)

Mina Attin first became interested in the underlying mechanisms that affected cardiac arrhythmias when she worked as a nurse treating patients in an invasive cardiac electrophysiology unit. She decided she wanted to learn more about patients' persistent symptoms, but she was too busy in the clinical environment to investigate.

She completed a PhD at UCLA's School of Nursing in Nursing Science.

Attin received a pre-doctoral and post-doctoral fellowship from the National Institute of Nursing Research. She studied calcium ion channels to understand the mechanisms underlying ventricular fibrillation, a cause of sudden death.

In 2002, Attin, with other researchers, studied healthcare professionals knowledge of pulse oximetry. They identified pulse oximetry as the most important clinical issue affecting patients of all ages and specialties.

The researchers circulated a questionnaire to a sample of nurses, physicians, and respiratory therapists. They determined all three disciplines required more education. All the professionals knowledge of pulse oximetry improved significantly after additional training.

She published several articles on ventricular arrhythmias, atrial fibrillation, and other cardiac electrophysiological issues. Attin said nurses were just beginning to become involved in physiology research. [38]

After receiving her doctorate in 2005, Attin successively joined the faculties of CSU, Bakersfield; San Diego State University; the University of Rochester; and the University of Nevada, Las Vegas.

In 2018, the American Heart Association awarded her the Young Investigator Award for her work to improve the odds of patients with pacemakers and implantable defibrillators. [39]

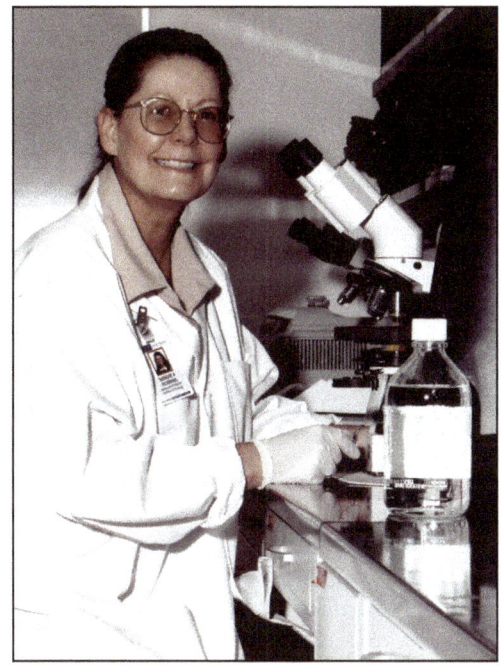

Figure 11.17. Wendie Robbins at UCLA, 2005. (Photo by Yvette Roman)

Wendie Robbins worked as a nurse practitioner in rural areas of Arizona and Texas in the 1980s.

On her drive through the desert, to one clinic she noticed smoke from the copper smelter drifting over the homes. She wondered if patient outcomes could be related to the smelter.

She decided to contribute her knowledge to help prevent reproductive tragedies.

Robbins examined the effects of organophosphate pesticides, air pollution, tobacco smoke, alcohol, caffeine, chemotherapeutics, and antiretroviral agents used to treat HIV. She earned her PhD in Epidemiology at UC Berkeley. During her doctoral studies, she evaluated human sperm cells.

Robbins learned that after treatment, certain chemotherapy drugs caused an increase in an abnormal number of chromosomes in sperm cells. Fortunately, the chromosomes returned to pre-treatment levels within six months after chemotherapy. She also examined oxidative damage in sperm cells.

She headed a group in China that studied sperm cells in relation to occupational boron exposure. Her findings showed that male boron workers experienced a decreased ratio of Y-bearing versus X-bearing sperm compared to men who did not work in the boron industry. A shift in gender ratios of their offspring occurred at birth—boron workers had proportionally fewer sons at birth compared with the control group. [40]

Robbins became program director of the Occupational and Environmental Health Nursing Program within the Southern California Education and Research Center—a training grant funded by the CDC National Institute for Occupational Safety and Health. The grant provided financial and research support for PhD and master's-level trainees at UCLA and UC Irvine. Her funded projects explored work as a social determinant of health in communities following disasters. [41]

Chapter Eleven

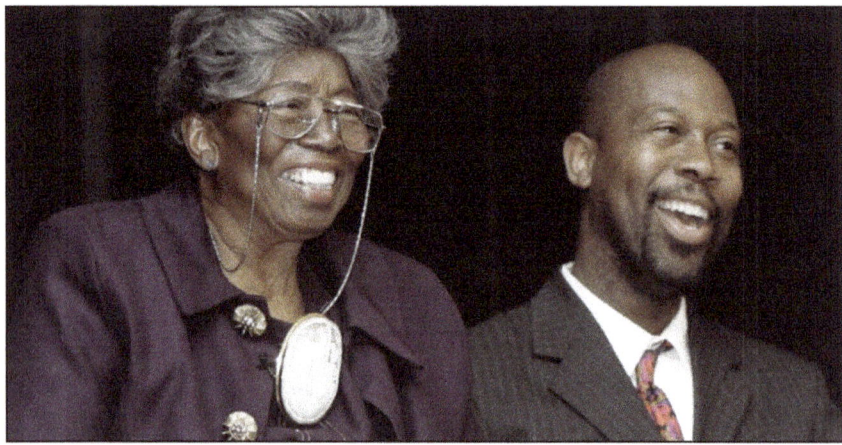

Figure 11.18. Courtney Lyder, right, with Mary Starke Harper on Diversity Day at the University of Virginia, 2005. (Courtesy of Courtney Lyder)

Courtney Lyder developed a love for elderly people while living with his grandparents in Trinidad and Tobago. He moved to Manhattan at age five. He graduated with degrees in psychology and biology. At Rush University, he attended a lecture about the skin by Professor Mildred Kemp, who had doctorates in nursing and physiology. Kemp became his mentor. She taught him skin assessment and told him he would specialize in wound care.

He completed a BSN, a Master of Gerontology, a Doctor of Geropsychiatry, and a Gerontological Nurse Practitioner degree. He received fellowships on aging from the National Institute on Aging, the Brookdale Foundation, the Summer Institute on Research, and the American Association of Colleges of Nursing Leadership for Academic Nursing Program.

Lyder traveled the world lecturing on wound care. He worked as a clinical instructor, a geropsych and gerontological nurse practitioner, a nurse clinician, an associate professor, a director of wound care programs, and a gerontologic nurse consultant.

He became the first nurse awarded a million-dollar grant from the National Institute of Health. Luther Christman, founder of the National Male Nurses Association and first male dean of a school of nursing, mentored Lyder. He followed with his own first: the first Black male nurse appointed dean of a school of nursing (UCLA). His UCLA term spanned from 2008 to 2015.

Lyder said nurse scientists should be clinicians because important questions are gained from clinical experience. He believed nurses should switch from race-based assessments to culture-based assessments. He maintained cultural factors influence health concerns more than race or place of birth. [42-43]

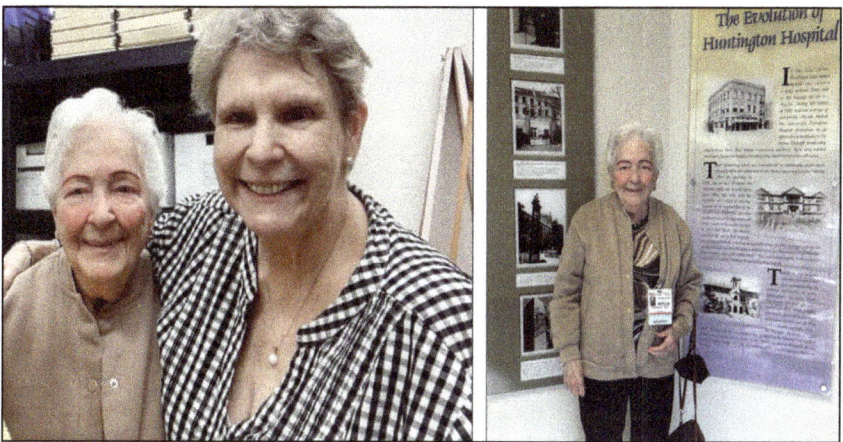

Figure 11.19. Phyllis Esslinger, president (left), and Diane Harris-Hara, vice president of the Western Conservancy of Nursing History. The photo on the right is Esslinger in the nursing history hall display she created in 2004 at Huntington Hospital in Pasadena, 2024. (Photos by Diane Harris-Hara)

In 1993 Phyllis Esslinger, an Azusa Pacific University (APU) professor emeritus, heard that Huntington Hospital had disposed of their school of nursing records. She hurried to retrieve them. As she stored the boxes, she imagined other disbanded schools of nursing would suffer a similar fate. She wanted to preserve the histories of previous nursing generations for future nurses and historians. She hoped to collect nursing artifacts and documents from Western states for interpretation, scholarly pursuits, and displays. [44]

Esslinger gathered a team of dedicated nurses. Together with Diane Harris-Hara and many volunteers, they established the Western Conservancy of Nursing History (WCNH). They gained nonprofit status. The Iota Chapter of Sigma Theta Tau International contributed funds to launch the project; the WIN Foundation gave $10,000; Kaiser Permanente donated $40,000. APU provided rooms for the collections. The group hatched many plans, including an oral history project, but they need donated funds for that and for an archivist to organize and maintain the collections.

WCNH received materials from APU Assistant Nursing Professor Pamela Cone: items from her aunt Edwin Todd, a POW Navy nurse interred in the Philippines during WWII. They obtained collections from California, Hollywood Presbyterian, and Methodist Hospital Schools of Nursing. When St. Vincent's Medical Center closed, the Sisters donated their nursing archives. They've amassed over 1,000 nursing history books and textbooks. [45]

Their ultimate goal is to house the archives and create museum displays in a dedicated space. However, a special benefactor is needed to achieve that goal.

Chapter Eleven

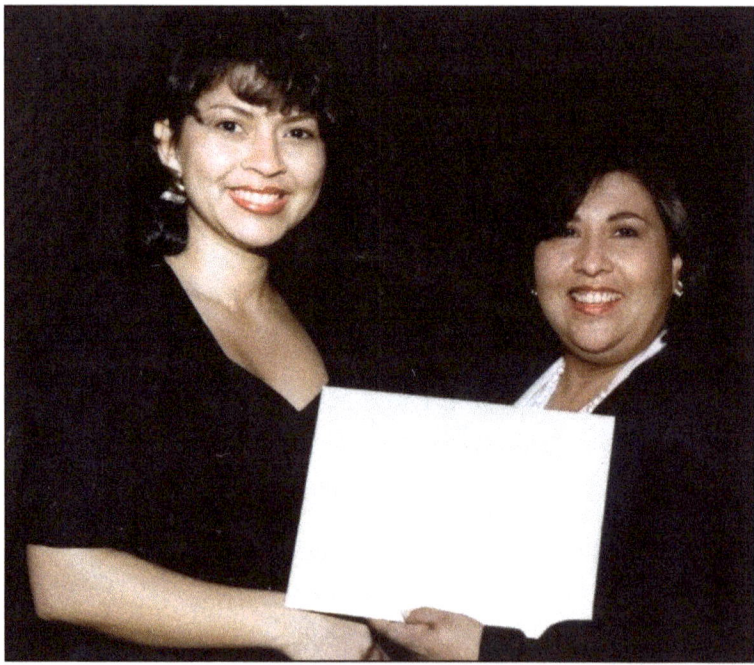

Figure 11.19. Anissa Perez, left, with Gloria Molena presenting a nursing scholarship to Perez, 1993. C. (Courtesy of Anissa Perez)

The Department of Health provided scholarships to Hispanic nurses in 1993. Perez was one of seventeen who received a check. In 1991, Molena became the first Latina to be elected to the Los Angeles County Board of Supervisors.

Anissa Perez was a bookkeeper in a comfortable office. One night she had to stay late because she could not account for three pennies in the book. She said, "This is ridiculous. I cannot spend my life stuck in an office worrying about three cents." She considered what to do next. She remembered how she admired nurses who helped her during the birth of her child. She decided to become a nurse.

The application process at East Los Angeles College required a handwritten essay and letters of recommendation from doctors and nurses; she considered it a privilege when she received her letter of acceptance into the ELAC nursing program.

Perez worked in the emergency room for ten years. She obtained a BSN and MSN from the University of Phoenix. She worked in a challenging nurse practitioner job; however, when she accepted an educational position in 2004, she knew she would stay in education. In 2009 American Career College, in Los Angeles, promoted her to the director of nursing. [46-47]

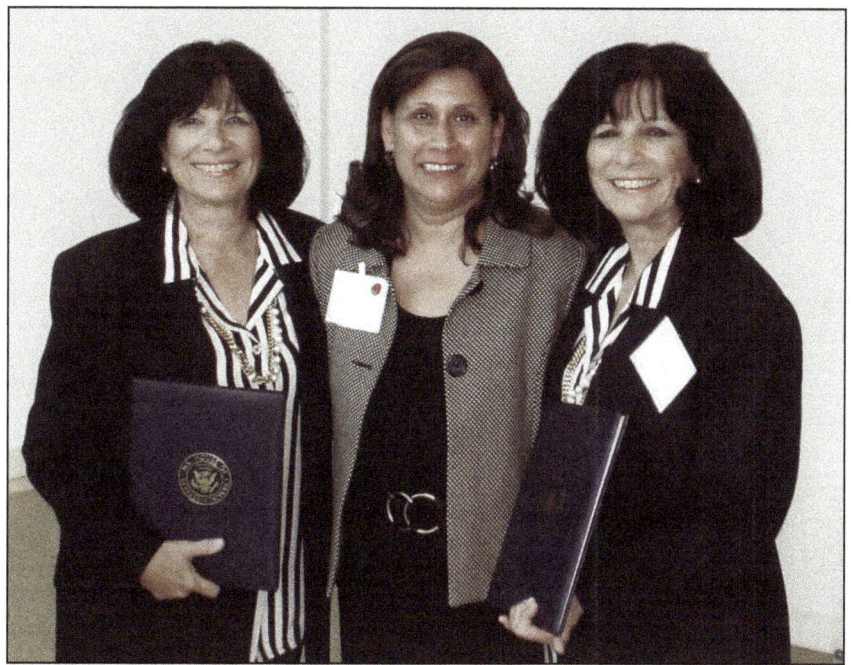

Figure 11.20. Angie Millan, center, with Carol and Carolyn Bloch at the annual LA NAHN Professional Nursing Conference at the California Endowment Center, 2009. The Blochs were nursing faculty at Los Angeles County School of Nursing; at the conference they received recognition from Congresswoman Grace Napolitano for their contribution to the community as teachers. (Courtesy of Angie Millan)

The National Association of Hispanic Nurses (NAHN) was founded in 1979. The NAHN evolved from the Spanish Speaking/Surnamed Nurses Caucus formed at the ANA convention in 1974. The Los Angeles Chapter of the NAHN (LA NAHN) began in 1990. [48]

Millan became a member of LA NAHN in the 1990s, was president for six years, and was president of NAHN in 2010. She received a nursing diploma from L.A. County Hospital in 1986, an ADN in 1995, a BSN and an MSN from CSULA, an NP certificate from WHCNPP at Harbor-UCLA, and a Doctor of Nursing Practice from Western University of Health Sciences.

Millan was the nursing director at L.A. County Dept. of Public Health, Children's Medical Services Department—she supervised 160 nurses in three divisions. She was a nursing instructor at East Los Angeles College, a member of the Chamberlain University Board of Trustees, and a fellow of the American Nursing Academy. In 2015 she received the NAHN Nurse of the Year award and the 22nd Senate Woman of the Year award. [49-50]

Chapter Eleven

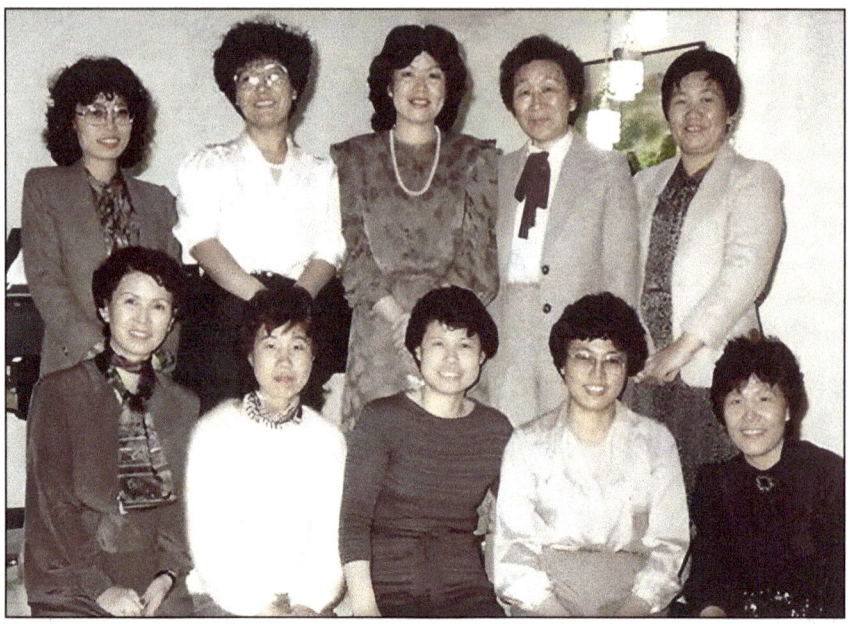

Figure 11.21. Members of the Korean Nurses Association of Southern California, founded in 1970. C. (Courtesy of the Korean Nurses Association of Southern California)

The original goals of the association included making Korean nurses more effective so they could deliver the highest quality care to Korean Americans. When Korean nurses immigrated, they needed to learn the American healthcare system. Difficulties could occur because of language barriers and philosophical differences between Korean nursing and nursing in the United States. The organization included student nurses, LVNs, RNs, and NPs.

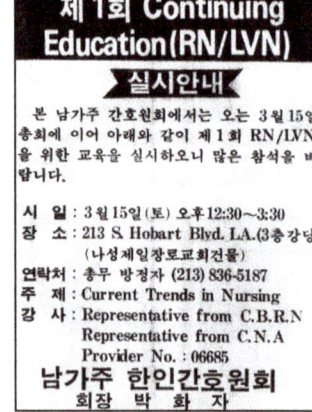

Figure 11.22. Announcement of the first Continuing Education Seminar that the association offered. They conducted educational programs to assist in the acculturation process and obtain required credits. The group also offered community services, scholarships, a Nurse of the Year award, and international nursing consultation and education. [51]

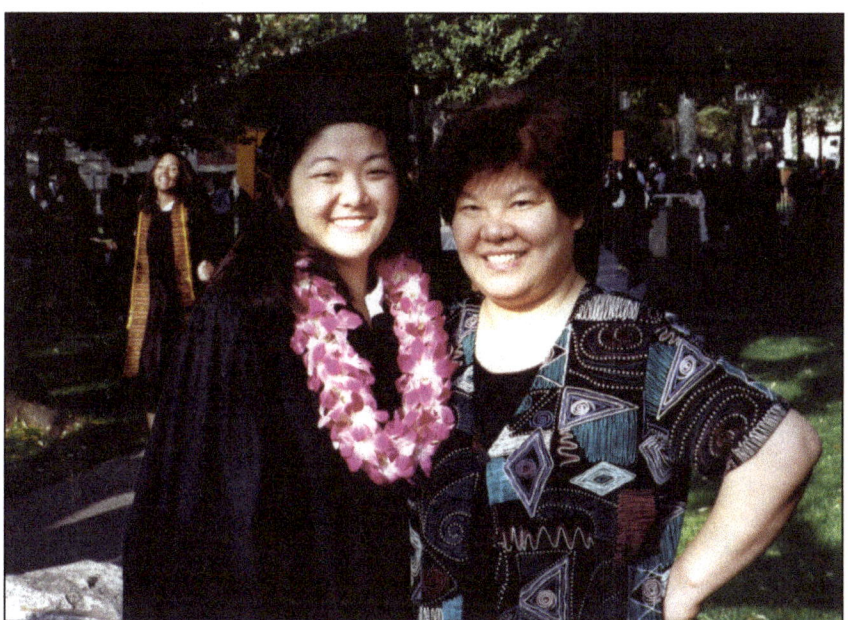

Figure 11.23. Nurses Aimie Pak, left, and Oknyu Pak at Aimie's BSN graduation ceremony. (Courtesy of Aimie Pak)

Oknyu Pak did not know what to study in college, but she knew she wanted to see the world. Nurses were one of the few professions that could emigrate from South Korea, so her father told her to become a nurse. She graduated from Ewha Woman's University in 1970 and was recruited to work in Los Angeles. She worked twenty-two years in the operating room at Olive View.

Oknyu wasn't happy when her daughter, Aimie Pak, said she wanted to be a nurse—she wanted Aimie to have more freedom—but Aimie had friends who couldn't find a job after college. She did not want that. Oknyu agreed.

When Aimie graduated from USC with a BSN in 1999, Oknyu was disappointed the college did not give her a nurse's cap. Oknyu thought it was a symbol of identity. Aimie's nursing school experience was different from Oknyu's; Aimie's student uniforms were khaki-colored scrubs.

Aimie worked in the ICU and OR, then decided to try something different. She obtained an MBA but learned she did not like money-hungry bankers. She joined a USC program that offered a Master in Social Work to nurses. The Veterans Administration (VA) hired her in their community care program; she found they didn't really understand her hybrid capabilities. Was she a nurse or a social worker? However, she liked the VA system. She decided to help others, as her mother had been helped, and she became a recruiter.[52]

Chapter Eleven

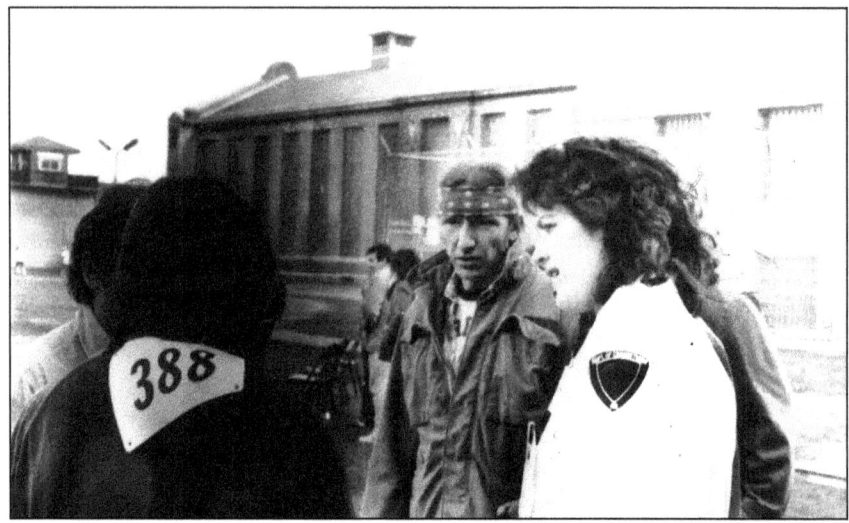

Figure 11.24. Ellen Kane, right, with inmate-runners at a prison muscular dystrophy fundraiser, 1987. C. (Courtesy of Ellen Kane)

Ellen Kane was an occupational therapy assistant and felt frustrated because she couldn't administer pain medication. She first obtained an LPN, then an Associate in Nursing in 1985, and a Bachelor in Health Care Management.

The Minnesota Correction Facility was less than a mile from her home in Stillwater. People in Stillwater called prison work "a good state job." She applied. She worked the night shift her first year—the only nurse for 1,400 inmates. She learned about every illness because inmates had them all: cancer, kidney failure, mental illnesses, AIDS, and heart disease. She ran cardiac codes and managed fifty patients with diabetes. The prisoners repaired buses and made farm implements, so accidents were frequent emergencies.

Kane accompanied prisoners for in-town doctor visits. The time and location were highly confidential; however, one day an inmate's friend learned of a scheduled appointment. The friend arrived at the office to break the inmate out of prison. Guns were fired. The inmate died; the shooter was incarcerated.

When inmates wanted aspirin, they lined up for a nurse who handed it to them in a small envelope. Kane thought many lined up just to see a smile or feel the touch of the nurse's hand. She thought this because when guards searched the cells during contraband shake-downs, they often found stacks of unopened pill envelopes. Ten years later, Kane's knowledge of AIDS led her to research. Research—and the sunshine—led her to Los Angeles in 2009.

In 2019 she wrote a memoir, *Prison Nurse: Mayhem, Murder, and Medicine*.[53]

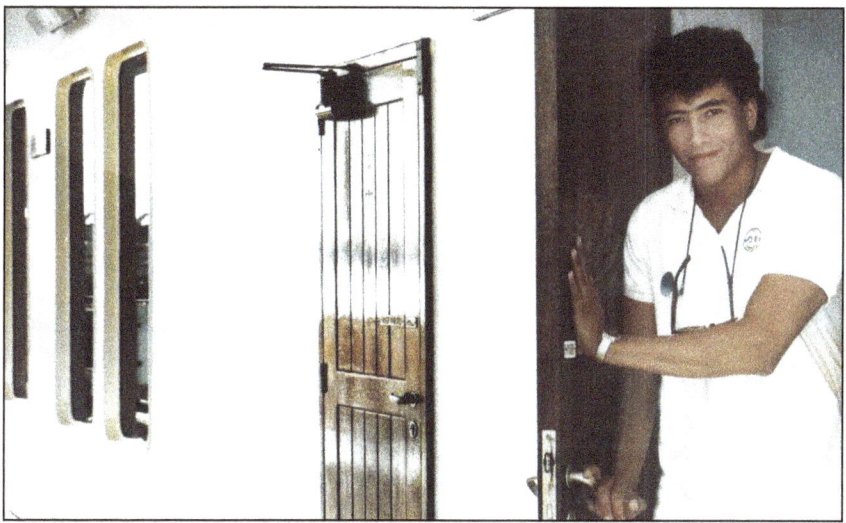

Figure 11.25. Eduardo Barreto on the deck of the *Sky Princess*, in the Caribbean, 1991. C. (Courtesy of Eduardo Barreto)

Eduardo Barreto worked as a cytotechnologist in Mexico City in 1990. He wanted an adventure, so he joined Princess Cruise Lines. He thought he would find it; he didn't know he would find much more. While working on the deck of the ship in 1991, Barreto saw Los Angeles nurse Cynthia taking photographs of the sunset. He stopped to talk.

Five years later he had married her, moved to Los Angeles, and graduated from LVN school. In 2000 he completed an ADN. In 2002, KTLA-TV featured him in a news segment about male registered nurses. He worked as a clinical instructor and in other areas, but mainly he's used his decades-long expertise and knowledge in his role as a pediatric oncology nurse. [54]

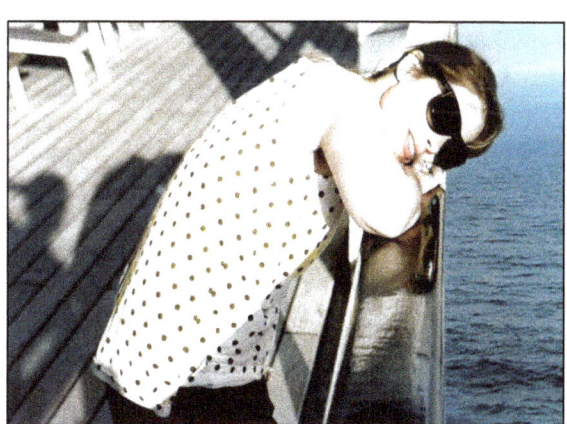

Figure 11.26. Cynthia, waiting for a sunset that day in 1991. C. (Photo by Robert Sutton)

Anniversaries and Roses: 1997-2013

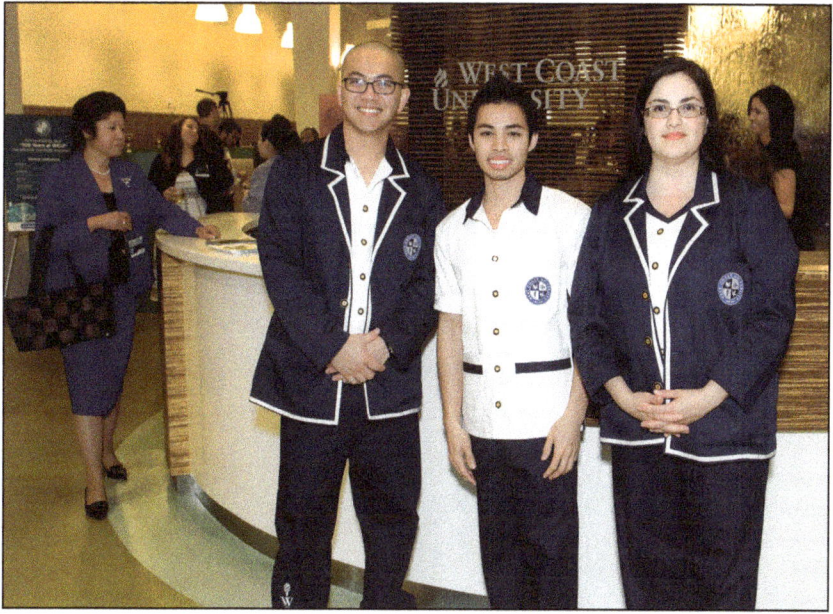

Figure 12.01. West Coast University nursing students, left to right: Marco Munar, Clark Pineda, and Ofelia Cortez at the opening of the North Hollywood campus. Dean of Nursing Nancy Hoff, of the Orange County campus, stands at the far left, 2009. (Courtesy of West Coast University)

In 1997, Los Angeles celebrated two anniversaries: one hundred years since the first nurses graduated (College Training School for Nurses) and one hundred and forty years since nurses organized the first hospital (Los Angeles Infirmary/Sisters Hospital). Nurses advanced from training programs to the breadth of degrees available to other professions. Nurse practitioners proliferated, clinical specialists adapted, and nurse-scientists researched.

West Coast University became the first private, for-profit school to achieve CCNE accreditation and a pre-licensure BSN program in 2008.[1] Some academics disparaged the expensive private, for-profit nursing schools. Students, however, viewed them as a method to begin school without a lottery or years on a list. Many private, for-profit schools have opened since 2008.

Minimal entrance requirements and lower passing rates on the National Council Licensure Examination (NCLEX) were among the criticisms. True for some but not all. California required schools to transmit their NCLEX results; potential students could evaluate the scores on the BRN website.[2]

Chapter Twelve

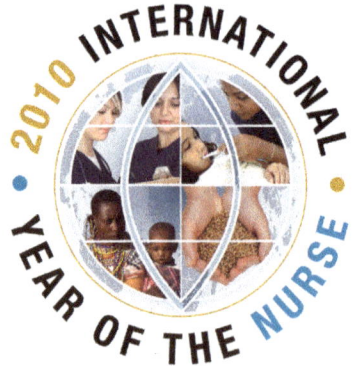

Figure 12.02. Organizers established 2010 as the first Year of the Nurse to involve nurses in a worldwide celebration and bring health to their communities.

Sigma Theta Tau International, the Nightingale Initiative for Global Health, and the Nightingale Museum created the 2010 initiative, which included an event at the National Cathedral in Washington, D.C., on 25 April 2010.[3] In 2020, groups celebrated again as the International Year of the Nurse and the Midwife.[4]

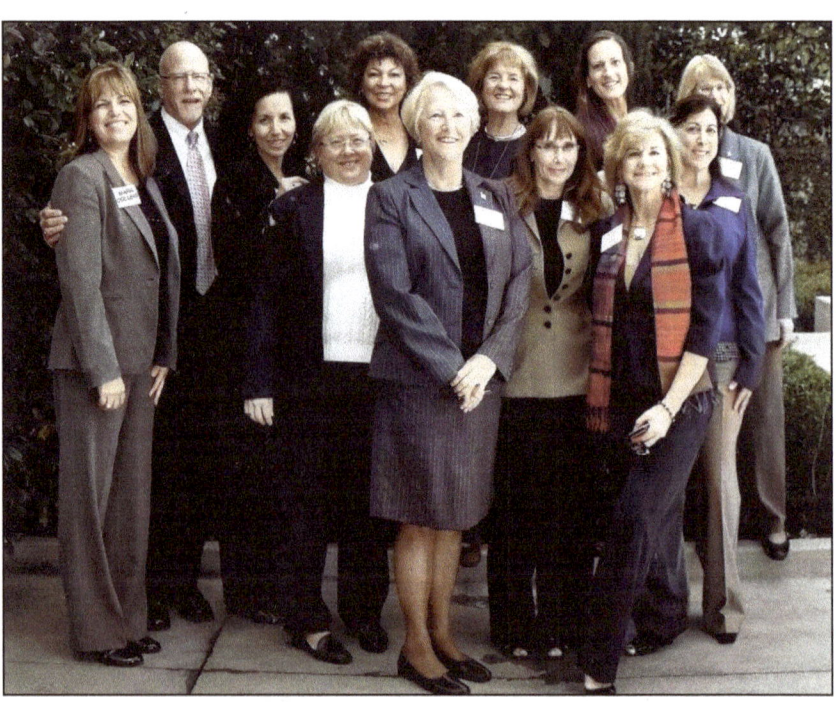

Figure 12.03. 2010 Sigma Theta Tau, Gamma Tau, Executive Board members at the new member's induction ceremony, 2009. Mara Collins, Peter Anderson, Erin Core, Anna Dermenchyan, Virginia Erickson, Bonnie Faherty, Leah Fitzgerald, Teresa Haley, Martha Highfield, Mary Alice Melwak, Isabel Purdy, and Choi Siegel. (Courtesy of Bonnie Faherty)

The first Sigma Theta Tau, Gamma Tau, Los Angeles chapter began at UCLA in 1978.[5] In 2007, CSU Northridge joined UCLA—it became Sigma Theta Tau, Gamma Tau-at-large. CSU Channel Islands joined them in 2020.[6]

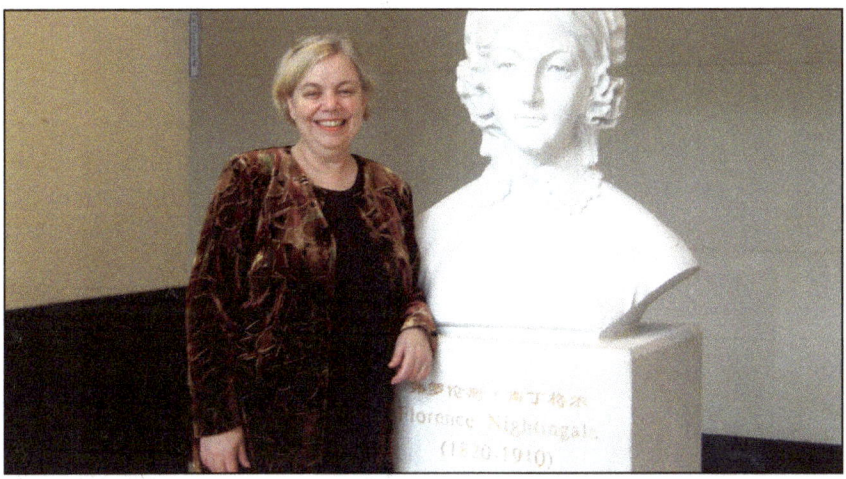

Figure 12.04. Deva-Marie Beck beside a bust of Nightingale at Shandong University School of Nursing in Jinan, China, 2008. (Deva-Marie Beck)

Deva-Marie Beck was born in Los Angeles. Two of her aunts were nurses: one attended training at White Memorial in the 1920s. Her other aunt had a starched-white image that didn't suit Beck's creative mind; she said she'd never be a nurse. At age sixteen Beck spent three weeks at Childrens Hospital with a ruptured appendix. She experienced a nurse style she could emulate.

She received an ADN in San Diego in 1976 and worked in critical care. She enjoyed the mountains and nature hikes and practiced holistic nursing wherever she worked; she taught her techniques to nurses. In 1991 she experienced an epiphany, a life-changing idea: she would become a global activist. She would improve world health.

Beck had no experience in world health, no savings, and had only traveled a few times. How would she do it? Questioning did not stop her. She first moved to Washington, D.C., and then to Ottawa, Canada, where she met networks of global activists. She traveled to China, Istanbul, Brazil, and other countries—always learning. [7]

In 1992 she discovered Florence Nightingale's focus on health-nursing, communication, and education. Nightingale had the model Beck needed. She obtained a PhD; in 2005 she co-authored *Florence Nightingale Today*, using her thesis. Beck and co-author, Barbara Dossey, started the Nightingale Initiative for Global Health to increase global public awareness of health.

When they realized 2010 would be the centennial year of Nightingale's death, they organized with Sigma Theta Tau International and the Nightingale Museum to celebrate 2010 as the first International Year of the Nurse. [8]

Chapter Twelve

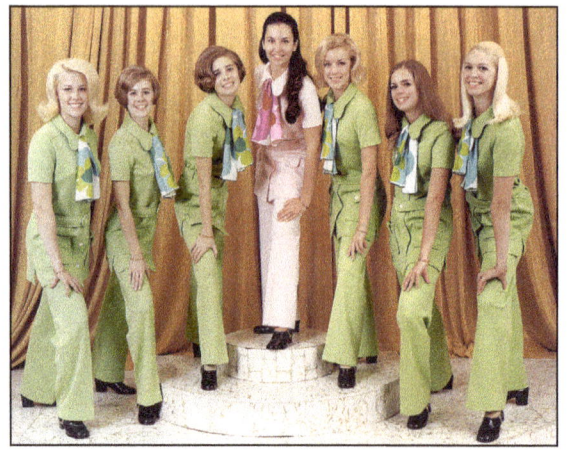

Figure 12.05. Cindy Coleman Jones (second from left) posing with the Queen and the Royal Court, 1970. (Courtesy of the Tournament of Roses Archives)

During her first year of nursing school, in 1970, Cindy Coleman Jones received the letter she'd waited months for—she had secured a place on the Royal Court. The judges had chosen her as a princess for the Pasadena Tournament of Roses.

Pasadena City College allowed her time off, but not much. She traveled to the scheduled public functions of a princess, and then the Rose Parade limo dropped her off at the hospital. She would race inside, nursing uniform in hand, to arrive just in time for her hospital clinicals. Sally, Judy, Marna, and Monica (fellow nursing students) helped by sharing the lecture notes they had taken with carbon paper. After graduation, Jones worked in labor and delivery, as a health assistant (school nurse) for fifteen years, and then in a post-anesthesia care unit.[9]

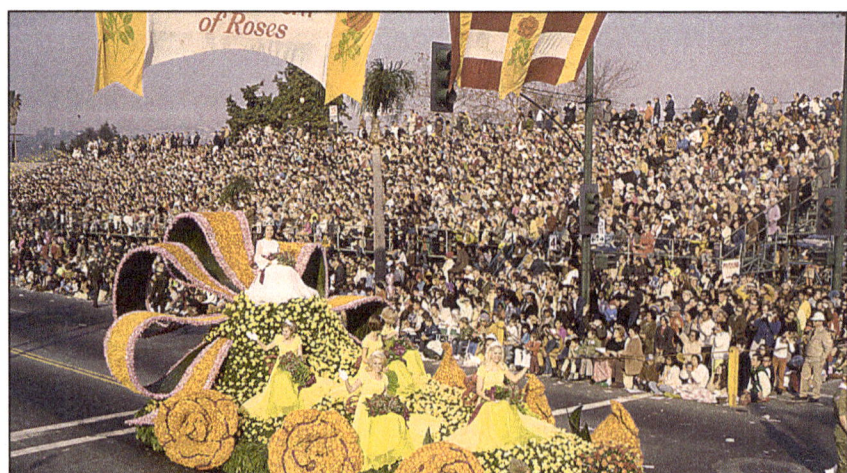

Figure 12.06. The Court Float, January 1, 1971. (Courtesy of the Tournament of Roses Archives)

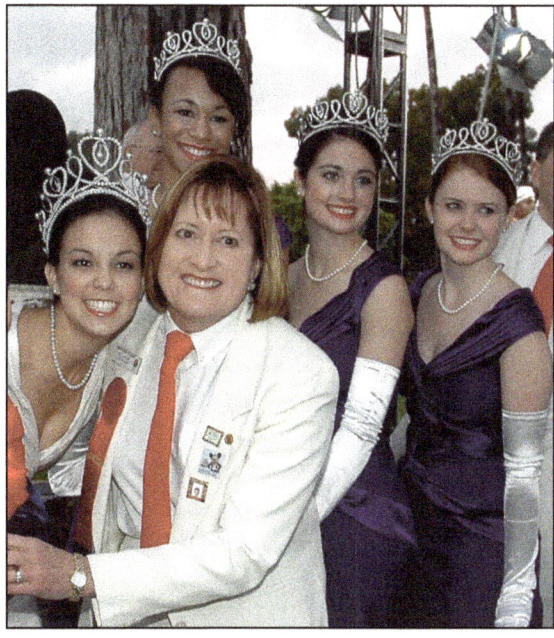

Figure 12.07. Sally M. Bixby, in white, with the Royal Court, as Chair of the Queen and Court committee, January 1, 2005. (Tournament of Roses Archives)

Sally M. Bixby grew up in California, a second-generation native, living in a home at the end of the route for the Rose Parade. On New Year's Day her family set up two ladders, stretched a plank of wood between them, and watched the parade from their perch above the spectators who had camped out all night for the perfect spot.

Bixby received an ADN from Pasadena City College in 1972. She decided almost immediately to become an operating room nurse. She first worked as a circulating nurse and a scrub nurse. Eventually, they promoted her to director of surgical services; later she became a consultant. She obtained a Bachelor of Health and Safety and a Master of Health Care Management.

She remained active in the Association of Operating Room Nurses (AORN), and she was equally active as a volunteer for the Pasadena Tournament of Roses organization. While at Pasadena City College in the seventies, Bixby's fellow nursing student, Cindy Coleman Jones, was nominated as a Rose Court princess. This presented an opportunity that led Bixby to her lifelong commitment with the Tournament of Roses organization.

When Bixby's AORN colleagues heard she would be the president of the Tournament of Roses in 2013, they told her, "Nurses should have a float."

In 2007 those five nurses, Monica Weisbrich, Judy Dahle, Paul Wafer, Pat Spongberg, and Suzanne War, began two endeavors: the Bare Root Inc. organization to raise money to fund the float and a website to organize nurses to decorate it. [10] Los Angeles nurses heard the call—they arrived every day to decorate the float that would honor their profession. [11]

Chapter Twelve

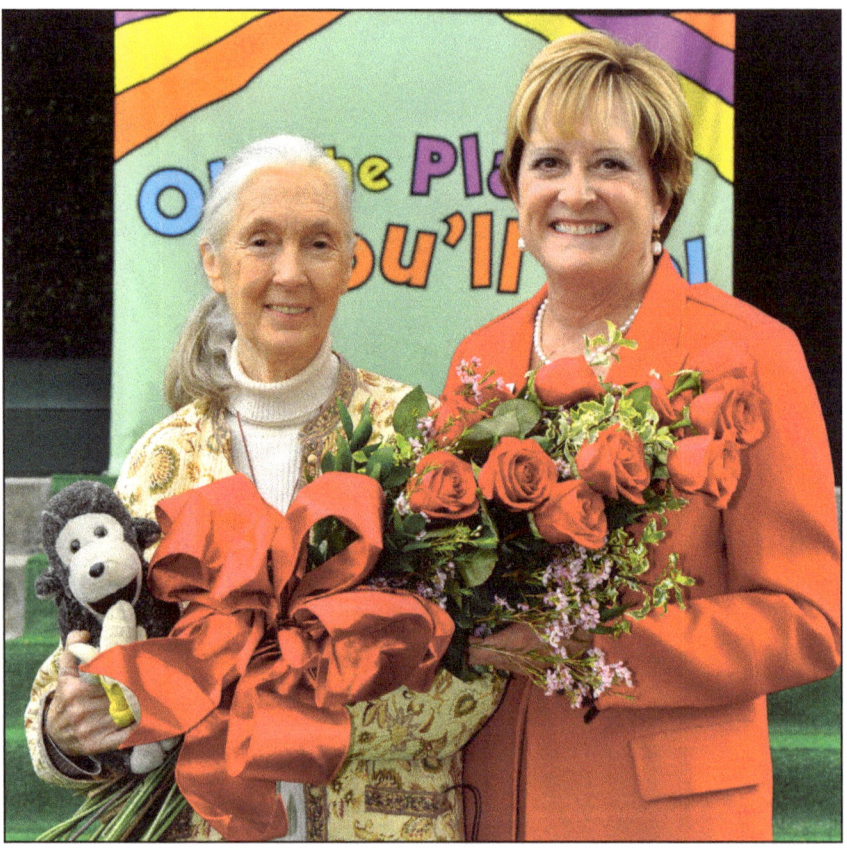

Figure 12.08. Grand Marshall Jane Goodall with President Sally Bixby—the first nurse chosen as president for the Pasadena Tournament of Roses, January 1, 2013. (Courtesy of the Tournament of Roses Archives)

On 25 April 2012, the Pasadena Tournament of Roses announced Dr. Jane Goodall, DBE, would serve as Grand Marshall of the 2013 Tournament of Roses parade. They chose the theme, "Oh, the Places You'll Go!" [12]

In 1960, at the age of twenty-six, Goodall moved from England to Tanzania, Africa, to research the life of chimpanzees. The world knew very little about chimpanzees when Goodall entered the forest of Gombe with barely more than a notebook, binoculars, and her endless fascination.

She observed their society, long-term bonds, and emotions. She learned they constructed and used tools—one of her greatest discoveries and scholarly documentations. [13] Goodall established the Jane Goodall Institute in 1977 to support continued research and demonstrate the urgent need to protect chimpanzees from extinction. [14]

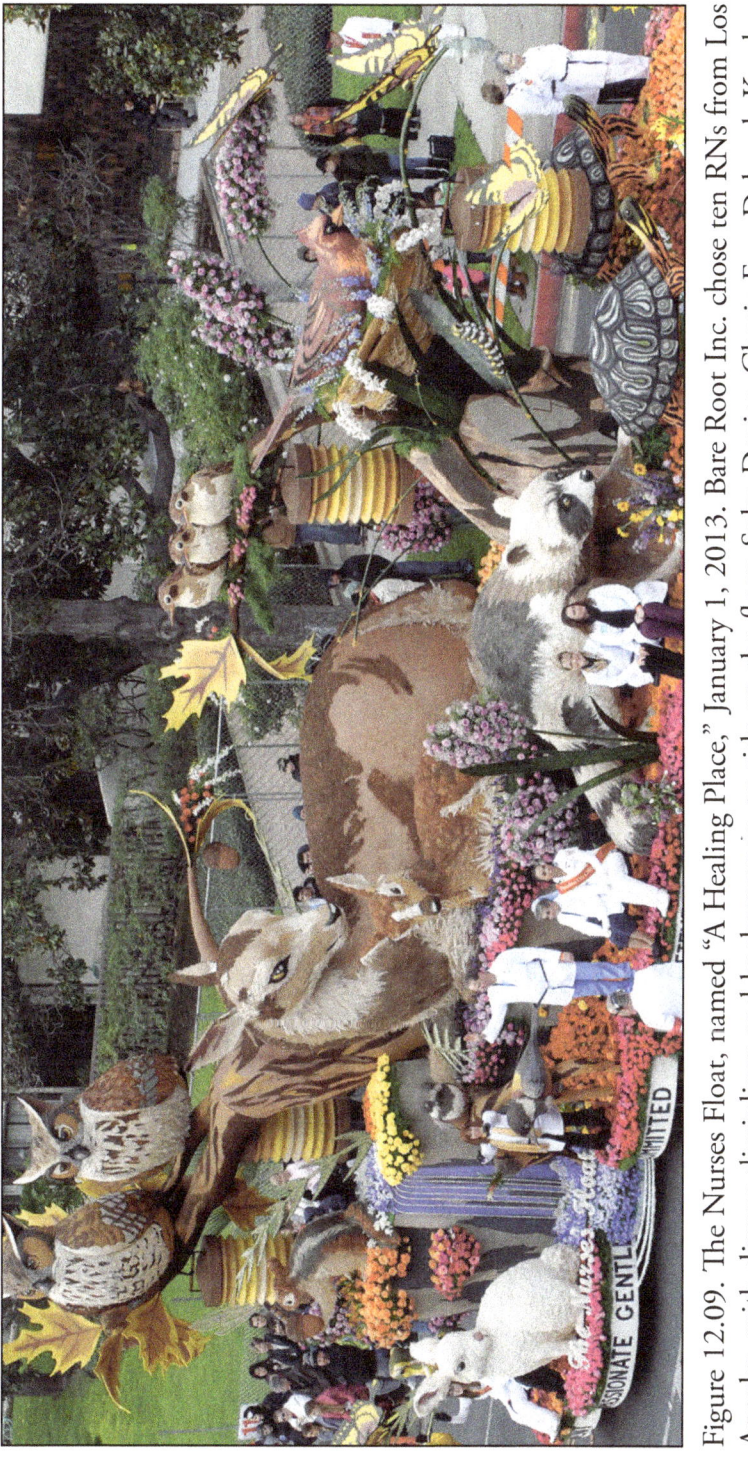

Figure 12.09. The Nurses Float, named "A Healing Place," January 1, 2013. Bare Root Inc. chose ten RNs from Los Angeles, with diverse disciplines and backgrounds, to ride on the float: Suko Davies, Cherie Fox, Deborah Keasler, Sister Terrence Landini, Maureen Latham, Bob Patterson, Priscilla Taylor, Cathy Rodgers Ward; two nursing students from Pasadena City College, Ariel Eby and Nicole Brown, also rode.[15] (Courtesy of Phoenix Decorating Company)

Los Angeles Schools of Nursing and Graduate Pins: 1897-2024

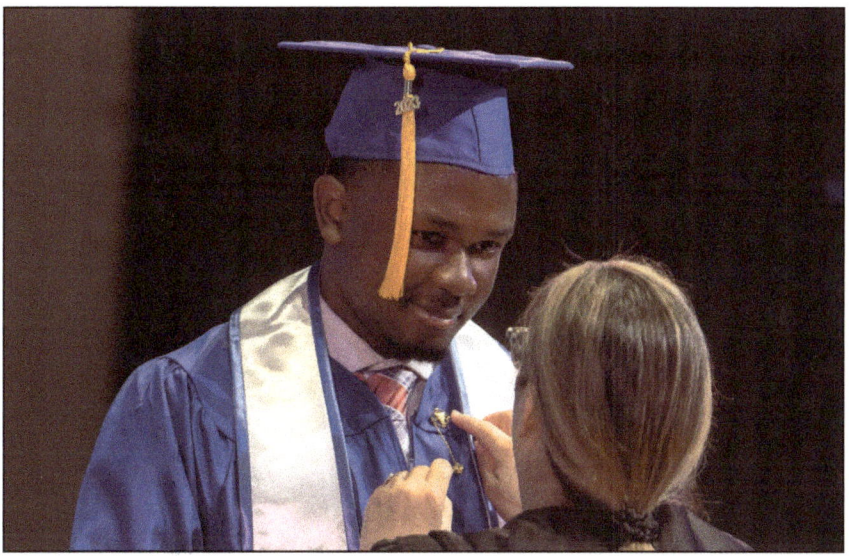

Figure 13.01. An El Camino College instructor pins a nursing graduate at their graduation ceremony, June 5, 2023. (Courtesy of El Camino College)

Uniforms changed, and nursing caps were abandoned since the first schools of nursing began. However, graduate pins and pinning ceremonies remained.

Sources point to the 1860s as the origin of the pinning ceremony—Queen Victoria pinned the Royal Red Cross on Florence Nightingale in recognition of her Crimean War service. Nightingale awarded badges to the best students in her school. However, there was no documentation of a first ceremony. In the U.S., the first pinning occurred at Bellevue Hospital in 1880.[1]

Most nursing schools organized and graduates attended pinning events. Some schools eliminated it, calling the custom outdated; others allowed it but required students to raise the money and plan the ceremony themselves.[2]

Schools are listed here **chronologically by the first year of their first degree conferred** (most schools now confer multiple degrees) and grouped: diploma, baccalaureate, MEPN, RN to BSN, and ADN. An inaugural-year pin was used when available. If a pin photo could not be obtained, a recreated pin from an image, a school's patch-as-a-pin, or a generic pin was substituted.

Read Chapter Three for historical origins of graduate pins and their shapes.

Chapter Thirteen

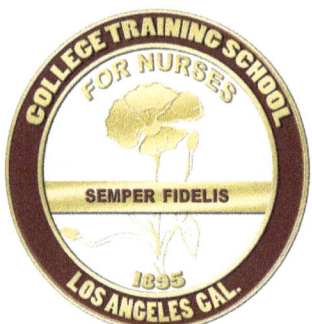

Figure 13.02. **1897 Graduation**, College Training School for Nurses at the Medical College, Buena Vista Street, L.A. Diploma.[3]

A gold and white pin with red enamel and the Latin phrase *Semper Fidelis* (always faithful), a frequently used motto in the early days. This is an artist's recreated pin, drawn from the school's seal and a written description.[4]

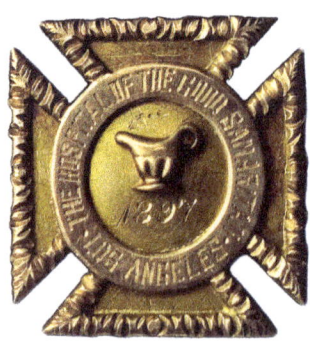

Figure 13.03. **1898 Graduation,** Training School for Nurses at the Good Samaritan Hospital, Los Angeles. Diploma.[5]

A Formée Pattée cross with a lamp of learning in the center. Hospital records state nurses began training in 1896 and graduated in 1898, but this first-year pin is engraved in the center with 1897. In 1929, they renamed the school Bishop Johnson School of Nursing.

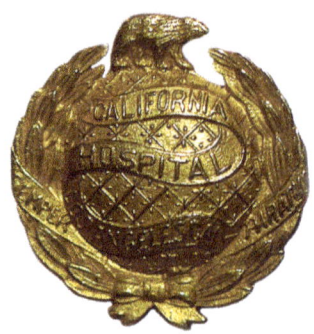

Figure 13.04 **1899 Graduation**, California Hospital Training School for Nurses, Los Angeles. Diploma.[6]

A bear on top, laurel wreaths circling a bulbous coin shape. *Semper Paratus* (always ready) is inscribed on the wreath, and the band says California Hospital Los Angeles. Before 1898, California Hospital student nurses attended the College Training School for Nurses.

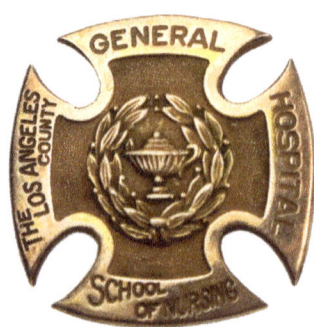

Figure 13.05. **1899 Graduation,** Los Angeles County Hospital, Training School for Nurses, at County Hospital, L.A. Diploma.[7]

An Alisee Patée cross with laurel leaves encircling a lamp of knowledge. This pin is from 1936; the style remained similar throughout the school's early years. Before 1898, County Hospital students attended the College Training School for Nurses.

Los Angeles Schools Nursing and Graduate Pins

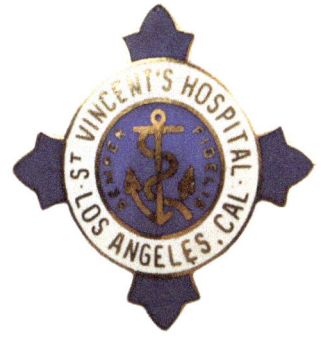

Figure 13.06. **1901 Graduation**, the Los Angeles Infirmary Training School for Nurses, Los Angeles. Diploma. [8]

A Vatican Cross shape with an anchor (an ancient Christian symbol) in the center and the phrase *Semper Fidelis*. The school began in 1899. Later, they called the school St. Vincent's Hospital School of Nursing.

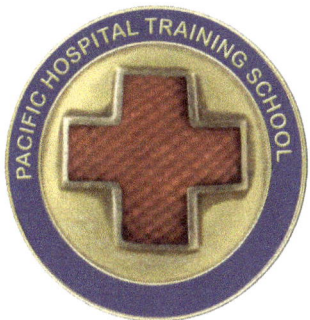

Figure 13.07. **1901 Graduation**, Pacific Hospital Training School for Nurses, Los Angeles. Diploma. [9]

A coin shape with a red Greek Cross at the center. The class included the first male student nurse to graduate from a training school in Los Angeles. Recreated pin.

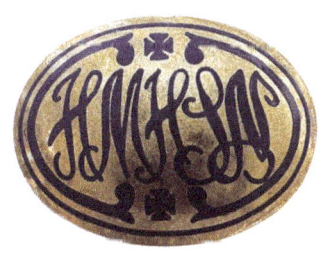

Figure 13.08. **1904 Graduation,** Pasadena Hospital School of Nursing. Diploma. [10]

In 1932, students began to earn a college certificate, simultaneously, from Pasadena City College. [11] The name changed to Huntington Memorial Hospital School of Nursing in 1935 (HMHSN is scrolled on this 1953 pin). In 1958, they opened one of the first intensive care units in the U.S.

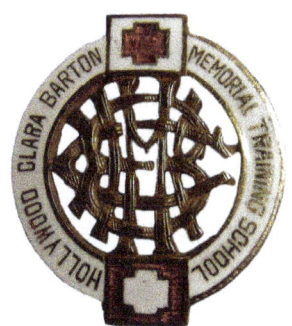

Figure 13.09. **1905 Graduation**, the first Clara Barton Training School for Nurses, Hollywood. Diploma. [12]

Filigree initials with red and white Greek crosses for Barton's creation of the Red Cross organization. In 1926, the Clara Barton Hospital moved and merged with Hollywood Hospital and became the Hollywood Clara Barton Memorial Training School. [13]

Chapter Thirteen

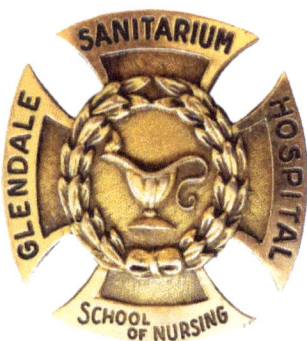

Figure 13.10. **1906 Graduation,** Glendale Sanitarium Training School for Missionary Nurses, Glendale. Diploma. [14]

An Alisee Patée cross with laurel leaves circling a lamp of learning. The *bacca laureate* (Latin for laurel berries) marked the first graduation ceremonies when Greeks and Romans awarded laurels to scholars. Eventually, "baccalaureate" signified a degree.

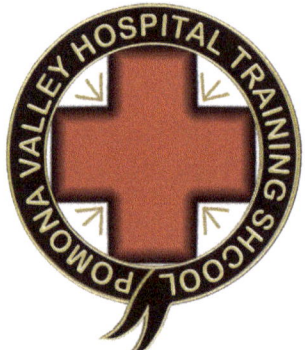

Figure 13.11. **1907 Graduation**, Pomona Valley Hospital Training School. Diploma. [15]

Pomona Valley Hospital, Pomona's first hospital, opened in 1903 with 12 patients after a 1899 train crash demonstrated the need for a community facility. [16] The school of nursing began in 1905 with three students. [17] Recreated pin.

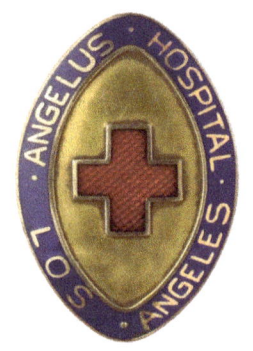

Figure 13.12. **1908 Graduation**, the Angelus Hospital, School of Nursing, in the city of Los Angeles. Diploma. [18] †

A shield with a red Greek cross in the center. The colors for the ceremony of the first five graduates were blue and gold, mirroring the pin colors. Although not written on the pin, the class motto was *Semper Paratus*.

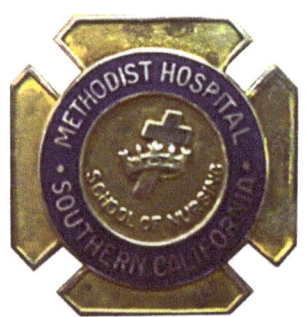

Figure 13.13. **1915 Graduation**, Methodist Hospital of Southern California, School of Nursing, started in Los Angeles, and then the school moved to Arcadia. Diploma. [19]

Formee Patée Cross variant. Methodist Hospital lauded the first air-conditioned operating rooms and featured the first postoperative recovery room in 1953. The final class graduated in 1958. [20]

Los Angeles Schools Nursing and Graduate Pins

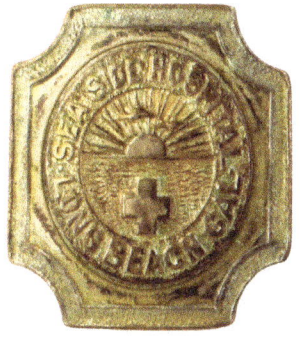

Figure 13.14. **1920 Graduation,** Seaside Hospital, Long Beach. Diploma. [21] †

Dr. Harriman Jones opened the Seaside Hospital in 1913, in West Long Beach, after the closure of Long Beach Hospital. The School of Nursing opened in 1918—the same year the Spanish Flu began. When Seaside opened, it was one of the first nursing schools in the Long Beach area.

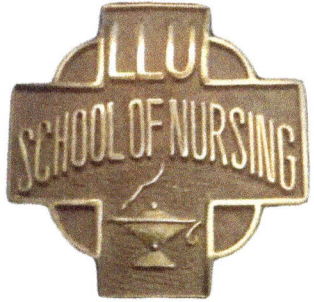

Figure 13.15. **1926 Graduation**, White Memorial, School of Nursing, first in Los Angeles then in Loma Linda. Diploma. [22]

A Greek cross with a lamp of learning. The White Memorial School of Nursing began in Los Angeles but moved to the city of Loma Linda in 1948. In 1961, the name became Loma Linda University School of Nursing. [23]

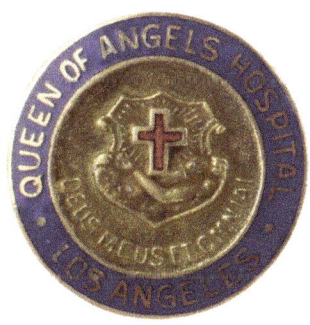

Figure 13.16. **1928 Graduation,** Queen of Angels, School of Nursing, in the city of Los Angeles. Diploma. [24] †

In the center is the Franciscan Order coat of arms and *Dues Meus et Omnia* (My God and My All). In 1989 Queen of Angels Hospital closed, merged with, and moved to Hollywood Presbyterian Medical Center to become Queen of Angels-Hollywood Presbyterian Medical Center. [25]

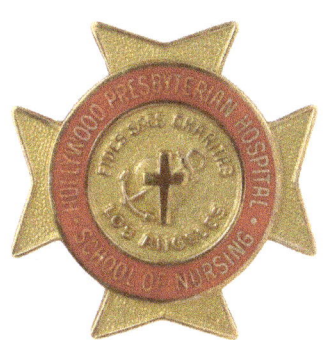

Figure 13.17. **1947 Graduation,** the Hollywood Presbyterian School of Nursing, Hollywood. Diploma. [26] †

Double-Fitched shape. *Fides Spes Cahritas* (Faith, Hope, and Charity) was written in the center above a Latin Cross (symbol for faith), an anchor (symbol for hope), and a heart (symbol for charity). [27-28] The school of nursing closed in 1975. [29]

Chapter Thirteen

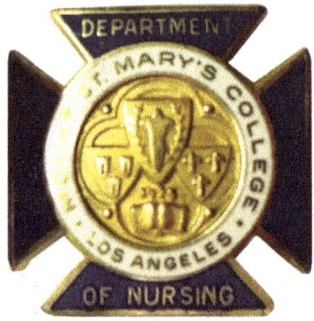

Figure 13.18. **1952 Graduation**, Mount St. Mary's College, School of Nursing, Brentwood. Baccalaureate Degree. [30]

A Cross Patée shape. The private Catholic nonprofit university graduated the first five women to earn a BSN in Los Angeles. Among them were a Japanese American, an African American, an Irish American, and a French American graduate nurse. [31]

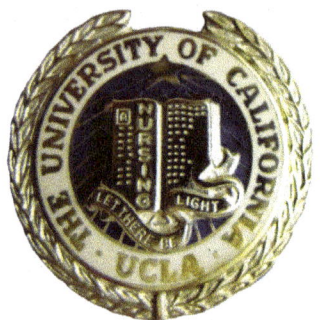

Figure 13.19. **1954 Graduation**, UCLA, SON, Westwood. Baccalaureate Degree. [32]

A laurel wreath, an open book with the word Nursing, and the phrase Let There Be Light on a banner. Classes began in 1949. Due to a delay, the first group did not graduate until 1954. The program closed to undergraduate nurses in 1995 because of state budget cuts; it reopened in 2006. [33-34]

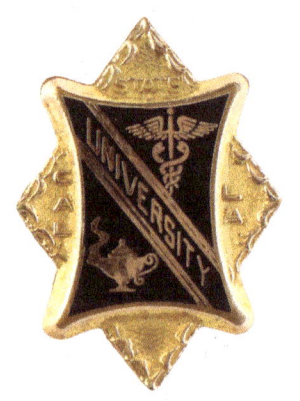

Figure 13.20. **1960 Graduation,** Patricia A. Chin, SON, California State University, Los Angeles. Baccalaureate Degree. [35]

A lamp of learning and a caduceus. The school began as California State College, Los Angeles. After obtaining university status in 1972, the school became California State University, Los Angeles. When former faculty member Patricia Chin, donated 7 million dollars to the School of Nursing in 2018, they renamed it in her honor.

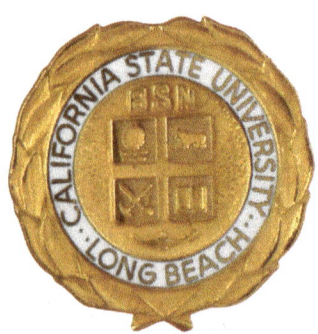

Figure 13.21. **1965 Graduation,** California State University, Long Beach, in Long Beach. Baccalaureate Degree [36] †

A laurel wreath encircling a coin shape and BSN above the seal. The university's seal in the center included a sun and sea symbol, the California bear, a pick and shovel, and a book denoting scholarship. A lamp of learning below it. The seal originated in 1964. [37]

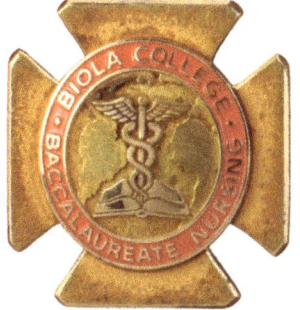

Figure 13.22. **1971 Graduation**, Biola College, in the city of La Mirada. Baccalaureate Degree. [38] †

A caduceus, a Bible, and a world continent to reflect their missionary work. A private, nonprofit Christian college. From 1969 to 1970, graduate nursing students qualified for the NCLEX and received a Bachelor of Science in Biology from Biola College. [39] †

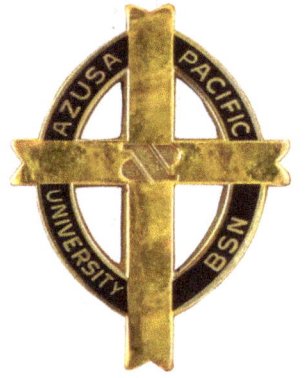

Figure 13.23. **1977 Graduation,** Azusa Pacific University. Baccalaureate Degree. [40] †

A private, nonprofit Christian college. At a conference in 1993, in Russia, eight Azusa Pacific faculty nurses presented their nursing curriculum to Russian nurse educators: "New Nurses for a New Russia." After that, the nurses wrote Russia's first pediatric/maternal child and medical/surgical textbooks. [41]

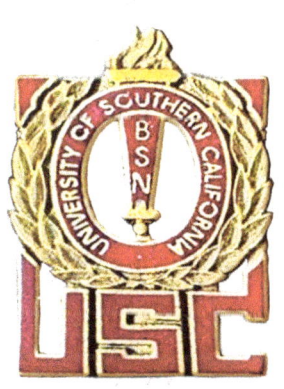

Figure 13.24. **1984 Graduation,** the University of Southern California, in Los Angeles. Baccalaureate Degree. [42]

Despite the program's early successes, the nursing department closed in 2004 due to budget decisions: the Department of Nursing's concept differed from those involved in the financial administration of the University. In 2024 USC eliminated their unique MSN for nurses within the School of Social Work; Spring 2025 would be the final cohort. [43]

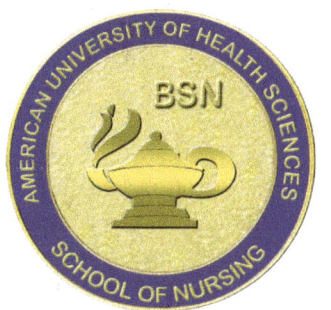

Figure 13.25. **2009 Graduation,** American University of Health Sciences, SON, Signal Hill. Baccalaureate Degree. [44]

BSN and a lamp of learning. A Christian-based, private for-profit, thirty-nine-month accelerated program with a traditional on-campus classroom style of instruction. The university opened in 1994; the School of Nursing began in 2003. Recreated pin.

Chapter Thirteen

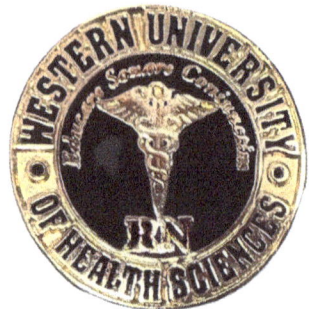

Figure 13.26. **2004 Graduation**, Western Univ. of Health Sciences, College of Graduate Nursing, Pomona. MSNE, Masters Degree. [45]

Private, nonprofit, graduate-level school. Established California's first Masters School of Nursing Entry (MSNE) in 2004 [46] and the first online FNP in 1997. The MSNE/RN pin included the Latin phrase *Educare Sanare, Coniunctim* (To Teach, To Heal, Together).

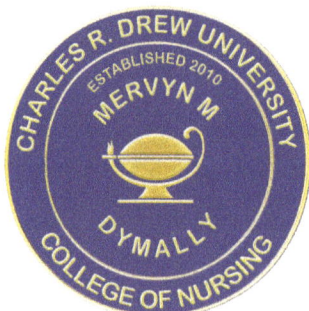

Figure 13.27. **2012 Graduation**, Mervyn M. Dymally College of Nursing, Charles R. Drew University of Medicine and Science, Los Angeles. ELM, Masters Degree. [47]

Private, nonprofit, academic nursing school named in honor of the politician, Mervyn M. Dymally, who advocated for CDU to open a nursing school. [48] The first RN class was an entry-level master's (ELM). The pin is of the school's patch; the school had no pin.

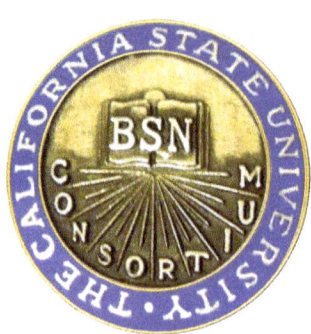

Figure 13.28. **1983 Graduation**, California State Univ. Consortium, Statewide Nursing Program. RN to Baccalaureate Degree. [49]

The unique Statewide Nursing Program began in 1981 as a student-fee-supported system, administered by the CSU Chancellor in Long Beach. The State did not fund the program, but in 1987 CSU, Dominquez Hills, began administering the program, and then the State contributed funds. [50]

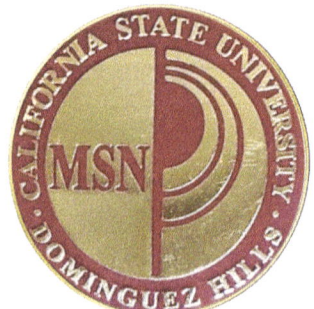

Figure 13.29. **1987 Graduation,** California State University, Dominguez Hills, Carson. RN to Baccalaureate Degree and MSN. [51]

CSUDH assumed the Statewide Nursing Programs in 1987. They added more degrees. By 2000, all programs were internet-based, except for a short-lived masters entry program. In 1980 55% of RNs held a diploma, 22% a BSN, and 18% an ADN. [52]

Los Angeles Schools Nursing and Graduate Pins

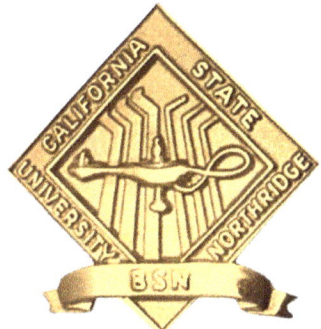

Figure 13.30. **1996 Graduation,** California State University, Northridge, in Northridge. RN to Baccalaureate Degree. [53]

In 1965 the ANA published the controversial "position paper:" a BSN should be the entry into nursing. [54] By 1996, 24% of nurses held a diploma, 31% a BSN, and 34% an ADN. [55] By 2022, 70% held a BSN. [56] In 2024, many hospitals required a BSN for new hires.

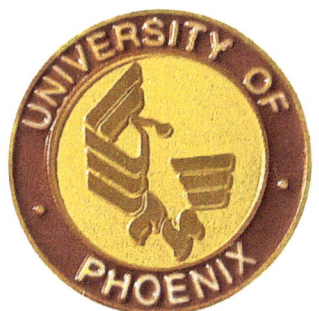

Figure 13.31. **1997 Graduation,** the University of Phoenix/Aspen University, Pasadena. An RN to Baccalaureate Degree. [57]

In the 1990s, UOPX offered an RN to BSN evening/weekend in-classroom program; in the 2000s it switched to online. [58] Various issues caused their Los Angeles schools to close in 2021. UOPX said most U.S. schools would close by 2025. [59]

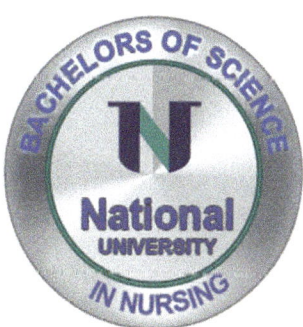

Figure 13.32. **2009 Graduation**, National University, in the city of Los Angeles. RN to Baccalaureate Degree. [60]

Private for-profit school. Included a hybrid of online and classroom study. Like many private for-profit schools, they eventually added a pre-licensure BSN to their program. Recreated pin.

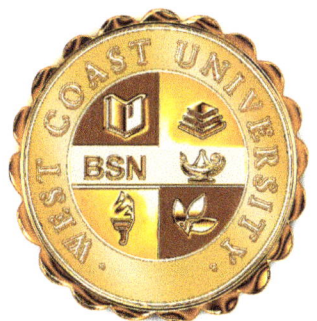

Figure 13.33. **2011 Graduation,** West Coast University, in North Hollywood. RN to Baccalaureate Degree. [61]

The West Coast University nursing program began the first private for-profit nursing school to achieve CCNE accreditation and a pre-licensure BSN program at its opening in 2009. [62] They have grown considerably. Recreated pin.

Chapter Thirteen

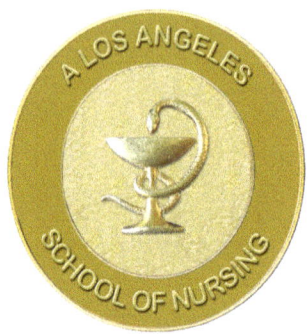

Figure 13.34. **2016 Graduation**, Homestead Schools Inc., in Torrance. An RN to Baccalaureate Degree. [63]

Homestead Schools, a private-for-profit school with online, campus, and hybrid options. The MSN program included a classroom option. Their banner motto: "Committed to Livelong Learning." The school had no pin. Generic pin referencing Hygieia & PBBSON.

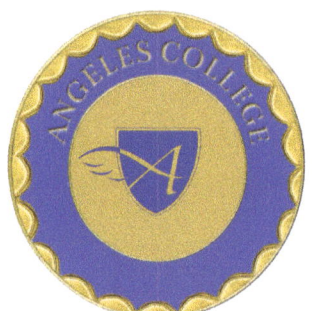

Figure 13.35. **2017 Graduation,** the Angeles College, in the city of Los Angeles, RN to Baccalaureate Degree. [64]

An RN to BSN program completed online. Their Los Angeles campus added a three-year accelerated pre-licensure BSN program, classroom required. Recreated pin.

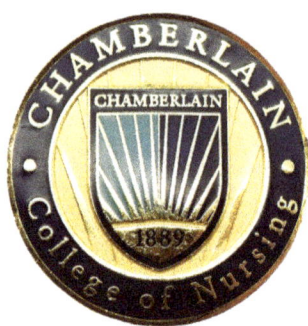

Figure 13.36. **2024 Graduation**, the Chamberlain University College of Nursing, Irwindale. RN to Baccalaureate Degree. [65]

Chamberlain, a private-for-profit college, said it's "the largest nursing school in the US." [66] They also developed a pre-licensure, classroom-based, year-round, accelerated BSN program.

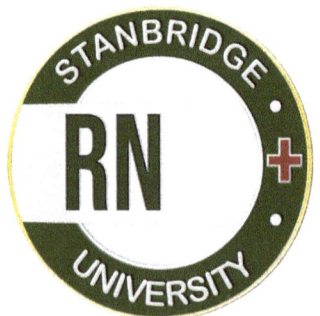

Figure 13.37. **2024 Graduation**, Stanbridge University, City of Alhambra. An RN to Baccalaureate Degree. [67]

Stanbridge University started one of the newest private for-profit RN to BSN programs. The school utilized a hybrid system: some lectures are online and some in the classroom. The clinical training used both their lab and community settings. Recreated pin.

Los Angeles Schools Nursing and Graduate Pins

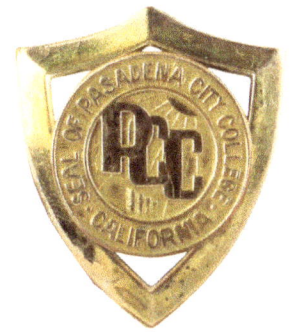

Figure 13.38. **1956 Graduation,** Pasadena City College. Associate Degree. [68] †

In 1953 Columbia University chose PCC as one of six community colleges in the U.S. to pilot a new college degree for RNs—the Associate Degree in Nursing. [69] The ADN program continued after the pilot ended, making it the first and the oldest ADN program in Los Angeles.

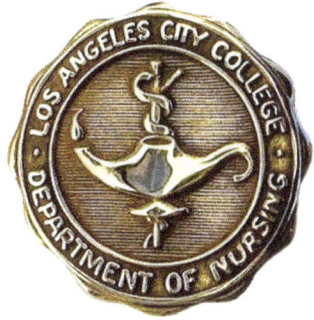

Figure 13.39. **1960 Graduation**, Los Angeles City College. Associate Degree. [70]

Despite the urgent need for nurses, the LACC Nursing Department closed in 1986 due to budget cuts. [71] The department opened again in 2004, with 20-40 nursing students accepted into the fall and spring semesters. [72]

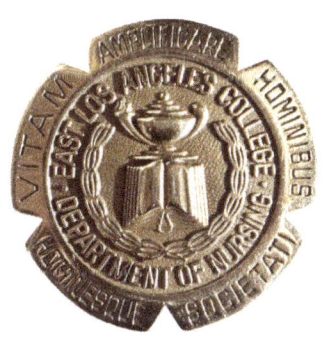

Figure 13.40. **1960 Graduation**, East Los Angeles College, City of Monterey Park. An Associate Degree. [73]

In 1950, nurses from County Hospital studied at ELAC and received both a diploma from County Hospital and an Associate of Arts from ELAC. When ELAC began an ADN program in 1958, the ELAC nursing students used County Hospital for their clinical site. [74]

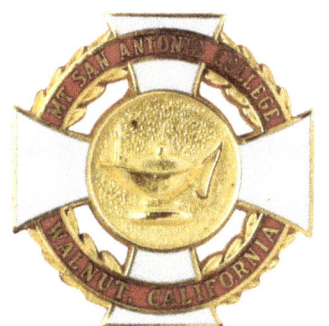

Figure 13.41. **1960 Graduation**, Mount San Antonio College, in the city of Walnut. Associate Degree. [75] †

Located in the eastern part of Los Angeles County. The city and college were small in 1958, yet they started one of the first ADN programs—at the same time as the larger and better-known areas of L.A. County. [76] The college has supplied many nurses for the area.

Chapter Thirteen

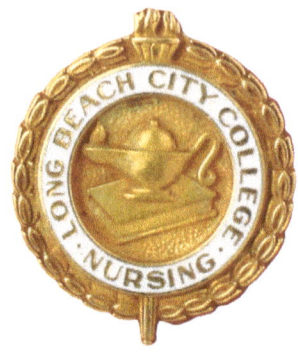

Figure 13.42. **1961 Graduation**, Long Beach City College. Associate Degree. [77] †

A lamp of learning and a book. The first graduates designed the pin to symbolize the achievement of becoming a nurse. The LBCC nursing department is a member of the School of Health, Science, and Mathematics. The school has served San Pedro, Catalina Island, Long Beach, Lakewood, and Signal Hill. [78]

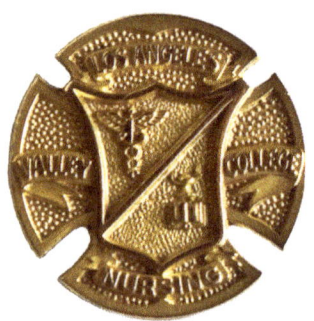

Figure 13.43. **1962 Graduation,** Los Angeles Valley College, Valley Glen. Assoc. Degree. [79]

The program began as a project of the UCLA School of Nursing on 1 July 1959. They admitted the first class of thirty students in September of 1960, and all the students graduated in June of 1962. [80]

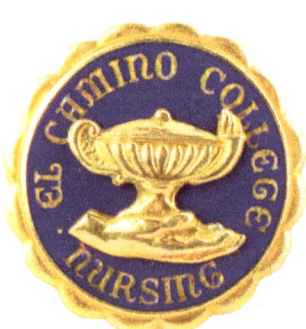

Figure 13.44. **1964 Graduation**, El Camino College, Alondra Park. Associate Degree. [81] †

In 2006, El Camino partnered with Compton College to provide a unique El Camillo College Associate Degree Nursing program at both El Camino and Compton College campuses. [82] The dual campus concluded in 2019 when Compton College received its independent accreditation. [83]

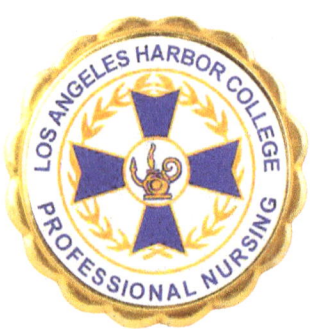

Figure 13.45. **1965 Graduation**, Los Angeles Harbor College, City of Wilmington. An Associate Degree. [84]

California ADN schools required students to complete various science, English, psychology, and math prerequisites, plus electives and co-requisites. They also needed to pass a national nursing exam: Test of Essential Academic Skills (TEAS test). [85] Pin of school patch.

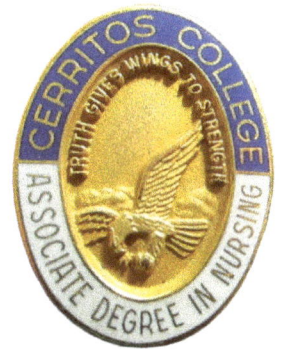

Figure 13.46. **1966 Graduation**, Cerritos College, Norwalk. Associate Degree. [86]

An eagle flies in the center of the pin with the Roman philosopher's saying: *Candor Dat Viribus Alas,* or "Sincerity Gives Wings to Strength." The program began with seventeen students. A traditional single campus with no satellite locations, no weekend options, and no online instruction as of 2024. [87-88]

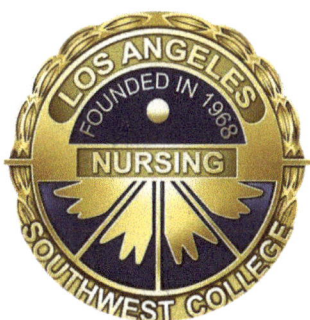

Figure 13.47. **1970 Graduation**, the Los Angeles Southwest College, West Athens. Associate Degree. [89-90]

In 1973, SWC began the first Twilight Program; they held lectures and clinicals in the evening. In 1997, the lectures moved to daytime because of budget constraints. [91]

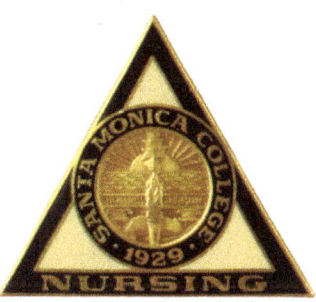

Figure 13.48. **1970 Graduation**. Santa Monica College, City of Santa Monica. Associate Degree. [92] †

SMC's nursing program began training LVNs in 1966, using funds from the 1963 Manpower Development and Training Act and the Federal Vocational Education Act. [93-94] In 1967 the program expanded to include the ADN program. [95]

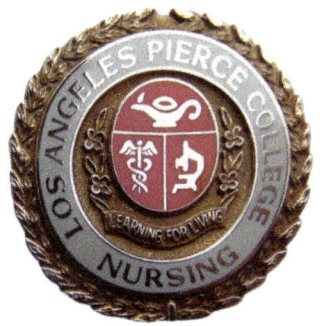

Figure 13.49. **1971 Graduation**, Pierce College, City of Woodland Hills. An Associate Degree. [96]

A lamp of learning, a Caduceus, a microscope, and a floral-held banner with the phrase "Learning for Living," a phrase previously used in adult education settings. The original college began in 1947 through the efforts of Clarence Pierce, MD.

Chapter Thirteen

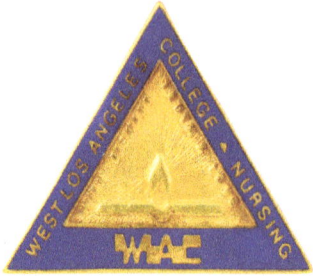

Figure 13.51. **1972 Graduation,** West Los Angeles College, Culver City. Associate Degree. [97] †

An open book, a flame, and the words Dignity, Truth, and Love in the center. WLAC opened in 1969. [98] In 1986 the county closed the nursing program because of budget issues. [99] It never restarted.

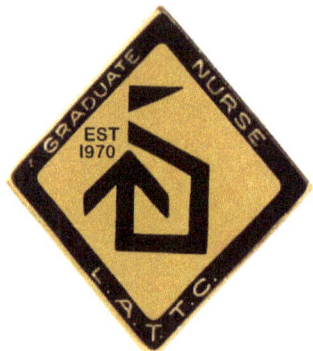

Figure 13.50. **1972 Graduation,** Los Angeles Trade Technical College, Los Angeles. Associate Degree. [100] †

Los Angeles Trade Tech established an ADN program in 1970, just one year after the college joined the Los Angeles Community College District as one of nine colleges. A few years before, in 1966, LATTC had merged with Metropolitan College. [101]

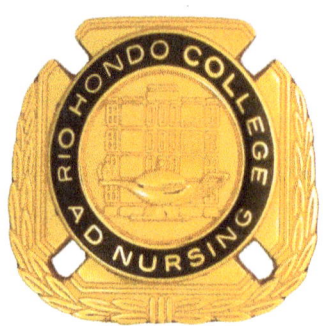

Figure 13.52. **1972 Graduation**, Rio Hondo College, Whittier. Associate Degree. [102]

A building and a lamp of learning encircled with laurel leaves. The college has supported the large geographic, open-access community in Los Angeles County, containing nine cities and four unincorporated communities. [103]

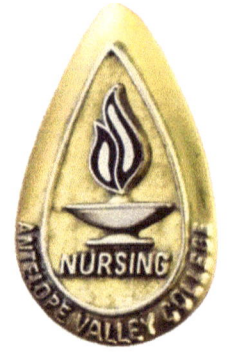

Figure 13.53. **1975 Graduation,** Antelope Valley College, Lancaster. Associate Degree. [104]

After Rae Yoshida left internment in Poston (a Japanese WWII camp), she studied nursing at Columbia University. Then she moved to Antelope Valley. In 1974 the college recruited her as the first director of their new ADN program. She became dean in 1975 and VP of Academic Affairs in 1981. The Applied Arts building is named in her honor. [105]

Los Angeles Schools Nursing and Graduate Pins

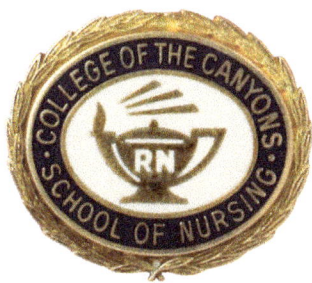

Figure 13.54. **1980 Graduation**, College of the Canyons, Santa Clarita and Valencia Campuses. Associate Degree. [106] †

COC was the first ADN program in California to gain charter membership in the Associate Degree Nurse Honor Society, Alpha Delta Nu. They named it the Gamma Eta Chapter. [107]

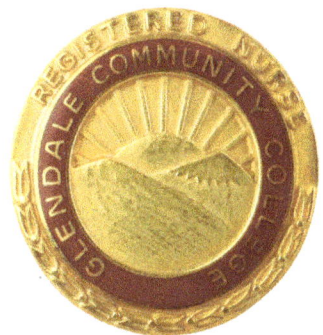

Figure 13.55. **1985 Graduation**, Glendale Community College, City of Glendale. Associate Degree. [108] †

GCC began as an LVN program in the 1950s, changed to an LVN to RN ladder program in the 1980s, and soon switched to an ADN program. [109] They also provided advanced placement services for transfer and foreign nurse graduates. [110]

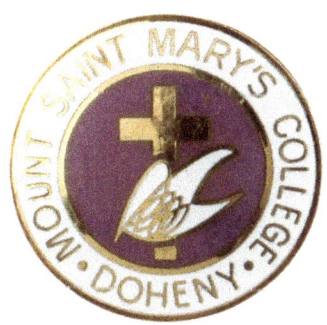

Figure 13.56. **1994 Graduation**, Mount Saint Mary's College, Doheny Campus in Los Angeles. Associate Degree. [111] †

The Dohney Campus ADN program opened in 1992 for working adults—one of three programs in Southern California that offered evening classes and weekend clinicals. [112] The author taught weekend clinicals at the school from 1994 to 1995.

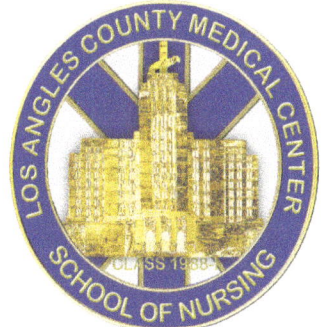

Figure 13.57. **1997 Graduation**, Los Angeles County College of Nursing & Allied Health, L.A. Associate Degree. [113]

The Los Angeles County Medical Center's diploma program existed from 1901 to 1995. In 1995, the County Dept. of Health began an ADN program as the College of Nursing & Allied Health. [114] They created many pins. This 1988 version, with the 1933 hospital building, was most unique. Recreated pin.

Chapter Thirteen

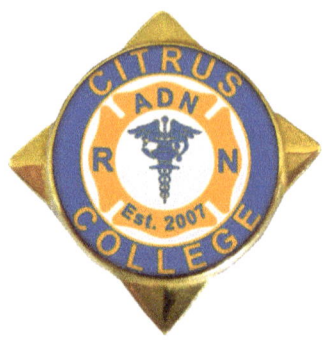

Figure 13.58. **2010 Graduation**, Citrus College, Glendora. Associate Degree. [115]

Citrus College, in the Citrus Community College District, has served the east side cities of Azusa, Claremont, Duarte, Glendora, and Monrovia. The program has had an advanced placement California-licensed LVN to ADN program and a generic ADN. Pin created with the school patch.

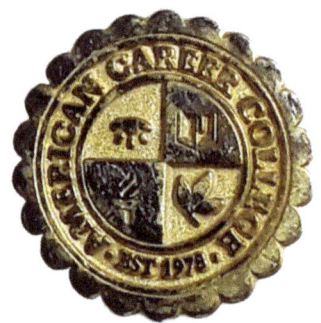

Figure 13.59. **2017 Graduation**, American Career College, at the Los Angeles Campus. Associate Degree. [116]

The private for-profit college began in 1978 as the American College of Optics. While they still offered an optics course, the business refocused on diplomas in the allied medical field and associate nursing degrees. [117]

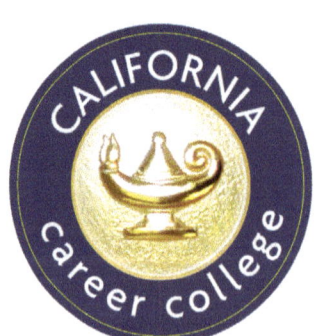

Figure 13.60. **2018 Graduation**, California Career College, Canoga Park Campus. Associate Degree. [118]

Private for-profit school. The HESI test (Health Education System Inc.) emphasized seven areas, including healthcare-specific topics; the TEAS examined science, math, reading, and English. Some nursing programs required both entrance exams. Recreated pin.

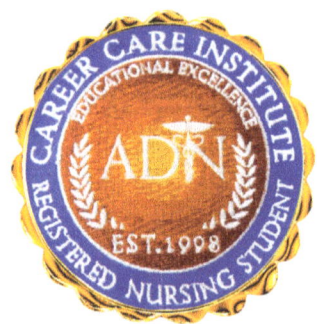

Figure. 13.61. **2019 Graduation**, Career Care Institute, in Lancaster. Associate Degree. [119]

Private, for-profit school educating nurses and other allied healthcare students using a traditional classroom and clinical educational model. Pin created with the school patch.

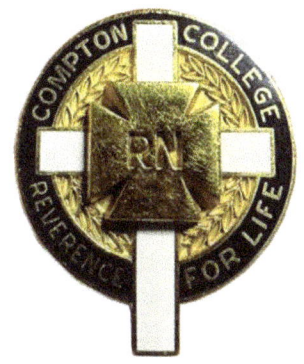

Figure 13.62. **2019 Graduation,** Compton College, in Compton. Associate Degree. [120]

From 2006-2019, Compton College operated under El Camino College's accreditation but attended classes on Compton's campus. In June 2019, Compton College and the nursing program received accreditation and graduated an independent, fully accredited, nursing class. [121]

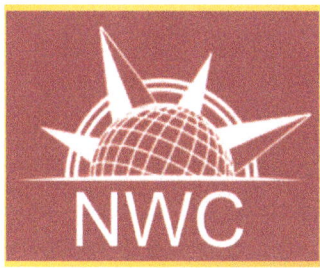

Figure 13.63. **2019 Graduation,** Marsha Fuerst SON, Glendale, & North-West College, West Covina. Associate Degree. [122]

In 1966 Marsha Fuerst opened private, for-profit allied health colleges named Success Education Colleges. In 2008 the company acquired Glendale Career College [123] and then North-West College. Pin of the school's patch.

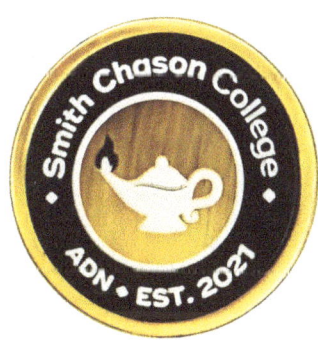

Figure 13.64. **2023 Graduation,** Smith Chason College, Los Angeles Campus. Associate Degree. [124]

Neville Smith, MD, and Myra Chason, RN, opened a small, private, for-profit ultrasound college in Beverly Hills in 1998. They expanded across the West to offer imaging and nursing degrees. [125] Students could complete an ADN in twenty-four months.

In Development, University of LaVerne, John A. Ware School of Nursing.

LaVerne alumna Frances Bever Ware and her late husband John donated 2.3 million dollars; the endowment funded a new college and its nursing program. The Wares dedicated their lives to education and healthcare. Frances said they "wanted to give back in a way that would leave a lasting impact with students." [126]

Many learning options were available for pre-licensure students to obtain an RN and for post-licensure RNs to advance to higher degrees. The term pre-licensure referred to students who were not yet RNs. In 2014 California Senate Bill 850 authorized community colleges to offer pilot baccalaureate degree programs; no pilot BSN programs existed as of 2024. [127] Educational opportunities included several choices in 2024:

- traditional classroom ADN/BSN/MSN/PhD/DNP
- online RN to BSN/MSN/PhD/DNP (APRNs required clinicals)
- hybrid classroom/online RN to BSN/MSN/PhD/DNP
- classroom and hybrid LVN 30 unit option and LVN to ADN/BSN
- Masters Entry Program in Nursing (classroom and clinicals required)

In 1969, California enacted Business and Profession Code #2736.3, requiring all BRN-approved programs to offer an educational track for LVNs to achieve eligibility for the NCLEX exam that did not require more than 30 semester or 45 quarter units of nursing courses (guidelines set by the BRN, Section 1429). They would not receive a college degree or wear the school pin. [128]

One of the newest pre-licensure programs created was the Masters Entry Program in Nursing for non-RNs who held a bachelor's degree in other disciplines. Students graduated with an MSN and qualified for the NCLEX exam. Many MEPN graduates pursued a nurse practitioner or other advanced practice registered nurse certifications after graduation.

The Department of Education has set standards to ensure higher education providers meet quality criteria but relied on private educational associations (regional and national) to act as the accrediting agencies (i.e., ACCJC, WSCUC, CHEA, USDE). Nursing programs also sought accreditation; however, they contracted with different accrediting agencies (ACEN, CCNE).

The BRN must approve all pre-licensure programs; however, accreditation was always voluntary. The Accreditation Commission for Education in Nursing (ACEN) and the Commission of the Collegiate Nursing Education (CCNE) accredited the programs. Both established academic and outcome-based standards for nursing schools. They conducted curriculum reviews to ensure accredited programs met or exceeded standards.

ACEN, the older accrediting body, has evaluated all nursing education levels. The CCNE accredited only bachelor's, master's, post-graduate APRN certificate programs, and entry-to-practice residencies for nurses. [129]

In 2020, 100 percent of L.A. County BSN (generic) granting programs achieved CCNE accreditation standards; approximately 35 percent of ADN granting programs (as the highest degree) achieved ACEN accreditation. [130]

Los Angeles Schools Nursing and Graduate Pins

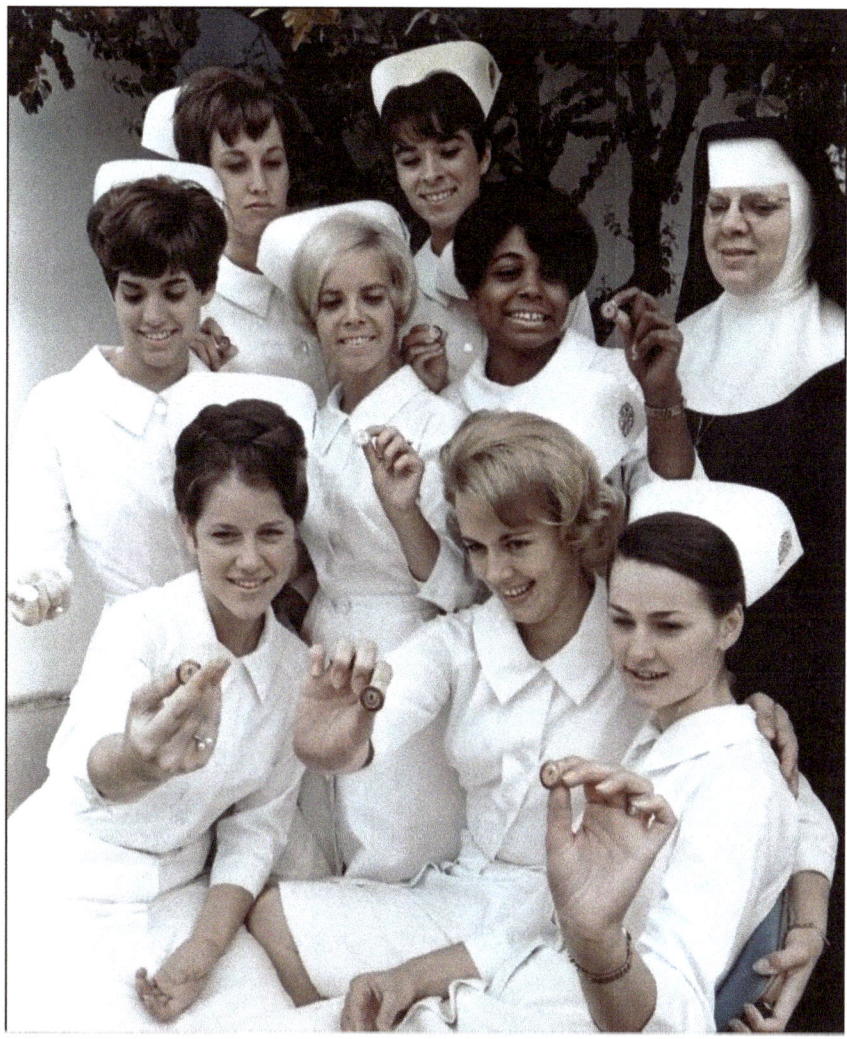

Figure 13.65. Sister Pauline looks on as eight Queen of Angels School of Nursing graduates display their new pins, June 1967. C. (Department of Special Collections, Charles Young Research Library, UCLA)

† Denotes photos courtesy of Dittrick Medical History Center, Case Western Reserve University.

RN Magazine (1937-2009) collected more than a thousand U.S. graduate nurse pins, printed photos yearly in December issues, and created calendars. Dittrick Medical History Center received a donation of these pins; their provenance does not state *RN Magazine*, but the photos are identical. Without this collection, many Los Angeles County graduate nurse pins would be lost.

Notes

Preface

1. "Trained Nurses," *Los Angeles Times*, 9 Jun 1897, 5.

Introduction

1. The Seventh Census of the United States: 1850.
2. www.waterandpower.org/museum/Main_Street_300_Block.html (accessed 2008).
3. *An Illustrated History of Southern California* (The Lewis Publishing Company, Chicago, 1890), 746.
4. Engh, Michael, "Soldiers of Christ, Angels of Mercy: The Daughters of Charity in Los Angeles, 1856–1888," *Vincentian Heritage Journal*, vol. 15, iss. 1 (1994): 25-50.
5. Newark, Harris, *Sixty Years in Southern California*, (NY, 1916), 190.
6. *Los Angeles Star,* 12 Jan 1885, 6.
7. www.daughtersofcharity.com/who-we-are/heritage/los-angeles (accessed 5 Oct 2008).
8. Newark.

Chapter 1

1. Dirvin, Joseph, *Mrs. Seton: Foundress of the American Sisters of Charity.* (New York: Farrar, Straus and Giraux, 1975).
2. www.daughtersofcharity.com/who-we-are/heritage/los-angeles.
3. Engh, 25-50.
4. *Los Angeles Star,* 20 August 1870.
5. Dirvin.
6. Coste, Pierre, *The Life and Works of Saint Vincent de Paul,* (Newman Press, 1952).
7. www.waterandpower.org/museum/Victor_Heights.html.
8. Bostridge, Mark, *Florence Nightingale: The Making of an Icon.* (Farrar, Straus, and Giroux, 2008).
9. Gill, Christopher "Nightingale in Scutari: her legacy reexamined," *Clinical Infectious Diseases,* vol. 40, no. 12 (15 June 2005): 1799–1805.
10. "Unveiling of Florence Nightingale Statue," *Program Booklet*, (Los Angeles County Library, 1937).
11. "Competition," *Los Angeles Times*, 16 May 1974, A3.
12. "Accord Reached in Dispute Over Statue," *Los Angeles Times,* 10 May 1974, B2.
13. Author's interview with Diane Harris-Hara, 19 Feb 2024.
14. www.publicartinpublicplaces.info/florence-nightingale-1937-by-

david-p-edstrom (accessed 20 Oct 2024).

15. https://www.florence-nightingale.co.uk (accessed 4 May 2008).

16. Richards, Linda, *Reminiscences of Linda Richards, America's First Trained Nurse*, (Boston, Whitcomb & Barrows, 1911), 32-46.

17. "C-9A/C Nightingale," https://amcmuseum.org/at-the-museum/aircraft/c-9ac-nightingale (accessed 05 May 2007).

18. "USS Florence Nightingale (AP-70), www.navsource.org/archives/09/22/22070.htm (accessed 05 May 2007).

19. Bostridge.

20. Seacole, Mary, *Wonderful Adventures of Mrs. Seacole in Many Lands*. (London, 1857), 3-6.

21. Ibid, 77-82.

22. Ibid, 90-91.

23. "Mary Seacole's Grave Restored in London," *Jamaica Newsletter*, (London, 26 Nov 1973).

24. www.maryseacoletrust.org.uk/maryseacoleawards (accessed 4 June 2007).

25. "The J. Paul Getty Museum Journal," (Getty, vol. 24, 1996).

26. Beasley, Delilah, *Negro Trail Blazers of California*, (Los Angeles, CA, Times mirror printing and binding house, 1919).

27. Ibid.

28. www.nps.gov/people/biddymason.html (accessed 6 Apr 2009).

29. Hayden, D., *Urban Landscapes Public History*, (MIT Press, 1995).

30. www.laconservancy.org/learn/historic-places/biddy-mason-memorial-park (accessed 6 Apr 2009).

31. Mary Holland, *Our Army Nurses*, (Boston, B. Wilkins & Co. 1895), 90.

32. "Margaret Hayes," *Jefferson City Post-Tribune*, 11 Dec 1933.

33. Holland, 90.

34. "Army Nurses With Us Now," *Los Angeles Times*, 1904.

35. "Construction for Nurses Home," *Los Angeles Times*, 10 Sep 1906.

36. Plante, Trevor K. "The National Home for Disabled Volunteer Soldiers," *Genealogy Notes*, vol. 36, no. 1 (Spring 2004).

37. Dumke, Glenn, "The Boom of the 1880s in Southern California," *Southern California Quarterly*, vol. 76, no. 1 (1994): 99-114.

38. Richards, 20.

39. Ibid.

40. Nordland, Ole J., *History of the Coachella Valley Water District*, (Desert Printing Co. Inc. Indio, CA, 1968), 66.

41. Patterson, Tom, "Dr. June Hill Robertson McCarroll," *1997 Periscope*, 3 Mar 1997, (Valley Historical Society, Indio, CA, Coachella).

42. Ibid.

43. Shannon Starr, "Woman credited for highway center lines: Dr. June McCarroll of Indio will be honored with signs on Interstate 10," *Press-Enterprise*, 6 Apr 2002, B3.

Chapter 2

1. Anderson, N., "Historical Development of American Nursing Education," *Occupational Health Nursing*, vol. 29 no. 10 (1981): 14-26.
2. "With the Destitute," *Los Angeles Times*, 8 Oct 1895.
3. "Trained Nurses," *Los Angeles Times*, 9 Jun 1897, 5.
4. www.nursing.upenn.edu/nhhc/nursing-through-time/1870-1899 (accessed 23 Feb 2024).
5. Meiding, Virginia, *Los Angeles County Medical Center School, Looking Back a Century of Nursing*, (Centennial Book Committee Los Angeles County, Jan 2000).
6. "Trained Nurses," *Los Angeles Times*, 9 Jun 1897, 5.
7. Letter from the Recording Secretary to the Board of the College Training School for Nurses, 13 Jan 1898, Dr. Walter Lindley Scrapbook, Claremont Colleges.
8. "Election of Officers," *Los Angeles Times*, 14 Jan 1898, 16.
9. "The College Training School for Nurses," *Brochure for Opening Exercises*, 5 Oct 1897.
10. "Article I & II, Name and Object," *College Training School for Nurses By-Laws*, 1-2.
11. "Knowledge for Nurses," *Los Angeles Times*, 7 Oct 1896.
12. Ibid.
13. Ibid
14. "The College Training School for Nurses," *Brochure for Opening Exercises*, 5 Oct 1897.
15. Cope, Z., "Joseph Lister, 1827-1912," *British Medical Journal*, (Apr 1967): 7–8.
16. https://dekalbhistory.org/blog-posts/medical-history-of-dekalb-part-ii (accessed 23 Feb 2024).
17. Haynes, Francis L., "Surgical Nursing," *Southern California Practitioner*, vol. XIV, (1899): 50
18. *Los Angeles County Medical Center School, Looking Back a Century of Nursing*.
19. "Trained Nurses," *Los Angeles Times*, 9 Jun 1897, 5.
20. Heidland A, et al., "Neuromuscular electrostimulation techniques: historical aspects and current possibilities in treatment of pain and muscle waisting." *Clinical Nephrol.*, vol. 79, supp. 1 (Jan 2013): S12-23.
21. Hampton, Isabel A., *Nursing: Its Principles and Practice*, 1893.
22. Ibid.
23. "A Los Angeles Home for the Sick and Convalescent, The California Hospital," *Brochure*, n.d., Lindley Scrapbook.
24. Ibid.
25. "A Heritage of Commitment and Caring," *Pacemaker*, Good Samaritan Hospital Archives, n.d.
26. Ibid.

27. Clark, David, *A History of Good Samaritan Hospital in Los Angeles: 1885-2010 A Tradition of Caring*, (Good Samaritan Hospital, L.A., 2010).

28. Pahl, Harriet, "Training School Announcement," Nov 1904, Good Samaritan Medical Center Archives.

29. Ibid.

30. Clark.

31. www.lacsonalumni.org/about-us (accessed 6 Dec 2023).

32. "Trained Nurses are Graduated," *Los Angeles Herald*, 28 Mar 1905.

33. www.daughtersofcharity.com/who-we-are/heritage/los-angeles (accessed 27 Feb 2024).

34. "The French Hospital," *Associated Historical Societies of Los Angeles County*, Apr 1988.

35. https://frenchtownconfidential.blogspot.com/2018/07/hang-in-there-joan.html (accessed 24 Feb 2024).

36. "Obituaries." *American Journal of Nursing 37*, no. 7 (1937): 819.

37. Koslow, Jennifer, *Cultivating Health: Los Angeles Women and Public Health Reform*, (Rutgers University Press, 13 Jul 2009), 20.

38. Ibid.

39. Chisholm, Hugh, "Zymotic Diseases," *Encyclopedia Britannica*, 11th ed., (Cambridge University Press, 1911).

40. Potemkina, Antonia, "Margaret Sirch," *The Trained Nurse and Hospital Review*, Volumes 100-101, (Lakeside Publishing Company, 1938).

41. Ibid.

42. "The Pacific Hospital," *Los Angeles Herald*, no. 82, 22 Dec 1899.

43. "New Pacific Hospital Has Formal Opening," *Los Angeles Times*, 10 Sep 1902, 12.

44. https://pcad.lib.washington.edu/building/22206 (accessed 7 Dec 2023).

45. "Report of the Housing Commission of the City of Los Angeles," 1906-1908, 3.

46. Koslow, 34.

47. Ibid.

48. "Youngest Manager of Hospital Work," *Los Angeles Times*, 6 Dec 1903, A1.

49. Ibid.

50. McGroarty, John Steven, *Los Angeles From the Mountains to the Sea*, (American Historical Society, 1921), 777.

51. www.rn.ca.gov/about_us/history.shtml (accessed 5 May 2008).

52. Nordhoff, Charles, *California, for Health, Pleasure, and Residence*, (Harper, New York, 1875).

53. "Southern California a Mecca for Sick Pilgrims," *Los Angeles Times*, 1 Jan 1887, 12.

54. Schwarz, Richard W., *John Harvey Kellogg, M.D.: pioneering health reformer*, (Hagerstown, MD: Review and Herald Pub. Assoc., 2006).

55. Kellogg, John Harvey, "Breakfast Cereals," *The New Dietetics: What*

to Eat and How, (The Modern Medicine Publishing Co., Battle Creek, MI, 1921), 256-258.

56. "Infirmary Consumptives," *San Francisco Call,* 13 Oct 1901, 14.

57. Barlow, John F., "Barlow Genealogy 1998-2005," *Who's Who in Los Angeles,* (Barlow Foundation).

58. Ibid.

59. https://www.laparks.org/sites/default/files/facility/elysian/pdf/1992_UCLA/ElysianPK_UCLA_Chp5.pdf (accessed 10 Oct 2008).

60. "Brochure," Glendale Adventist Medical Center Archives, 1905.

61. Ibid.

62. Newest of Hospitals," *Los Angeles Times,* 10 Dec 1903, A1.

63. "Busy Hospital," *Los Angeles Times,* 15 Jun 1904, A1.

64. "Clara Barton Alumni Association Minutes, 1991," History & Special Collections Division, Louise Darling Biomedical Library, UCLA.

65. Clara Barton Hospital School of Nursing, 1910-1989, OAC, https://oac.cdlib.org/findaid/ark:/13030/tf009n99t3/entire_text (accessed 20 Apr 2024).

66. "Alumni minutes," Clara Barton School of Nursing Alumnae Association, May 1991.

67. Davis, Margaret Leslie, *Childrens Hospital and the Leaders of Los Angeles: The First 100 Years,* (Childrens Hospital Los Angeles, 2002).

68. "Large Funds Provided for Children's Good," *Los Angeles Times,* 25 Sep, 1912, II1.

69. Walter Lindley letter to the president of Children's Hospital, Claremont Colleges, Dr. Walter Lindley Scrapbooks, California Hospital, Box 3, 177.

70. "Letters to the Editor," *The American Journal of Nursing,* vol. 15, no. 8 (May 1915): 678-679.

71. Ibid.

72. Ibid.

73. "Childrens Hospital to Celebrate," *Los Angeles Times,* 27 Apr 1927, A10.

74. Information on Santa Fe Coastline Hospital Postcard, 1907.

75. "Miss Hively's anger rising; war of nurses grows apace," *Los Angeles Examiner,* 2 Sep 1905.

76. "Angelus Hospital, building of Grecian design, will be notable for fireproof arrangements," *Los Angeles Examiner,* 4, Jul 1904.

77. "Angelus Hospital is Open for Inspection," *Los Angeles Herald,* 15 May 1906, 5.

78. "Two-Hundred Thousand Dollar Hospital," *Los Angeles Times,* 10 May 1906, 17.

79. "Many See Angelus Nurses Graduate," *Los Angeles Examiner,* 28 Jul 1908.

80. McGroarty, John Steven, *Los Angeles from the Mountains to the Sea,* (Chicago, American Historical Society, 1921).

81. Williamson, Anne, *50 Years in Starch*, (Murray & Gee, 1948).
82. Ibid.
83. *Los Angeles Herald*, 23, 1910.
84. Interviewed by Sherna Berger Gluck, n.d. "Women's History: Professionals and Entrepreneurs. The Virtual Oral/Aural History Archive, California State University, Long Beach," Interview 1a. Segment 1.
85. Methodist Hospital Archives, 2009.
86. "Unit For Anesthesia Recovery Saves Lives," *Los Angeles Times*, 17 Jul 1953, A7.
87. Methodist Hospital Archives, 2009.
88. Newmark, Marco R. "Pioneer Merchants of Los Angeles," *The Quarterly: Historical Society of Southern California*, vol. 24, no. 1-2 (Mar 1943): 4-65.
89. Harris, N.A.; Hunziker-Dean, J. Florence; Henderson. "The art of open-drop ether," *Nurs Hist Rev.* (Jan 2001):159-84.
90. Ibid, 177.
91. Ibid, 178.
92. Ibid, 180.
93. "Suit Filed to Restrain Nurse's Act," *Los Angeles Times*, 13 Jul 1934, A9.
94. "The Life and Trial of Dagmar Nelson-Part 1," *AANA Journal* vol. 74, no. 3, (June 2006): 183-7.
95. Ibid.
96. Ibid.
97. "Sophie Winton," *AANA News Bulletin*, vol. 38, no. 11 (Nov 1984): 5-7.
98. Ibid.
99. Ibid

Chapter 3

1. Foster, Michael, "History of the Maltese Cross, as used by the Order of St John of Jerusalem," (2004), www.lishfd.org/History/history_of_the_maltese_cross.htm (accessed 7 Oct 2008).
2. Iveson-Iveson J., "History of Nursing, Knight Nurse," *Nursing Mirror* (Apr 1982): 28-30.
3. Seymour, W., *The Cross in Tradition History and Art*, 1898.
4. "The Coat of Arms," *Annual Journal of the Heraldry Society, Series 4*, vol. 4, no. 238, (4Wrd Ltd.): 2021.
5. Seymour.
6. Frank, Charles Marie, *Historical Development of Nursing*, (W.B. Saunders Company, 1953).
7. Rode, M.W. "The nursing pin: Symbol of 1,000 years of service," *Nursing Forum* vol. 24, no. 1 (1989): 15-17.
8. Frank.

9. Cook E.T., *The Life of Florence Nightingale*, (London, Macmillan and Co., 1913).
10. https://honours.cabinetoffice.gov.uk/about/orders-and-medals (accessed 9 May 2008).
11. https://collection.nam.ac.uk/detail.php?acc=1963-10-54-3 (accessed 4 May 2008).
12. Ibid.
13. https://collection.nam.ac.uk/detail.php?acc=1963-10-54-2 (accessed 9 May 2008).
14. Frank, Charles Marie, *Historical Development of Nursing*.
15. https://archives.med.nyu.edu/collections/bellevue-school-of-nursing (accessed 9 May 2008).
16. Ibid.
17. Nightingale, Florence, "Sick-Nursing and Health-Nursing," 1893.
18. Karen Buhler-Wilkerson, "Bringing Care to the People: Lillian Wald's Legacy to Public Health Nursing," *American Journal of Public Health*, 83 (Dec 1993): 1778-86.
19. Koslow, 20.
20. Wright, Florence Swift, *Industrial Nursing*, (New York: Macmillan Company, 1920).
21. Ibid.
22. June 25, 1948, ch. 645, 62 Stat. 732; May 24, 1949, ch. 139, §17, 63 Stat. 92; Pub. L. 103-322, title XXXIII, §330016(1)(E), Sept. 13, 1994, 108 Stat. 2146.
23. Gurowitz, Margaret, "The Red Cross," 10 Aug 2007.
24. www.nursingworld.org/ana/about-ana/history (accessed 23 Apr 2024).
25. www.nps.gov (accessed 23 Apr 2024).

Chapter 4

1. Budreau, Lisa M., Prior, Richard M., *Answering The Call: The U.S. Army Nurse Corps, 1917-1919: A Commemorative Tribute to Military Nursing in World War I*. (Gov. Printing Office, 10 Nov. 2008).
2. "Equal Suffrage," Address of the President of the United States, 30 Sep 1918, (Washington Gov. Printing Office, 1918).
3. Rueda, Nimfa, "Red Cross Honors Unsung Heroine," 6 Oct, 2006 www.specialtoredcross.org (accessed Nov 2008).
4. Blackstock, Joe, "She doesn't deserve to be forgotten," *Inland Valley Daily Bulletin*, 2005.
5. Ibid.
6. "Grace Williams Major," 3. Archives at Good Samaritan Hospital.
7. Ibid.
8. "Great Parade to Usher in Red Cross Drive," *Los Angeles Times*, 18 May 1918, II1.

9. Ibid.
10. Adair, Birdie May, "Collection pertaining to the Training Camp at Vassar College, 1918," Louise M. Darling Biomedical Library History and Science Collections, UCLA.
11. *White Task Force: the story of the Nurse Corps, United States Navy.* (NAVMED 939 1945), 21-22.
12. Ferrell, Robert H., *The Strange Deaths of President Harding*, (University of Missouri Press, (16 Sep 1998), 47.
13. *White Task Force.*
14. "Nurse Gets War Cross," *Los Angeles Times*, 5 Jan 1931, A8.
15. Flood, Marylyn, "Proclaiming our Work A Science," https://nursing.ucsf.edu/sites/nursing.ucsf.edu/files/pdfs/ourwrk.pdf (accessed 11 Mar 2024).
16. Bryan, Edith S., R.N., PhD, "Read at the general session of the National League of Nursing Education," San Antonio, TX, 14 Apr 1932.
17. Bryan, Edith S., R.N., PhD, "Methods of Research and Study," vol. XXXII, no. 7749, (July 1932).
18. Flood, Marylyn, "Proclaiming our Work A Science."
19. *Annual Report of the Surgeon General*, (U.S. Navy 1919), 368.
20. "City Council Plans New 'Flu' Law," *Los Angeles Evening Herald*, 31 Oct 1918, 3.
21. "Annual Report of the Department of Health, City of Los Angeles, California, for the Year Ended June 30, 1919," (Los Angeles, 1919), 6.
22. "May Soon Lift Closing Order," *Los Angeles Times*, 11 Oct 1918, 1.
23. "Annual Report of the Department of Health of the City of Los Angeles, California."
24. "To Establish Influenza Hospital For City," *Los Angeles Evening Herald*, 6 Nov 1918, 3.
25. "Stay At Home," *Los Angeles Times*, 26 Nov 1918, 1-2.
26. "Red Cross War Begin on Pest," *Los Angeles Times*, 8 Oct 1918, 13.
27. "Influenza Declining Rapidly Here," *Los Angeles Evening Herald*, 9 Nov 1918, 3.
28. "All Schools To Open In City Tomorrow," *Los Angeles Evening Herald*, 5 Feb 1919.
29. Markel H, Lipman HB, Navarro JA, et al., "Nonpharmaceutical interventions implemented by U.S. cities during the 1918-1919 influenza pandemic," *JAMA*, vol. 298, no. 6, (8 Aug 2007): 644-654.
30. "Says Hospital Faces Crisis," *Los Angeles Times*, 16 Oct 1918.
31. *Los Angeles County Medical Center School, Looking Back a Century of Nursing.*
32. *The Annual, Army School of Nursing*, (Walter Reed General Hospital in Washington, DC, 1921).
33. https://history.army.mil/books/anc-highlights/chrono.htm (accessed 5 May 2007).
34. *The Annual, Army School of Nursing.*

35. https://atdnursing.org/Home/membership, (accessed Mar 2024).

36. Treacy, Jane, *Vision of 75 years: An anniversary celebration, 1922-1997* (1997): 56-57.

37. Ibid.

38. "Who's Who in Los Angeles," *Los Angeles Times*, 4 Feb 1935, 7.

39. Dietrich, Ella, "How Los Angeles Nurses Financed Their Club," *American Journal of Nursing*, Apr 1924.

40. Kothe, Vivian, "Los Angeles Club in Use," *American Journal of Nursing*, (Apr 1925): 267-269.

41. "Nurses Open Own Home," *Los Angeles Times*, 27 Jul 1924, 28.

42. Author's tour of the building, 2009.

43. National Register of Historic Places, (National Park Service, 15 Apr 2008).

44. Gann, Dan M., *At Forty: The Queen of Angels Hospital Story*, (Queen of Angels, 1967).

45. Vorspan, Max, and Gartner, Lloyd, *History of the Jews of Los Angeles*, (Jewish Publication Society of America, 1970).

46. "Screen Stars, Civic Leader to Appear at Mt. Sinai Nurses, Home Ceremony," *California Jewish Review*, (12 Mar 1937).

47. White Memorial Hospital Collection, (Loma Linda University, Loma Linda, CA, 2009).

48. Ibid.

49. *Hands of Healing In The City of Angels—90 Years, 1913-2003*, (White Memorial Medical Center), 4.

50. Reynolds, Keld J. *Outreach: Loma Linda University, 1905-1967*, (Loma Linda, CA, Loma Linda University, 1968), 41.

Chapter 5

1. Schimmoler, Lauretta, "And They Said It Wouldn't Be Done," unpublished manuscript at Bucyrus Historical Society, Bucyrus, Ohio.

2. "Aerial Nurse Corps Wins Place in Sun," *Los Angeles Times*, 8 Feb 1942, D7.

3. "Flying Angels Seek Recruits," *Los Angeles Times*, 18 Feb 1941, 11.

4. Schimmoler.

5. Pearce, Carol A. "Amelia Earhart," *Facts on File*, (New York, 1988).

6. "Start Work On New Hanger, *The Marion Star*, 27 Apr 1931, 13.

7. "Ex-Bucyrus Airport Manager Turns to Movies," *Mansfield News-Journal*, 16 Aug 1942.

8. "Private Planes Except Airliners Are Grounded," *Washington Evening Star*, 8 Dec 1941.

9. Broze, Cynthia, *Aerial Nurse Corps of America*, (Semper Publishing, 2023), 110-111.

10. Schimmoler.

11. "Miss Schimmoler Awarded Honorary Flight Nurse Certificate and

Wings," *Aerospace Medicine* (July 1966).

12. "World's First Air Hostess," *Mason City Globe-Gazette*, 14 Mar 1939, 16.

13. "Reminiscence of Ellen Church," Oral History Office, Columbia University, 1960.

14. "In Richest Mans' Employ," Los Angeles Bureau, back of photo information, #LA 13885, 2 April 1938.

15. Linebach L., "The Railroad Stewardess-Nurse: a Step Toward Autonomy in Nursing Practice," *History Nursing Bulletin* (1988): 17-35.

16. Ibid.

17. https://www.kshs.org/index.php?url=km/items/view/307501 (accessed 20 Mar 2024).

18. Keeling, Kirchgessner, Hehman, *History of Professional Nursing in the United States*, (Springer, 1 Sept 2017).

19. Kansas State Historical Society papers.

20. "Phillips Highway Hostess," ConocoPhillips Magazine quoted in Katz, Micheal, *American Gas Station Station*, (Motorbooks 1992), 107-111.

21. Wallis, Michael, Route 66: *The Mother Road*, (Macmillan, 1990).

22. https://tessa2.lapl.org/digital/collection/photos/id/5429 (accessed 18 Mar 2024).

23. Author's interview with Jim French, 5 Mar 2008.

24. "Nurses Open Meet Today," *Los Angeles Times*, 20 Jun 1936, A1.

25. "Nurses Here for Meeting," *Los Angeles Times*, 19 Jun 1936, A3.

26. "Kay Francis Loves the Role of Angel," *Los Angeles Times*, 28 Jun 1936, C3.

27. "Nurses Will Pay Tribute," *Los Angeles Times*, 17 Jun 1936, A5.

28. "Nurses Open Meet Today," A1.

29. "Convention Assisted by Boy Scouts," *Los Angeles Times*, 25 Jun 1936, A2.

30. "Fit Family Life Urged," *Los Angeles Times*, 24 Jun 1936, A2.

31. Gilford, Steve, "Remembering Betty Runyen: How Dr. Garfield's First Nurse Helped Mold the Principles of Permanente Medicine," *Permanente Journal* (2001 Summer): 68–69.

32. Ibid.

33. https://www.marchofdimes.org (accessed 12 Mar 2008).

34. Halvorsen, Helen, "One District and Its Disabled Members," *American Journal of Nursing*, vol. 38, no. 5 (May 1938): 549-553.

35. Ibid.

36. "School of Friendship Book, Personal Journal of Helen Ackley," 1929-1931 (author's collection).

37. Ibid.

38. Author's interview with Margaret Freed, 2009.

39. *RX: The Los Angeles County General Hospital School of Nursing Annual*, 1933.

40. "Barlow Volunteer Honored for 60 Years of Service," *Barlow*

Foundation News, 2006.

Chapter 6

1. "Sunbrite Junior Nurse Corps News," vol. 1 no. 8 (1938 Feb).
2. "The Sunbrite Junior Nurse Corps Manual," (Swift & Co, 1936).
3. www.netwrx1.com/CherryAmes/index.html (accessed 1 Oct 2006).
4. "Nurses Three Cut-outs," (Whitman Company, 1964).
5. "Nurses Three Cut-outs," (Whitman Company, 1965).

Chapter 7

1. www.med-dept.com (accessed 05 Mar 2010).
2. Speck, Jane, *The Trained Nurse and Hospital Review* (Dec 1942): 414-415.
3. Danner, Dorothy Still, *What a Way to Spend a War: Navy Nurse POWs in the Philippines* (Naval Inst. Press, Jan 1995).
4. Broze, Cynthia, *Aerial Nurse Corps of America* (Semper Publishing, 1 Dec 2023), 246.
5. Danner.
6. Bullough, V. and Sentz, L., *American Nursing: A Biographical Dictionary, Volume 3* (Springer Publishing, 2004), 24-26.
7. McLellan, Dennis, "Ruby Bradley, 94; Army Nurse Was 'Angel in Fatigues' for POWs," *Los Angeles Times*, 2 June 2002.
8. Bullough, V. and Sentz, L.
9. McLellan.
10. Galvani, William, "The Perseverance of Lieutenant Nash," *Naval History*, (Apr 2023).
11. Fessler, Diane, *No Time for Fear: Voices of American Military Nurses in World War II* (Michigan State University Press, 1996), 99.
12. Ibid.
13. Norman, Elizabeth M., *We Band of Angels: The Untold Story of American Nurses on Bataan* (Random House, 1999).
14. Ibid.
15. Ibid.
16. Brehm, Connie, "Next Reenactment is Captain C. Edwina Todd, WWII Navy Nurse," *Western Conservancy of Nursing History Newsletter*, vol. 1, iss. 1 (Spring 2001).
17. Norman, E.M., "Maude Campbell Davison," quoted in Bullough, V. and Sentz, L., *American Nursing: A biographical dictionary, Volume 3* (Springer Publishing 2004), 66.
18 www.uswarmemorials.org/html/people_details.php?PeopleID=24888 (accessed 10 Nov 2024).
19. Norman, *"We Band of Angels."*
20. Ibid.

21. Norman, Elizabeth, "How Did They All Survive: An Analysis of American Nurses' Experience in Japanese Prisoner-of-War-Camps, *Nursing History Review,* (University of Pennsylvania Press for the American Association for the History of Nursing, 1995), 105–127.

22. "Ontario-born Girl Among Army Nurses Back from Manila," *Ottawa Journal,* 26 Feb 1945, 2.

23. Deiss, Henshaw Gwendolyn, "Army Nurse Corps Oral History Program Interviews, Transcript," Dept. of the Army Center for Military History, Washington D.C., 1984.

24. Proclamation 5031, National P.O.W.-M.I.A. Recognition Day, (Filed with the Office of the Federal Register, 10:57 a.m., 15 Mar 1983).

25. Deiss.

26. https://navylog.navymemorial.org/yetter-dris (access 5 May 2024).

27. "Freed Los Banos Nurses Elect to Stay on Duty," *Los Angeles Times,* 28 Feb 1945, 5.

28. https://www.tinker.af.mil/News/Article-Display/Article/1225055/air-force-history-capt-lillian-kinkella-keil-af-hero (accessed 10 Oct 2008).

29. https://militaryhallofhonor.com/honoree-record.php?id=2696 (accessed 10 Oct 2008).

30. Merl, Jean, "Post Office Named After Nurse," *Los Angeles Times,* 29 Oct 2006.

31. Nelson, Valerie "Lillian Kinkella Keil, 88; 'an Airborne Florence Nightingale,'" *Los Angeles Times,* 10 July 2005.

32. www.loc.gov/collections/ansel-adams-manzanar/about-this-collection (accessed 4 May 2009).

33. Adams, Ansel, *Born Free and Equal: Photographs of the Loyal Japanese-Americans at Manzanar Relocation Center,* Inyo County, CA, (U.S. Camera, New York, 1944).

34. www.archives.gov/education/lessons/japanese-relocation#background (accessed 5 May 2009).

35. Robinson, Thelman M., *Nisei Cadet Nurse of World War II: Patriotism in Spite of Prejudice* (Black Swan Mill Press, Jan 2005).

36. Feldman, Harriet R., *Nursing Leadership: A Concise Encyclopedia,* (Springer Publishing Company, 25 Feb 2008).

37. Petry, Lucile, "U. S. Cadet Nurse Corps: Established under the Bolton Act." *American Journal of Nursing,* vol. 43, no. 8 (1943): 704-708.

38. Andrus, Ethel Percy "High School Victory Corps," *The Journal of Educational Sociology,* vol. 16, no. 4, (1942): 231–240.

39. Santa Monica Public Library Image Archives caption.

40. www.smithsonianmag.com/history/armys-first-black-nurses-had-tend-to-german-prisoners-war-180969069 (accessed 1 Apr 2024).

41. "A Brief History of Letterman General Hospital," *Letterman Army Hospital,* 27 June 1951.

42. "Army Nurse Assigned to Van Nuys Hospital," *Los Angeles Times,* 7 Feb 1944, A2.

43. "First Wounded Men Enter New Hospital Here," *Los Angeles Times*, 29 Feb 1944, 1.
44. "Alice Sterling Turner," Charles Young Research Library, UCLA.
45. Ibid.
46. https://militarymuseum.org/BirminghamGenHosp.html (accessed 9 Jun 2009).
47. "Ensign Dorothy Olsen," Special Collections, Charles E. Young Research Library, UCLA.
48. Ibid.
49. Author's interview with Edith Shain, 29 May 2007.
50. "Who is Kissing Sailor?" *Life*, Oct 1980.
51. "Celebrating the V-J Day Kiss Seen Round the World," *Los Angeles Times*, 14 Aug 2005.
52. Brandenburg, David A.,"WWII Commemorative Statue Unveiled in San Diego," Story # NNS070216-14, 16 Feb 2007, Navy.mil (accessed 10 Aug 2007).
53. www.npr.org/2005/08/13/4799520/a-kiss-a-photo-a-statue-and-a-memory (accessed 15 Aug 2007).
54. Author's interview with Edith Shain.
55. Ibid.

Chapter 8

1. "Visiting Nurses Association Sponsored for Los Angeles," *Los Angeles Times*, 24 Jan 1940, A2.
2. Moore, Zeanette, "Reporter Finds Trouble Rife on Nurse's Tour," *Los Angeles Times*, 14 Oct 1946, A1.
3. Wilson, Bess, "Elizabeth Hill Spurs Home Nursing Service," *Los Angeles Times*, 24 Mar 1940, D8.
4. Moore.
5. "Nursing Services Increase," *Los Angeles Times*, 30 May 1943, D5.
6. Fisher, Sara, "Big care providers pushing into home health industry," *Los Angeles Business Journal*, vol. 19 no. 45, (10 Nov 1997): 34.
7. https://alpv.org/history (accessed 3 May 2024).
8. Rasmussen, Cecilia, "God's Geese' Watched Over Flocks of Girls," *Los Angeles Times*, 29 June 1997.
9. "History," *Hollywood Presbyterian School of Nursing Booklet*, 4.
10. "Our New Director," Medicine Glass, vol 1, no.7, *Hollywood Presbyterian Hospital* (1 Nov 1944).
11. "Two Sawtelle Nurses Scholarship Winners, *Los Angeles Times*, 1 Sep 1947, 8.
12. Ibid.
13. "Twin Nurses Shun Navy," *Los Angeles Times*, 8 Dec 1947, 5.
14. https://npgallery.nps.gov/NRHP/SearchResults?view=list (assessed 20 Dec 2008).

15. www.laconservancy.org/learn/historic-places/hollenbeck-terrace (accessed 7 Apr 2024).16. Brown, Les, *New York Times Encyclopedia of Television* (Random House Inc, 1 Jan 1977).

17. "Study Course in Premature Babies Opens," *Los Angeles Times*, 2 April 1949, A1.

18. "200 Girls See St. Luke's Hospital Exhibition," *Los Angeles Times*, 14 May 1953, 31. and "Hospitals Prepare Disaster Action," *Los Angeles Times*, 6 May 1956, B1.

19. "National Nurses Week History," www.nursingworld.org/education-events/national-nurses-week/history (accessed 20 June 2024).

20. "Cedars-Sinai Medical Center," *Academic Medicine*, Jan 2003, 110.

21. Author's interview with Mary Tomassini, 8 Feb 2008.

22. www.dailybreeze.com/2016/12/15/ho-ho-ho-harbor-city-home-loves-christmas-all-year-long (accessed 4 Apr 2024).

23. Author's interview with Mary Tomassini.

24. Interview with Darren Williams Smith, 5 April 2008, quoted in https://spotdk.blogspot.com/2005/10/silva-family.html.

25. "The Rotarian," vol. 115, no. 6 (Dec 1969): 26.

26. "Nurses Sized Up For Names," *Los Angeles Times*, 30 June 1966.

27. York R, Bhuttarowas, "The Development of Nursing in Thailand," *American Journal of Maternal Child Nursing* (1999 May-Jun): abstract.

28. "Nurses' fashion: pants," *Los Angeles Times Archives*, 8 June 2006.

29. Coutant, Betty, "Katheryn Crosby," *Ledger Independent*, n.d.

30. Gordon, Stanley, "Mrs. Bing Crosby: Student Nurse," *Look*, 12 Mar 1963, 98-100.

31. Melchior, J. et al., "Fetal heart rate variability calculated by an external technique during pregnancy," *Fetal Physiological Measurements*, 1986, 254-255.

32. https://classictvhistory.wordpress.com/2013/10/16/the-nurses-of-ben-casey (accessed 8 Apr 2024).

33. Ibid.

34. Laird, J., Moser, J., Demian, M., "I Remember a Lemon Tree," *Ben Casey*, season 1, episode 4 (23 Oct 1961).

35. Mancino, Diane, "Breakthrough to Nursing," *Dean's Notes*, vol. 26, no. 1 (NSNA Imprint, 2004): 1-3.

36. https://oadn.org/alpha-delta-nu-honor-society, 7 May 2024.

37. Bernstein, Harry, "Brown Pledges Aid to Picketing Nurses on Wage Demands," *Los Angeles Times*, 14 Oct 1966, 3.

38. Cohen, Jerry, "The Future Comes too Late," *Los Angeles Times*, 29 Aug 1965, G1.

39. Murphy Jean, "Adults Succeed As Nursing Students," *Los Angeles Times*, 27 Jan 1968, B1.

40. "HPH Contributes Facilities for Refresher Nurse Program," *Holly Press*, vol. II, no. 8 (Oct 1967): 1.

41. De Wolfe, Evelyn, "Male Nurses: Slayers of Stereotypes," *Los*

Angeles Times, 30 Nov 1971, E1.

42. Ibid.

43. Hertel, Howard, "Woman Reservist Granted Injunction Barring Discharge," *Los Angeles Times*, 6 Oct 1970, A1.

44. De Wolfe, Evelyn, "Southland Alumni Who Broke the Mold," *Los Angeles Times*, 8 Jul 1970, E1.

45. Lilliston, Lynn, "School Nurse: Is She Just a Frill," *Los Angeles Times*, 11 May 1972, I1.

46. Ibid.

47. "Medical Corpsmen Earn Their RNs," *Holly Press*, Apr 1972, 2.

48. "The New Look Now in School—It's Men," *Holly Press*, 1970.

49. Stand Alone, *Los Angeles Times*, 6 Dec 1974, 1.

50. Stand Alone, *Los Angeles Times*, 11 Jan 1975, 26.

51. Jones, John C., MD, "Open-Heart Surgery Suing Deep Hypothermia Without an Oxygenator," *J. Thoracic and Cardiovas Surgery*, vol. 40, no. 6 (Dec 1960): 787-812.

52. Stand Alone, *Los Angeles Times*, 11 Jan 1975, 26.

53. Goffam Debbie, "5 Deaf Students Finish Nursing Course," *Los Angeles Times* 27 Jun 1976, C1.

54. Ibid, 5.

55. http://jonestown.sdsu.edu (accessed 13 Nov 2008).

56. www.nzherald.co.nz/world/three-tell-their-tales-of-how-they-survived-the-jonestown-massacre (accessed 9 Apr 2024).

57. Author's interview with Ray Duarte, 5 Jul 2008.

58. https://invention.si.edu/podcast-sharon-rogone-invents-preemies-part-1-2) accessed 29 Oct 2008).

59. Author's interview with Lynn Campanaro, 3 July 2008.

60. Author's interview with Fey Reichman, 19 Oct 2008.

61. www.vvmf.org/stories/Diane-Carlson-Evans (accessed 10 Feb 2009).

62. "Glenna Goodacre, Created the Vietnam Women's Memorial, Dies at 80," *New York Times*, 16 Apr 2020.

63. The *Vietnam Women's Memorial* booklet.

64. https://post3legion.org/Vietnam_Statistics.pdf (accessed 10 Feb 2009).

65. http://www.thebabylift.com (accessed 10 Feb 2009).

66. Biographies mailed to author from Women in Military Service for America Memorial Foundation.org/Military Women's Memorial.org.

67. Ibid.

68. Sterner, Doris, *In and Out of Harm's Way, A History of the Navy Nurse Corps*, (Peanut Butter Publishing, Seattle, 1997), 310.

69. Biographies mailed to author from Military Women's Memorial.

70. Ibid.

71. Ibid.

72. Ibid.

Chapter 9

1. McNeil, Mary Germaine, *History of Mount St. Mary's College, Los Angeles, 1925-1975* (Vantage Press, 1985).
2. "A Golden Celebration for a Jewel of a Program," The *Mount* (Spring 2002): 12.
3. "Sister Rebecca Doan," *Working Nurse*, May 2009.
4. McNeil.
5. Ibid.
6. Author's Interview with Maureen Boylan Scherzberg, 5 June 2007.
7. Hassenplug, Lulu Wolf, Hassenplug papers, Louise Darling Biomedical Library, UCLA, Los Angeles.
8. Gordon, Dan, *History of the UCLA School of Nursing* (UCLA Press, Jan 1999).
9. Ibid.
10. Jeanne Hackley Stevenson, "Mary Adelaide Nutting, 1858-1948," *Notable Maryland Women* (Maryland Tidewater Publishers, Cambridge, 1977), 256-262.
11. Hassenplug papers.
12. "The Florence Nightingale International Foundation." *American Journal of Nursing*, vol. 8, no. 9 (1938): 975–977.
13. https://resource.rockarch.org/story/the-women-pioneers-of-global-nursing-education-who-built-the-rockefeller-foundation-program (accessed 4 Apr 2024).
14. Rubenfeld, M. Gaie et al., "The Nurse Training Act: Yesterday, Today, And..." *American Journal of Nursing*," vol. 81, no. 6 (1981): 1202–4.
15. "Recognition for Continuing Education." *American Journal of Nursing*, vol. 74, no. 5, (May 1974): 878–80.
16. Squaires, Marjorie, box 7, UW-Milwaukee Faculty and Staff Biographical File.
17. Keighley, Tom, "Roy C. The Interview—Callista Roy," *Nursing Manager*, 4 Sep 1997.
18. Johnson, D. E. "The Behavioral System Model for Nursing," *Theoretical Basis for Nursing* (Lippincott Williams & Wilkins, 1980).
19. Bullough, V., Sentz, L., 149–151.
20. Author's interview of Betty Newman, 3 Mar 2008.
21. Gunter, L., Estes, C., *Education for Gerontic Nursing* (Springer Pub, New York, 1979).
22. Eberspoe, Pricilla, *Geriatric Nursing: Growth of a Specialty* (Springer Publishing, Feb 2006), 58.
23. Kolanowski, Ann, "An Interview with Dr. Laurie Gunter: A Pioneer Helping Gerontological Nurses Establish Educational Roots," *Journal of Gerontological Nursing*, vol. 32, no. 4 (Apr 2006): 7-8.
24. Kolanowski, Ann, "In memory: Laurie M. Gunter, PhD, RN, FAAN, March 5, 1922-June 15, 2015," *Journal of Gerontological Nursing*,

vol. 41, no. 9 (Sep 2015): 3.

25. "Bonnie Bullough; Initiated Nurse Practitioner Movement," *Los Angeles Times*, 20 Apr 1996.

26. Bullough, Bonnie, "Barriers to the Nurse Practitioner Movement: Problems of Women in a Woman's Field," *International Journal of Health Services*, vol. 2, no. 2 (1975): 225-233.

27. Bullough, Bonnie, "Professionalization of Nurse Practitioners," *Annual Review of Nursing Research*, vol. 13, no. 1 (Jan 1995): 239-265.

28. https://oac.cdlib.org/findaid/ark:/13030/c8g166bf/entire_text (accessed 20 Oct 2009).

29. Ibid.

30. "Vern L. Bullough, professor, sex researcher, author," *Buffalo News*, 5 Jul 2006, Obituary.

31. Bullough, V., "Bonnie Bullough," *American Nursing: A Biographical Dictionary: Volume 3* (Springer Publishing, Jan 2004), 36-38.

32. Cashion, Joan, "One Dreaming Nurse," *Mount St. Mary's Chalon Magazine* (Fall 1987): 15.

33. Author's interview with Joyce Kelly, 4 Apr 2009.

34. www.aana.com/membership/recognition/aana-awards/annual-recognition-awards/agatha-hodgins-award-for-outstanding-accomplishment (accessed 5 Apr 2009).

35. "Joyce Kelly Receives First Helen Lamb Award for Outstanding Educator," *AANA News Bulletin* (Oct/Nov 1980): 8-9.

36. Author's interview with Patricia Snyder, 21 Mar 2009.

37. Author's interview with Gertrude Hutchinson, 9 Sep 2008.

38. www.linkedin.com/in/gertrude-hutchinson (accessed 5 Apr 2024).

39. Porter, Nellie M. "Affiliations with Junior Colleges in California," *American Journal of Nursing*, vol. XXXII, no. 9. (Sep 1932): 976-982.

40. Ibid.

41. Montag, Mildred, "Experimental Programs in Nursing," *American Journal of Nursing*, vol. 55, no. 1 (Jan 1955): 45.

42. Ibid.

43. https://pasadena.edu/about/history.php (accessed 17 Apr 2024).

44. Hiatt, Wilma, "Associate Degree Nursing Programs in California," *American Journal of Nursing* (Oct 1961): 93-95.

45. Ibid.

46. Author's interview with Barbara Jury, 26 Feb 2010.

47. Author's interview with Joyce Jacobs, 26 Feb 2010.

48. "Los Angeles State College of Applied Arts and Science Bulletin 1956-1957," 209.

49. https://www.csulb.edu/historical/1964-1965 (accessed May 2008).

50. *Santa Monica Community College Annual*, 1968.

51. "Class for Registered Nurses Opens at SMCC, *Los Angeles Times*, 21 Sep 1967, WS2.

52. "Origins of the Program," *Funding for the California State*

Notes, Pages 288-299

University's Statewide Nursing Program: A Report to the Legislature in Response to Supplemental Language to the 1988-89 Budget Act, (Commission Report 89-28, Oct 1989).

53. "American Nurses' Association's First Position on Education for Nursing." The *American Journal of Nursing 65*, no. 12 (1965): 106–11.

54. "The Registered Nurse Population: Findings from the National Sample Survey of Registered Nurses," (Washington, DC: U.S. Department of Health and Human Services, 1995): 16.

55. *Funding for CSU's Statewide Nursing*, 25 (1).

56. Ibid, 39 (15).

57. Ibid, 69 (3).

58. Ibid, 30 (2).

59. Ibid, 31 (3).

60. Ibid, 1 (8).

61. "Substantive Change Report, Prepared for the Senior Accrediting Commission of the Western Association of Schools and Colleges," *Funding for the California State University's Statewide Nursing Program*, 67.

62. www.usinflationcalculator.com (accessed 7 July 2024).

63. "Substantive Change Report," 73 (7).

64. "Memorandum of Understanding," *Transfer of Consortium BS and MS Programs in Nursing*, 86-87 (1-2).

65. Ibid, 88 (3).

66. *Funding for the California State University's Statewide Nursing Program: A Report...*,18 (11).

67. "Memorandum of Understanding," 100 (4).

68. *Statewide Nursing Program, Spring Term Class Schedule*, 1991, 17.

69. "School of Nursing Cuts Ribbon on Clinical Skills Lab," *CSUDH Campus News Center*, 18 Nov 2010.

70. "Nursing, OT Skills Labs Receive Federal Appropriations for Upgrades," *CSUDH Campus News Center*, 5 May 2022.

71. Per records of Kathleen Chai, former CSUDH BSN & MSN graduate, tenured professor, and SON director, 12 July 2024.

72. www.calfac.org/contract-2022-2025 (accessed 13 July 2024).

Chapter 11

1. https://nursing.cuanschutz.edu/about/news-archives/loretta-ford (accessed 14 July 2024).

2. Reilly, Bernard, "The Nurse Practitioner: Development of a New Role in Medical Care," *Journal of Health and Human Resources Administration*, vol. 3, no. 1 (Aug 1980): 100-111.

3. Author's interview with Robert Bragonier, 5 May 2009.

4. www.legacy.com/us/obituaries/latimes/name/j-bragonier-bituary?id=31363060 (accessed 15 July 2024).

5. https://lundquist.org/whcc-archive (accessed 2 Jan 2024).

6. Author's interview with Elsie Fontanilla, 27 Feb 2010.
7. Ibid.
8. www.mypnasc.org/our-history (accessed 28 Feb 2010).
9. www.bw.edu (accessed 05 Apr 2024).
10. Author's interview with Betty Smith Williams, 10 Feb 2010.
11. Williams, B.S, et. al., *Providing Safe Nursing Care for Ethnic People of Color*, (Appleton-Century-Crofts 1976).
12. Littleton, Scott C., *Gods, Goddesses, and Mythology*, Vol 4. Marshall, (New York 2005), 474–476.
13. https://canainc.org (accessed 1 Jun 2009).
14. "USC Department of Nursing, BSN Student Handbook, 1994-1995," USC Archives.
15. Gray, Barbara B., MN, RN, "USC Student Nurses Save Four in Crash," *Nurseweek*, 11 Nov 1991, 1.
16. Sklar, Jeff, "Nursing Program May Be Dropped," *Daily Trojan*, 23 Apr 2001, 1.
17. Waugaman W., Schneiderman J., "The Demise of Nursing Education at a Major Research University, *Nursing Outlook*, vol. 52, no. 6 (Nov-Dec 2004): 304-10.
18. www.kpsan.org/school/history (accessed 2 Jan 2010).
19. Anson, Jack L., *Baird's Manual of American Fraternities*, (Baird's Manual Foundation, Inc., Indianapolis, IN, 1991), 10–11.
20. Richwald, Gary A., MD MPH; Potik, Renee, RN, NP, et al. "Effectiveness of the Cavity-Rim Cervical Cap: Results of a Large Clinical Study," *Obstetrics & Gynecology*, vol. 74, no. 2 (Aug 1989): 143-148.
21. Klitsch M., "FDA Approval Ends Cervical Cap's Marathon," *Family Planning Perspect*, (May-Jun 1988): 137-8.
22. Author's interview with Renee Potik, 21 Jul 2008.
23. Liddick, Betty, "A Special Delivery via Nurse-Midwife," *Los Angeles Times*, 26 May 1974, C1.
24. Greulich, Betsy, et all, "Twelve Years and More Than 30,000 Nurse Midwife Attended Births," *Journal of Nures-Midwifery*, vol. 39, no. 4 (July/Aug 1994): 185-196.
25. Noyes, Clara, "Training School for Midwives at Bellevue and Allied Hospitals," *The American Journal of Nursing*, vol. 12, no. 5 (Feb 1912): 417-422.
26. Poole, Ernest, *Nurses on Horseback*, (Macmillian Company, New York, NY, 1932).
27. www.midwife.org (accessed 8 Jun 2009).
28. Author's interview with Frances Hayes-Cushenberry, 3 May 2009.
29. https://minoritynurse.com/tag/midwifery-certified-nurse-midwife-cnm (accessed 10 Apr 2024).
30. https://www.linkedin.com/in/h-frances-hayes-cushenberry-373a0614 (accessed 10 Apr 2024).
31. Author's interview with Deborah Henderson, 9 May 2009.

32. www.presidency.ucsb.edu/documents/statement-the-resignation-national-aids-policy-coordinator-kristine-gebbie (accessed 5 May 2009).

33. Lee, Marietta, "Kristine Gebbie," *American Journal of Nursing*, (Feb 1995): 34-37.

34. DeBuono, Barbara, et al., "Applying Your Degree to Public Health Practice," The *Pfizer Guide to Careers in Public Health* (Pfizer Pharm. Group, 2002): 178-182.

35. "Mom at Center," *New York Times*, 16 Jul 1992.

36. Dicker, Shira, "Slowly, Midwives Gain a Niche in the County," *New York Times*, 7 June 1992.

37. Author's interview with Dianne S. Moore, 23 Feb 2010.

38. "Doctoral Students Go Back to Basics to Better Understand Clinical Problems," *UCLA Nursing*, vol. 19 (2002): 16.

39. "Attin Recognized by American Heart Association," *Nursing, University. Rochester School of Nursing*, vol. 1, (2018): 11.

40. "Wendie Robbins: Identifying Exposures That Increase Reproductive Risk," *UCLA Nursing*, vol. 19 (2002): 12.

41. https://ph.ucla.edu/about/faculty-staff-directory/wendie-robbins (accessed 14 Apr 2024).

42. Author's interview with Courtney Lyder, 1 Sep 2009.

43. "More About Lyder," *UCLA Newsroom*, August 2008.

44. Ruccione, Kathleen, PhD, MPH, RN, FAAN, "More Than Just an Old Brick," *Advance for Nurses, Southern California* (14 May 2007): 16.

45. Interviews with Diane Harris-Hara, RN, BSN, 13 June 2024, and Phyllis Esslinger, RN, PHN, MSN, 18 Nov 2024.

46. Author's interview with Anissa Perez, 2 Mar 2010.

47. Edwards, Bob "Gloria Molina Becomes New LA Supervisor," *NPR*, 20 Feb 1991, 1.

48. https://www.lanahn.com (accessed 24 Apr 2009).

49. Author's interview with Angie Millan, 22 April 2009.

50. www.chamberlain.edu/staff/angie-millan (accessed 14 Apr 2024).

51. www.kanasc.org (accessed 15 Apr 2024).

52. Author's interview with Aimie Pak, 25 Feb 2010.

53. Author's interview with Ellen Kane, 25 Jan 2010.

54. Author's interview with Eduardo Barreto, 25 Jan 2010.

Chapter 12

1. Moore, Dianne, "West Coast University," *Innovations in Professional Nursing Education Awards 2010 Call for Nominations* (February 2010).

2. www.rn.ca.gov/education/passrates.shtml (accessed 10 Apr 2024).

3. www.2010iyn.net (accessed 15 Apr 2010).

4. www.icn.ch/news/icn-calls-heads-state-back-year-nurse-and-midwife (accessed 15 Apr 2024).

5. "Vision of 75 Years," (Sigma Theta Tau International, Honor Society,

1997): 56-57, IC 087 Guide to Beta Beta Houston Records 1969-2011 (2019), box 6.

6. https://www.csuci.edu/news/releases/2020-nursing-honor-society.htm (accessed 17 Feb 2024).

7. Author's interview with Deva-Marie Beck, 31 Mar 2010.

8. Beck, Deva-Marie, et all, *Florence Nightingale Today: Healing, Leadership, Global Action* (American Nurses Association, 2005).

9. Author's interview with Cindy Coleman Jones, 10 Feb 2010.

10. Author's interview with Sally M. Bixby, 7 Feb 2010.

11. Author's experience decorating the Nurse's Float, 12 Dec 2012.

12. www.arching.com (accessed 17 Feb 2024).

13. https://janegoodall.org/our-story/about-jane (accessed Feb 2024).

14. https://janegoodall.org/wp-content/uploads/the-Jane-Goodall-Institute_Boilerplate.pdf (accessed 17 Feb 2024).

15. "Nurses' Float Announces Riders for 2013 Rose Parade,®" *Marketwired*, 26 Nov 2012.

Chapter 13

1. https://nursing.yale.edu/news/commencement-nursing-pins-signify-honor-and-tradition (accessed 26 Apr 2024).

2. "PUC to Eliminate Traditional Nurse Pining Ceremony," The *Times*, 23 Oct 2015, A3.

3. "The College Training School for Nurses first graduation program," 6 June 1897, *Lindley Scrapbooks*, Libraries of Claremont Colleges.

4. "Trained Nurses," *Los Angeles Times*, 9 Jun 1897, 5.

5. "Three Graduate from Good Samaritan Hospital Class," *Los Angeles Herald*, 21 July 1898.

6. "Invitation for the First Annual Commencement of the Training School for Nurses at the California Hospital," 29 June 1899, *Lindley Scrapbooks*, Libraries of Claremont Colleges.

7. www.lacsonalumni.org/about-us (accessed 6 Dec 2023).

8. www.stvincentmedicalcenter.com/about/history.htm (accessed 5 May 2007).

9. "They Are Full Fledged Nurses," *Los Angeles Herald*, 17 Dec 1901.

10. https://pasadenacf.org/funds/pcc-hmh-schools-of-nursing-alumni-association-endowment (accessed 20 Apr 2024).

11. Montag, Mildred, "Experimental Programs in Nursing," *American Journal of Nursing*, vol. 55, no. 1 (Jan 1955): 45.

12. Clara Barton Hospital School of Nursing, 1910-1989, OAC. https://oac.cdlib.org/findaid/ark:/13030/tf009n99t3/entire_text (accessed 20 Apr 2024).

13. Register of the Clara Barton Hospital School of Nursing Collection, 1910-1989, Louise M. Darling Biomedical Library, History and Special Collections Division, University of California, Los Angeles.

14. 1905 Brochure at Glendale Adventist Medical Center Archives.
15. "Pomona Nurses Graduate," *Los Angeles Times*, 28 Jun 1907, II, 10.
16. "Pomona Valley Hospital," *Daily Bulletin*, 3 Mar 2017, Opinion.
17. "Pomona Nurses Graduate," *Los Angeles Times*.
18. "Many See Angelus Nurses Graduate," The *Los Angeles Examiner*, 28 Jul 1908.
19. Information at Methodist Hospital Archives, 2009.
20. "Unit For Anesthesia Recovery Saves Lives," *Los Angeles Times*, 17 Jul 1953, A7.
21. Schipske Gerrie, "Historical Look at LB Hospitals," *Beachcomber*, 28 Mar 2019.
22. White Memorial Hospital Collection, (Loma Linda University, Loma Linda, CA, 2009).
23. Ibid.
24. Gann, Dan M. *At Forty: The Queen of Angels Hospital Story*, (Queen of Angels, 1967).
25. Ibid.
26. "History," *Hollywood Presbyterian School of Nursing Booklet*, 4. Hollywood Presbyterian Archives.
27. Ibid.
28. "Medical Corpsmen Earn Their RNs," *Holly Press*, Apr 1972, 2.
29. Clara Barton Hospital School of Nursing Collection, 1910-1989.
30. "The 50th Anniversary of the Mount's Nursing Program," *The Mount* (Spring 2002): 12-15.
31 Ibid.
32. Barnett, R., and Gordon, D., eds, UCLA School of Nursing Alumni Association. History Committee, *History of the UCLA School of Nursing*, (University of California, Jan 1999).
33. "UCLA to Bring Back Nursing Program," *Los Angeles Times*, 27 Nov 2005.
34. "Los Angeles State College of Applied Arts and Science Bulletin 1956-1957," 209.
35. Ibid.
36. "Graduate Student Handbook, 2020" (California State University, Long Beach School of Nursing), 6.
37. www.csulb.edu/historical/1964-1965 (accessed 22 Apr 2024).
38. Gewe, A. Fleeger, R. *50 Years of God's Faithfulness: the History of the Biola Department of Nursing, 1966-2016* (Biola University, Sep 2018).
39. Ibid, 11.
40. www.apu.edu/nursing/about/timeline (accessed 1 May 2024).
41. Ibid.
42. Waugaman W. and Schneiderman J., "The Demise of Nursing Education at a Major Research University, *Nursing Outlook*, vol. 52, no. 6 (Nov-Dec 2004): 304-10.
43. https://dworakpeck.usc.edu (accessed 13 Nov 2024).

44. "Statement of Accreditation Status American University of Health Sciences, 2023." www.wscuc.org/institutions/american-university-of-health-sciences/?print=pdf (accessed 24 Apr 2024).

45. Email from Olivia Solis, University Archivist, 3 Jul 2024.

46. Ibid.

47. www.cdrewu.edu/academics/college-of-nursing/history-con; www.cdrewu.edu/about/history (accessed 1 May 2024).

48. www.cdrewu.edu/academics (accessed 24 Apr 2024).

49. "Statewide Nursing Program Responses to Questions Raised," *Funding for the California State Univ. Statewide Nursing Program: A Report to the Legislature* (Oct 1989): 29 (3).

50. Ibid, 32 (4).

51. "Statewide Nursing Program Responses to Questions Raised," *Funding for the California State Univ. Statewide Nursing Program: A Report to the Legislature* (Oct 1989): 36 (9).

52. "The Registered Nurse Population: Findings from the National Sample Survey of Registered Nurses" (Washington, DC: U.S. Department of Health and Human Services, 1995): 16.

53. www.csun.edu/health-human-development/news/csun-nursing-celebrates-20-years (accessed 20 Apr 2024).

54. "American Nurses' Association's First Position on Education for Nursing." The *American Journal of Nursing, 65,* no. 12 (1965): 106–11.

55. "The Registered Nurse Population: Findings from the National Sample Survey of Registered Nurses" (U.S. Department of Health and Human Services, Mar 1996).

56. Smiley, R., et al., "The 2022 National Nursing Workforce Survey," *Journal of Nursing Regulation*, vol 14 (Apr 2023): Supplement.

57. www.britannica.com/topic/University-of-Phoenix (5 July 2024).

58. Handford, Emily, "The Story of the University of Phoenix," (American Public Media, n.d.).

59. Steele, David, "One University of Phoenix Campus Left After 2025," www.insidehighered.com (accessed 27 Apr 2022).

60. Email from Carol Marroquin, Nursing Operations Specialist, Los Angeles Nursing Department, National University, 24 Apr 2024.

61. Moore, Dianne, "West Coast University," *Innovations in Professional Nursing Education Awards 2010 Call for Nominations*, Feb 2010.

62. Ibid.

63. Interview with Director of Nurses, Adelisa Blanco, RN, June 2024.

64. "1.4 History," *Angeles College Catalog*, 2023-2024, 5.

65. Bond, Emily, "Chamberlain University Opens New Campus in Irwindale, California," 1 Mar 2021, www.chamberlain.edu/blog/chamberlain-university-opens-new-campus-in-irwindale-california (accessed 1 June 2024).

66. www.chamberlain.edu/nursing-school/illinois/addison (accessed 5 July 2024).

67. "Cheers to our inaugural LA campus BSN cohort BSNLA001," Stanbridge University, Facebook post, 22 Mar 2024 (accessed 6 Jul 2024).

68. Montag, Mildred, "Experimental Programs in Nursing," *American Journal of Nursing*, vol. 55, no. 1 (Jan 1955): 45.

69. Hiatt, Wilma, "Associate Degree Nursing Programs in California," *American Journal of Nursing* (Oct 1961): 93-95.

70. "News," *American Journal of Nursing* vol. 86, no. 12 (Dec 1986).

71. "Community College Layoffs," *Los Angeles Times*, 9 May 1986, 39.

72. "Registered Nursing Program Celebrates its Ten-Year Anniversary," *LACC Foundation Homepage News*, 23 Apr 2014.

73. *Los Angeles County Medical Center School, Looking Back a Century of Nursing*, (Centennial Book Committee Los Angeles County, 2000).

74. Ibid.

75. *Mt. San Antonio College First 50 Years*, (Mt. San Antonio College Library), n.d.

76. *Mt. San Antonio College Catalog, 1958-1959*. (Mt. San Antonio College Library), n.d.

77. Email from Marc Smith, v.p. of nursing, LBCC, 6 May 2024.

78. "Student Handbook," *Associate Degree Nursing 2023-2024*, Long Beach City College, Aug 2023, 44.

79. www.lavc.edu/academics/pathways/hps/hs-dept (accessed 26 Apr 2024).

80. Ibid.

81. "History of the El Camino College Associate Degree Nursing Program," *2020-2021 Student Handbook* (7-29-2020): 10.

82. Ibid.

83. www.ourweekly.com/2019/06/20/compton-college-nursing-program-has-received-state (accessed 2 May 2024).

84. "Nursing Information Session, Los Angeles Harbor College," Sep 2020, 4; www.lahc.edu/sites/lahc.edu/files/2023-02/January2023LAHCNursinginfo.pdf (accessed 2 May 2024).

85. Ibid.

86. "Cerritos College Program Review, Nursing Program," (Cerritos College, Spring 2019): 2.

87. Ibid.

88. https://mdharrismd.com/2014/10/26/useful-latin-sayings (accessed 2 May 2024).

89. www.lasc.edu/about/history (accessed 7 Jul 2024).

90. "Nursing Student Handbook," (Los Angeles Southwest College Department of Nursing, Feb 2009): 9.

91. Ibid.

92. "Class for Registered Nurses Opens at SMCC," *Los Angeles Times*, 21 Sept 1967, WS2.

93. www.dol.gov/general/aboutdol/history/mono-mdtatext (accessed 4 May 2014).

94. Steffes, Tracy, "Smith-Hughes Act," 1917, www.britannica.com/topic/Smith-Hughes-Act (accessed 30 Apr 2024).

95. "SMC Nursing Celebrates a 50 Year Calling, vol II, issue 1," (Santa Monica College, 9 Feb 2016) www.smc.edu/news/in-focus/2016/vol-ii-issue-1/01-04-smc-nursing.php (accessed 30 Apr 2024).

96. Email from Pierce Library via Nursing Dept. Chair, 20 Apr 2024.

97. Estimated graduation date based on opening of the college.

98. "History of the College," www.wlac.edu/about/college-history (accessed 30 Apr 2024).

99. "Community College Layoffs," *Los Angeles Times,* 9 May 1986.

100. "Los Angeles Trade-Tech. College," *2014-2016 General Catalog.*

101. Ibid.

102. Blumes, H., Harris L.,"Graduate of Rio Hondo Nursing Program Is also Mother of 9," *Los Angeles Times,* 10 Feb 1991.

103. "General Information About Rio Hondo College: History," *Rio Hondo College Catalog, 2019-2020,* 8.

104. Brady, David, "Rae Yoshida; Antelope Valley College Official," *Los Angeles Times,* 10 Dec 1994, VYB5.

105. Ibid.

106. Email from Tammy Bathke, PhD, RN, Nursing Program Director of College of the Canyons, 13 May 2024.

107. "Nursing Student Handbook," *College of the Canyons, Spring 2021,* 81.

108. https://campusguides.glendale.edu/chaparral2014-2015/chaparral23311 (accessed 18 Feb 2024).

109. Ibid.

110. www.glendale.edu/academics/academic-divisions/health-sciences-division/nursing/mission-and-philosophy (accessed 18 Feb 2024).

111. "A Golden Celebration for a Jewel of a Program," The *Mount, Spring, 2002,* 14.

112. Ibid.

113. Email from Herminina Honda, Dean of Research and Planning, Los Angeles County College of Nursing and Allied Health, 3 July 2024.

114. https://dhs.lacounty.gov/college-of-nursing-and-allied-health/home/who-we-are (accessed 5 May 2024).

115. www.citruscollege.edu/academics/programs/adn/Pages/default.aspx (accessed 3 May 2024).

116. "ACC to Offer First Associate Degree in Nursing Program at Los Angeles Campus," (27 Jan 2015) https://americancareercollege.edu/blog/acc_to_offer_first_associate_degree_in_nursing_program_at_its_los_angeles_campus (accessed 6 May 2024).

117. www.zippia.com/american-career-college-careers-679885/history (accessed 3 May 2024).

118. https://californiacareercollege.edu/associate-degree-in-nursing-program (accessed 29 Apr 2024).

119. "Career Care Institute, Student Catalog," (June 1, 2020-May 31, 2021, July 2020): 5.

120. "Compton College Nursing Program has Received State Accreditation," *Our Weekly, Los Angeles* (20 June 2019) www.ourweekly.com/2019/06/20/compton-college-nursing-program-has-received-state/ (accessed 5 June 2024).

121. Ibid.

122. www.nursingschoolsalmanac.com/rankings/california (accessed 5 May 2024).

123. https://mitchellfuerst.com/north-west-college-founder-marsha-fuerst-dies-79 (accessed 6 May 2024).

124. Smith Chason Nursing Instagram post, 24 Nov 2023, "A special shout out to our ADN graduates for being the first cohort to graduate in the history of Smith Chason College."

125. https://smithchason.com/blog/remembering-co-founder-dr-neville-smith (accessed 5 May 2004).

126. "University of La Verne Receives $2.3 Million Gift to Support New College of Health and Community Well-Being." *University of LaVerne* (11 May 2022) www.prweb.com/releases/university-of-la-verne-receives-2-3-million-gift-to-support-new-college-of-health-and-community-well-being-835715121.html (accessed 8 Sep 2024).

127. www.cccco.edu/About-Us/Chancellors-Office/Divisions/Educational-Services-and-Support/What-we-do/Curriculum-and-Instruction-Unit/Curriculum/Baccalaureate-Degree-Program (accessed 8 Sep 2024).

128. "LVN 30-unit option," *California BRN 2016 Supplemental Sunset Report* (California Board of Registered Nursing, 31 Dec 2016): 30.

129. https://nursinglicensemap.com/nursing-degrees/nursin,g-accreditation (accessed 6 May 2024).

130. "Accreditation, Attrition, and On-Time Completion Rates," www.rn.ca.gov/education/attrition.shtml (accessed 7 May 2024).

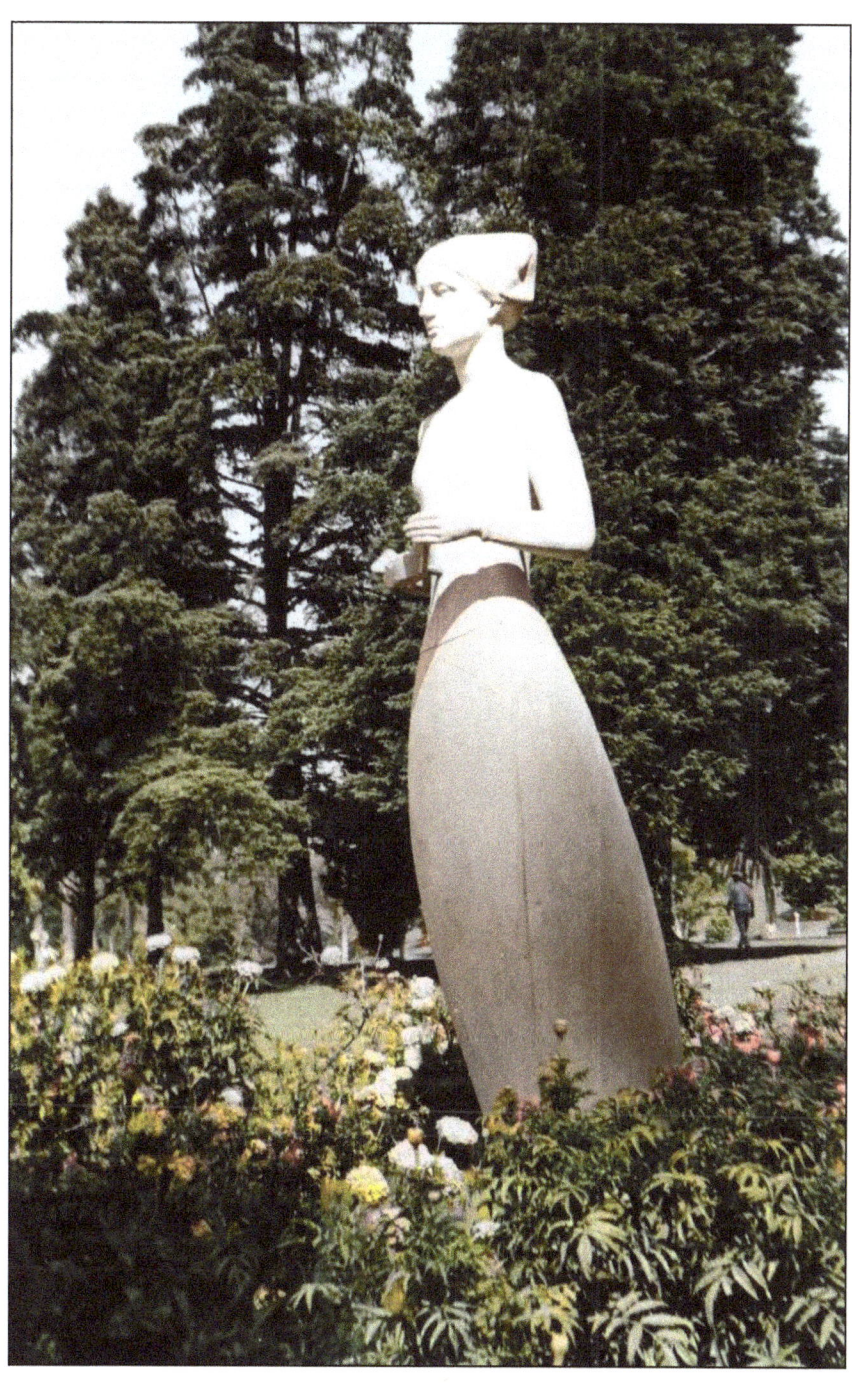

14.01. *Florence Nightingale* statue in Lincoln Park, Los Angeles, c. 1938. C.

Bibliography

1. Adams, Ansel, *Born Free and Equal: Photographs of the Loyal Japanese-Americans at Manzanar Relocation Center,* Inyo County, CA, U.S. Camera, 1944.
2. Allen County Public Library Genealogy Center, *An Illustrated History of Southern California,* The Lewis Publishing Company, 1890.
3. Barlow, John F., "Barlow Genealogy 1998-2005," *Who's Who in Los Angeles*, Barlow Foundation.
4. Beasley, Delilah, *Negro Tail Blazers of California*, California, 1919.
5. Beck, Deva-Marie, et al., *Florence Nightingale Today: Healing, Leadership, Global Action*, American Nurses Association, 2005.
6. Bostridge, Mark, *Florence Nightingale: The Making of an Icon,* Farrar, Straus, and Giroux, 2008.
7. Brown, Les, *The New York Times Encyclopedia of Television*, Random House Inc, 1977.
8. Budreau, Lisa M., Prior, Richard M., *Answering The Call: The U.S. Army Nurse Corps, 1917-1919: A Commemorative Tribute to Military Nursing in World War I*, Gov. Printing Office, 10 Nov. 2008.
9. Bullough, V. and Sentz, L., *American Nursing: A Biographical Dictionary, Volume 3*, Springer Publishing, 2004.
10. Clark, David, *A History of Good Samaritan Hospital in Los Angeles: 1885 -2010 A Tradition of Caring,* Good Samaritan Hospital, 2010.
11. Cook E.T., The Life of Florence Nightingale, London, UK: Macmillan and Co., 1913.
12. Coste, Pierre, *The Life and Works of Saint Vincent de Paul*, Newman Press, 1952.
13. Danner, Dorothy Still, *What a Way to Spend a War*, Maine: G.K. Hall & Co., 1995.
14. Davis, Margaret Leslie, *Childrens Hospital and the Leaders of Los Angeles: The First 100 Years*, Childrens Hospital Los Angeles, 2002.
15. Dirvin, Joseph, *Mrs. Seton: Foundress of the American Sisters of Charity.* Farrar, Straus and Giraux, 1975.
16. Dumke, Glenn, "The Boom of the 1880s in Southern California," *Southern California Quarterly*, vol. 76, no. 1, 1994.
17. Ellis, J.R. & Hartley, C.L. *Nursing in Today's World: Challenges, Issues and Trends*, 3rd Ed., Lippincott, 1988.
18. Engh, Michael, "Soldiers of Christ, Angels of Mercy: The Daughters of Charity in Los Angeles, 1856–1888," *Vincentian Heritage Journal*, vol. 15, iss. 1, 1994.
19. Ferrell, Robert H., The Strange Deaths of President Harding, University of Missouri Press, 1998.
20. Franks, Sr. C.M., *The Historical Development of Nursing*, W.B. Saunders Co., 1953.

21. Galvani, William, "The Perseverance of Lieutenant Nash," *Naval History* Apr 2023.

22. Gann, Dan M., *At Forty: The Queen of Angels Hospital Story*, Queen of Angels, 1967.

23. Gewe, A. Fleeger, R. *50 Years of God's Faithfulness: The History of the Biola Department of Nursing, 1966-2016*, Biola University, Sep 2018.

24. Gill, Christopher J "Nightingale in Scutari: her legacy reexamined," *Clinical Infectious Diseases,* vol. 40, no. 12, 15 June 2005.

25. Guerrero, Laura Zaragoza, "The Mount," 2002, vol. 19 no., 4.

26. Goodnow, Minnie, *Outlines in Nursing History*, W.B. Saunders Co., 1939.

27. Gutierrez, Gail, "Alice Jean Turner" *Women in the Military, Oral History Project,* California State University, Fullerton, May 9, 1987.

28. Hampton, Isabel A., *Nursing: Its Principles and Practice*, 1893.

29. Haynes, Francis L., "Surgical Nursing," *Southern California Practitioner,* vol. XIV, 1899.

30. *The History of the UCLA Nursing School, California*, History Committee of the UCLA School of Nursing Alumni Association, Regent of the University of California, 1999.

31. Holland, Mary, *Our Army Nurses*, Wilkins & Co., 1895.

32. Johnson, D. E. "The Behavioral System Model for Nursing," *Theoretical Basis for Nursing*, Lippincott Williams & Wilkins, 1980.

33. Kellogg, John Harvey, "Breakfast Cereals," *The New Dietetics: What to Eat and How*, Modern Medicine Publishing, 1921.

34. Keeling, Kirchgessner, Hehman, *History of Professional Nursing in the United States,* Springer, 2017.

35. Koslow, Jennifer, *Cultivating Health*, Rutgers Univ. Press, 2009.

36. Kress, George, *Medical Professions of Southern California*, 1910.

37. Martin, Helen, *The History of the Los Angeles County Hospital,* California, University of Southern California Press, 1979.

38. McGroarty, John Steven, *Los Angeles from the Mountains to the Sea,* American Historical Society, 1921.

39. McNeil, Mary Germaine, *History of Mount St. Mary's College, Los Angeles, 1925-1975,* Vantage Press, 1985.

40. Mieding, Virginia, *Los Angeles County Medical Center School, Looking Back a Century of Nursing*, Centennial Book Committee Los Angeles County, 2000.

41. Montag, M.L. "Experimental Programs in Nursing," *American Journal of Nursing,* Jan. 1955, vol. 55, no. 1, 45-46.

42. Newmark, Harris, *Sixty Years in Southern California, 1853–1913,* Knickerbocker Press, 1916.

43. Nordland, Ole J., *History of the Coachella Valley Water District*, Desert Printing Co. Inc., 1968.

44. Nordhoff, Charles, *California, for Health, Pleasure, and Residence*, Harper, 1875.

45. Norman, Elizabeth, *We Band of Angels*, Pocket Books, 1999.
46. Porter, Nellie, "Affiliates with Junior Colleges in California," *American Journal of Nursing*, September 1932, 975-982.
47. Potemkina, Antonia, "Margaret Sirch," *The Trained Nurse and Hospital Review*, Volumes 100-101, Lakeside Publishing Company, 1938.
48. Pagano, Penny, "Ex-POW Nurses Relive the Pain, Heroism in Philippines on a Day of Remembering," *Los Angeles Times*, April 10, 1983.
49. Patterson, Tom, "Dr. June Hill Robertson McCarroll," *The 1997 Periscope*, 3 Mar 1997, Valley Historical Society, Indio, CA, Coachella.
50. Poole, Ernest, *Nurses on Horseback*, Macmillian Company, 1932.
51. Potemkina, Antonia, "Meet the First Editor," *The Trained Nurse and Hospital Review*, vol. C, no. 4, Lakeside Publishing, 1938.
52. Reynolds, Keld J. *Outreach: Loma Linda University, 1905-1967*, Loma Linda University, 1968.
53. Richards, Linda, *Reminiscences of America's First Trained Nurse*, Whitcomb & Barrows, 1911.
54. Ringheim, Alice, "Nursing Education in Junior Colleges," *The American Journal of Nursing*: vol. 32, no. 9.
55. Robinson, Thelman M., *Nisei Cadet Nurse of World War II: Patriotism in Spite of Prejudice*, Black Swan Mill Press, 2005.
56. Seacole, Mary, *Wonderful Adventures of Mrs. Seacole in Many Lands*, Oxford University Press, 1988 (1857).
57. Seymour, Wm. W., The Cross in Tradition History and Art, 1898.
58. Smith, Jill Halcomb, *Dressed for Duty*, R.J. Bender, 2001.
Sterner, Doris, *In and Out of Harm's Way, A History of the Navy Nurse Corps*, Peanut Butter Publishing, 1997.
59. Treacy, Jane, *Vision of 75 years: An anniversary celebration, 1922-1997*, Center Nursing Press, 1997.
60. Van Nest, Ronald, "The Life and Trial of Dagmar Nelson," *American Nurse Anesthetist Journal,* August 2006.
61. Wallis, Michael, Route 66: *The Mother Road*, Macmillan, 1990.
62. Weatherford, Doris, *American Women and WWII*, Facts on File, 1990.
63. Williams, Betty Smith, "A Historical Review of Ethnic Nurse Associations," *Providing Safe Nursing for Ethnic People of Color*, Appleton Century Crofts, 1976.
64. Vorspan, Max, and Gartner, Lloyd, *History of the Jews of Los Angeles*, Jewish Publication Society of America, 1970.
65. Williamson, Anne, *50 Years in Starch*, Murray & Gee Inc., 1948.
66. Wright, Florence, Industrial Nursing, Macmillan Company, 1920.

Index

A

Adair, Birdie May, 112
advertisements, nurse, 296-297
Aerial Nurse Corps of America, 135-140, 165
Alpha Delta Nu, 225
Alpha Tau Delta, 120, 262, 305
American Career College, 316, 346
American Nurses Association (ANA), 105, 142, 148, 183, 213, 225, 273-274, 304
American University of Health Sciences, 337
Angeles College, 340
Angelus Hospital Training School for Nurses, 84-85, 124, 334
Antelope Valley College, 344
Arlington National Cemetery, 59, 167, 169, 178-179
Army Nurse Corps, 25, 59, 76, 96, 107, 114, 118-119, 141, 148, 163-167, 170-172, 183-189, 202, 232, 236, 248, 252-255, 260, 262, 308
Army School of Nursing, 118-119, 148, 202, 260
Assinesi, Tony, 227
Attin, Mina, 312
Aviation Meet, Los Angeles International, 87
Azusa Pacific University, 17, 121, 315, 337

B

Baccalaureate Degree (BSN), 257-262, 269-271, 284, 286, 288-291, 304, 323, 331, 334, 336-340, 348
Barber, Dr. D.C., ix, 33-34, 39, 55, 83
Barlow Sanatorium, 70-71, 156-157
Barreto, Eduardo, back cover photo, 321
Barton, Clara, 75-79, 86, 104, 225, 333
Beck, Deva-Marie, 325
Bella Union Hotel, 11
Bellevue Hospital School of Nursing, 34, 102, 242, 281, 307, 331
Biola University, 337
Birmingham Military Hospital, 172, 186-189
Bishop Johnson School of Nursing, 199, 332
Bixby, Sally M., 327-328
Black nurse groups, 20-23, 117, 183, 267, 302-303, 314
Bloch, Carol and Carolyn, 317
Board of Examiners, 42, 46, 95, 103
Bolton Act/Cadet Nurse Corps, 179-181, 183, 274, 278, 302

Borg, Martha, 132
Bradley, Colonel Ruby Grace, 167
Brotherton, Marie G., 238
Brown, Adeline, 238
Bryan, Edith, 115
Bullough, Bonnie and Vern, 274-275
Burgess, Vivian, 259, 276

C

California Career College, 346
California Hospital, 17, 37, 41, 45-51, 54, 59, 81, 86-87, 113, 213, 238, 284-285, 315, 332
California State University, Dominguez Hills, 121, 288-291, 338
California State University, Long Beach, 89, 121, 274, 278, 286, 288, 299, 302, 305, 336
California State University, Los Angeles, 120-121, 230, 285, 336
California State University, Northridge, 121, 274, 324, 339
California State University, Channel Islands, 121, 324
caps, history of, 14, 198, 216, 331
Career Care Institute, 346
Campanaro, Lynn, 246
Campiglia, Clementine, 182
Casey, Ben, 224
Cedars of Lebanon Hospital, 67, 192, 214-215, 226, 300
Cedars-Sinai Medical Center, 67, 131, 210, 215, 223, 242-243, 300
Cerritos College, 343
cervical cap, Prentif, 302
Chamberlain University, 317, 340
Cherry Ames, 160
Childrens Hospital, 57, 80-81, 128, 230, 238, 258, 325
Civil War, 24-26, 58, 95
Citrus College, 346
Clinton, Pat, 223
Clinton, President William (Bill), 310
Clos, Yvonne, 57
Coachella Valley, 30-31
College of the Canyons, 345
College Settlement, 60-63, 66
College Training School for Nurses, ix, 33-48, 55, 332
comics and art, nurses, 130, 161, 294-295
Comport, Mae, 67
Compton College, 308, 342, 347
Consortium, California State University, 288–291, 338
Continuing Education, original mandate, 267

Corns, Edith, 165, 173
Council of Black Nurses, 302-303
coxcomb graph/Rose Diagram, 18
Crimean War, 17-21, 89, 100-101, 331
Croix de Guerre (Cross of War), 96, 114
Crosby, Kathryn Grant and Bing, 216, 222
Cuddeback, Elizabeth, 88-89

D

Danner, Dorothy Still, 164, 168, 173
Daughters/Sisters of Charity, 11-17, 56, 58-59, 148, 198, 200, 333
Dauser, Sue, 113
Davison, Maude C., 170-171, 173
Deaconess Hospital, 75
deaf nurses, 240
Desert Shield/Desert Storm, 252
Doan, Sister Rebecca, 257-258, 276
Doctor of Nursing Science degree program, first in Los Angeles, 269
Duarte, Ray, 244

E

East Los Angeles College, 316-317, 341
Eclectic Medicine, 75
El Camino College, 308, 331, 342
Ellen White, 133, 147
Esslinger, Phyllis, 315
Ethnic Nurse Groups, 301-303, 317-318

F

first ambulance, Goodhew, 55
first school of nursing, Los Angeles, 33-46
first graduating class photos, 41, 49, 53, 65, 73, 76, 85, 90, 118, 127, 132, 199, 257, 282-287, 299, 305
first hospital, Los Angeles, 13-15
first Matron-Superintendent, Los Angeles, 37, 42
Filipino Nurses, POW, 172
Filipino Nurses Club, 301
Fontanilla, Elsie, 300-301
Freed, Margaret Anderson, 156-157
French, Francis Allen, 146-147
French Hospital, 57, 93
Future Nurses Club, 225

G

Gebbie, Kristine, 310
Glendale Community College, 345
Glendale Hospital, 206
Glendale Sanitarium, 72-74, 180, 334
Golden State Hospital, 146
gravesite/headstone, 21, 23, 63, 108, 178
great depression, vii, 107, 122, 133, 189
Good Samaritan Hospital, 37, 46, 52-54, 81, 112, 128-129, 180, 230, 332
golden shovel, 263
Gunter, Laurie, 273

H

Hamaguchi, Aiko, front cover photo, 176-177
Harbor-UCLA, 299, 306, 309, 317, 393
Harris-Hara, Diane, 17, 315
Hassenplug, Lulu Wolf, 214, 257, 260-266, 269-270
Hayes, Margaret, 24
Hayes-Cushenberry, Frances, 308
Henderson, Deborah Parkman, 309
Henderson, Florence, 92-93
Highway Hostess Nurses, 145
Hispanic Nurses, Association of National & Los Angeles, 317
Hollywood Bowl, 148-149
Hollywood Presbyterian Hospital, 77, 199, 228, 236-237, 280, 315, 335
Homestead Schools, 340
hospital ships, 18, 59, 113, 148, 163, 169, 173, 204-205
Hospital Week, 211-213
Hutchinson, Gertrude, 281

I

industrial nurses, 25, 103, 142, 196, 272
infant milk stations, 63
influenza of 1918, 116, 131, 189
International Year of the Nurse, 324-325
infection control nurse/nurse epidemiologist, 300

J

Jacob, Joyce, 17, 285
Japanese nurses interred, 176-177, 179
Joan of Arc Statue (Jeanne d'Arc), 57

Johnson, Major Lorraine., 232
Johnson, President Lyndon, 266
Jones, Cindy Coleman, 326-327
Jonestown, 241
Jury, Barbara, 284

K

Kaiser Permanente Hospital, 150-151, 278, 305, 315
Kane, Ellen, 320
Kaspare Cohn Hospital, 67
Keil, Lillian Kinkella, 174
Kelly, Joyce, 278-279
Kelly, Virginia Clinton, 310
Key, Nurses Home at Mount Sinai Home for Chronic Invalids, 131
Kiss, Times Square, 192-193
Knights Hospitaller/Crusaders/Knights Templar, 70, 99-101
Korean Nurses' Association of Southern California, 318
Korean War, 167, 169, 174, 259

L

Lackey, Anna Lois, 128-129
Lindley, Doctor Walter, 34-41, 46-47, 50
Lindley Hospital, Sixth Street Hospital, 34, 37, 39, 41, 45, 47, 50
Long Beach City College, 170, 342
Los Angeles City College, 112, 176, 286-287, 341
Los Angeles County General Hospital, ix, 17, 33-39, 41-42, 45-46, 55, 69, 83, 110-111, 117, 120, 152-156, 164-165, 172, 180, 210, 220, 224, 233, 244, 268, 277, 307, 317, 332
Los Angeles Harbor College, 342
Los Angeles Infirmary/Sister's Hospital, 13, 56, 67, 323, 333
Los Angeles Pierce College, 343
Los Angeles Southwest College, 343
Los Angeles Trade-Technical College, 344
Los Angeles Valley College, 342
Lyder, Courtney, 314

M

Male Nurses, 65, 74, 198, 221, 227-231, 236-237, 314, 333
Major, Grace Williams, 109
Manzanar War Relocation Center, 175-177
Mason, Biddy, 22-23
Masters Entry Into Nursing, 291, 302, 338

McCarroll, June Robertson, 30-31
Mervyn M. Dymally College of Nursing at CDU, 338
Messerly, Robert, 230
Methodist Hospital, 90-91, 150-151, 198, 219, 315, 334
Methodist Hospital, German, 75
Millan, Angie, 317
Moore, Annie, 241
Moore, Dianne Susan, 311
Mount San Antonio College, 197, 341
Mount St. Mary's College, 120-121, 201, 257-268, 276-277, 298, 336
Mount Sinai Home for the Incurables, 131
Mount Sinai Hospital, 42, 67, 131, 215, 223, 243

N

National Nurses Week, 18, 148, 213
National Student Nurses Association, 225, 263
National University, 339
Naval Hospitals, 113, 164, 168-169, 179, 190, 204-205, 251
Navy nurses, 107, 113-114, 148, 163-164, 166, 168-169, 173, 178-179, 189-191, 204, 232, 251, 315
Navy ship the USS Consolation AH-15 (US Hope), 169, 205
Neill, Sara, 40-41, 47-48
Nelson, Dagmar, 93-96
Neuman, Betty, 272
Nightingale, Florence, 14, 16-20, 34, 89, 100-102, 148-149, 154, 198, 225, 243, 262, 264-265, 324-325, 331, 377
Nightingale Jewel, 100
Nixon, President, 213
North-West College/Marsha Fuerst SON/Glendale Career College, 347
Nurse Anesthetists, 92-97, 278-279, 304-305, 304, 310
Nurse Midwives, 102, 247, 307, 311
Nurse Practitioners, 259, 274, 285, 299, 304, 313-317 323, 348, 393
Nurses Club & Apartments, 93, 124-125
Nurses Memorial, 58-59, 178-179, 248-249
Nutting, Adelaide, 262

O

Operation Babylift, Vietnam, 250

P

Pacific Hospital, 64-65, 333
Pahl, Harriet Waugh, 53, 85

Pak, Aimie and Oknyu, 319
Panama Canal, 89, 218
Parades, Nurses in, 110-112, 193, 238, 326-329
Parachute Nurse Movie, 138
Pasadena City College, 282-283, 309, 326-327, 329, 333, 341
Pasadena Tournament of Roses Parade, 326-329
Perez, Anissa, 316
Petrello, Colonel Judith, 253
Philippine Nurses Association, 301
Philippines, 163-172, 300-301, 315
pins (awards, badges, graduate nursing pins), 41, 76, 96, 99-105, 114, 118, 120-121, 123, 140, 144, 159, 170, 181, 225, 260, 262, 304, 331-349
polio, 152-153, 156, 202
Pomona Valley Hospital, 334
Pomona Valley Memorial Park, 108
Potik, Renee, 306
POW Nurses, 163-173, 315
public health, 60-61, 66, 103, 105, 115, 142, 148, 177, 180, 195, 214, 264-265, 273-274, 301-302, 317

Q

Queen for a Day, Nurses Day, 208-209
Queen of Angels Hospital, 77, 126-127, 180, 212-213, 221-222, 228, 258, 276, 335, 349

R

railway nurses (Courier Nurses), 142-144
Ransom, Eleanor, 25
Reagan, Ronald, Governor/President, 96, 172, 213, 226, 255, 267
Red Cross, American, 59, 77, 86, 93, 96-97, 104, 107-112, 116, 135-136, 172, 181, 185, 280, 333
Red Cross of St. George & Royal Red Cross, 100-101, 331
registration, nurses, 68
registry, nurses, 122-125
Reichman, Fey, 247
Reitz, Margaret, 42
Richards, Linda, 18, 29
Rio Hondo College, 344
Rodriguez, Alice, 224
Rogone, Sharon, 245
romance novels, nurses, 293, 296
Roy, Sister Callista, 268, 302

S

Salazar, Carmen, 184
San Francisco, 11, 17, 33-34, 41, 52, 116, 141, 170, 184, 226, 302
Santa Fe Coast Line Hospital & Railroad, 82, 142-144, 207
Santa Monica City College, 287, 343
sanitariums/sanatoriums, 37, 64, 67, 69-74, 156-157, 180, 334
Schimmoler, Lauretta, 135-140
Seacole, Mary, 20-21
Seaside Hospital, 267, 335
Sekiguchi, June, 250
Semper Fidelis & Semper Paratus, 41, 85, 332-334
Shain, Edith, 192-193
Shields, Patricia, 251
Sirch, Margaret Elliot Frances, 62-63
Sigma Theta Tau, 121, 273, 315, 324-325
Silva, Rosa, 218
Simmonds, Emily Louise, 108
Smith Chason School of Nursing, 347
Snyder, Patricia, 280
Soldiers Home/Military Home Hospital, 26-27
Soroptimist, organization, 267
Spanish-American War, 59, 86, 107
Squaires, Marjorie, 267
Stanbridge University, 340
St. John's Hospital, 215-216
Statewide Nursing Program/Consortium, 288-291, 338
statues/memorials, 14, 16-17, 20-21, 31, 57-59, 171, 178-179, 193, 24-249, 325, 377
Stapfer, Caroline, 29
Sterling, Alice, 188-189
strike, nurses 226
St. Vincent's Hospital, 13-15, 56, 67, 93-95, 180, 214, 258, 315, 333
Sunbrite Junior Nurse Corps, 159
Superintendent of Nursing/Matron, 26, 29, 34, 37-38, 42, 48, 51-53, 57-59, 63, 67, 75, 80-81, 83, 85, 90, 110-114, 120, 122, 132
Sisters/Daughters/Nuns, 11-17, 56-59, 126-127, 148, 200-201, 257-259, 268

T

Todd, Edwina, 168-169, 173, 205, 315
Tomassini, Mary, 216-217
Traynor, Yoshiko Taigawa, 179
Tuberculosis, 30-31, 63, 69-71, 82, 156-157, 196
Turner, Alice Sterling, 188-189

Tulley, Barbetta Jackson, 79, 305

U

University of California, Los Angeles (UCLA), 79, 112, 121, 148, 199, 214, 257, 260-274, 302, 305, 310-314, 324, 336, 342
University of LaVerne, 347
University of Phoenix/Aspen University, 339
University of Southern California (USC), 33-34, 120-121, 274, 276, 284-285, 304, 337

V

Vanderbilt University School of Nursing, 221, 265, 269-271
Vassar College, 112
Velasquez, Mila, 301
Victory Corps, 181
Vietnam War, 248-251, 297
Visiting Nurse Association (VNA), 60-61, 195-197

W

Wald, Lillian, 60
Welfare and Health Department, 63
West Coast University, 121, 311, 323, 339
West Los Angeles College, 344
Western University of Health Sciences, 338
Weston, Maude Foster, 60
White Memorial Hospital, 132-133, 147, 180, 325, 335
Wickham, Anna Lackey, 128-129
Williams, Betty Smith, 302-303
Williamson, Anne A., 86-87
Williamson, First Lieutenant Anne, 118
Winton, Sophie, 96-97
Women's Health Nurse Practitioner Program (WHCNPP), 299, 306, 317
Wood, Sister Mary, 52
World War I (WWI), 26, 91, 93, 96-97, 107-114, 264
World War II (WWII), 18, 104, 136, 139, 141, 143, 147, 163-193, 202, 219, 251, 284, 315, 344

Y

Year of the Nurse, International, 324-325
Yetter, Doris, 173
Yoshida, Rae, 344

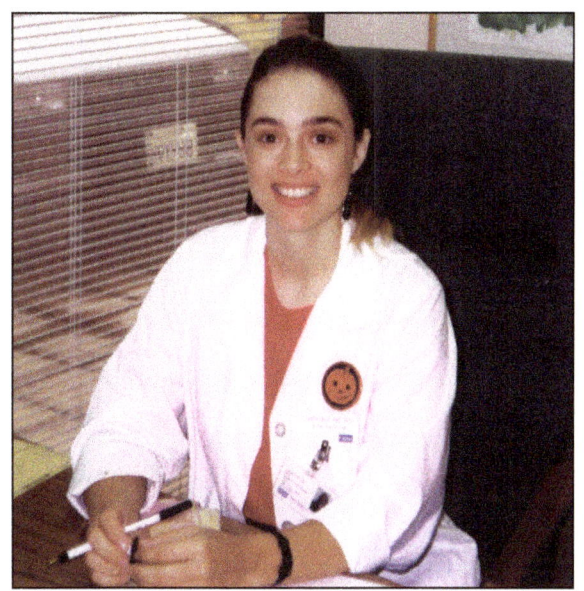

Cynthia Broze, feeling more nervous than she appears in this photo because this was the first week of life as a new Nurse Practitioner, October 31, 1992.

Cynthia Broze is a writer and nurse practitioner. She's published two history books: *Nurses of Los Angeles* and the *Aerial Nurse Corps of America*. Both were non-traditional history books as she included hundreds of photos in each one. For Broze, photographs are as historically interesting as words. To find them, she scoured archives for years in many states, looking through collections for documents and images.

When someone asks what college she graduated from, she usually answers, "Which one?" because she attended many. She moved to different states grabbing degrees, and certifications, and working in various specialties. She began as a nurse's aide and LPN in Illinois; she earned a massage therapy certification in Oregon. After a few years in the Peace Corps in the Philippines, she appeared in Colorado, where she obtained an ADN, followed by a BSN from a school in New York. Too cold. Hello Los Angeles and a neonatal intensive care nurse certification, a Master of Science from California State University, Long Beach, with a nurse practitioner specialization from the Women's Healthcare Nurse Practitioner Program at Harbor-UCLA: her highest academic degree and favorite vocation.

Then writing called, as it always had, and UCLA accepted her into their master novel writing program. She began by writing about history, but her novel completions are on the horizon.

Visit cynthiabroze.com

www.ingramcontent.com/pod-product-compliance
Lightning Source LLC
Chambersburg PA
CBHW062055290426
44110CB00022B/2603